Methodology for Genetic Studies
of Twins and Families

NATO ASI Series

Advanced Science Institutes Series

A Series presenting the results of activities sponsored by the NATO Science Committee, which aims at the dissemination of advanced scientific and technological knowledge, with a view to strengthening links between scientific communities.

The Series is published by an international board of publishers in conjunction with the NATO Scientific Affairs Division

A Life Sciences	Plenum Publishing Corporation
B Physics	London and New York
C Mathematical	Kluwer Academic Publishers
and Physical Sciences	Dordrecht, Boston and London
D Behavioural and Social Sciences	
E Applied Sciences	
F Computer and Systems Sciences	Springer-Verlag
G Ecological Sciences	Berlin, Heidelberg, New York, London,
H Cell Biology	Paris and Tokyo
I Global Environmental Change	

NATO-PCO-DATA BASE

The electronic index to the NATO ASI Series provides full bibliographical references (with keywords and/or abstracts) to more than 30000 contributions from international scientists published in all sections of the NATO ASI Series.
Access to the NATO-PCO-DATA BASE is possible in two ways:

– via online FILE 128 (NATO-PCO-DATA BASE) hosted by ESRIN,
Via Galileo Galilei, I-00044 Frascati, Italy.

– via CD-ROM "NATO-PCO-DATA BASE" with user-friendly retrieval software in English, French and German (© WTV GmbH and DATAWARE Technologies Inc. 1989).

The CD-ROM can be ordered through any member of the Board of Publishers or through NATO-PCO, Overijse, Belgium.

Series D: Behavioural and Social Sciences - Vol. 67

Methodology for Genetic Studies of Twins and Families

by

Michael C. Neale

Department of Human Genetics,
Medical College of Virginia,
Virginia Commonwealth University,
Richmond, Virginia, U.S.A.

and

Lon R. Cardon

Institute for Behavioral Genetics,
University of Colorado,
Boulder, Colorado, U.S.A.

Kluwer Academic Publishers

Dordrecht / Boston / London

Published in cooperation with NATO Scientific Affairs Division

Based on NATO, NFWO and NIMH funded Workshops
taught in Leuven, Belgium (1987, 1989 and 1991)
and Boulder, Colorado, U.S.A. (1990)

ISBN 0-7923-1874-9

Published by Kluwer Academic Publishers,
P.O. Box 17, 3300 AA Dordrecht, The Netherlands.

Kluwer Academic Publishers incorporates the publishing programmes of
D. Reidel, Martinus Nijhoff, Dr W. Junk and MTP Press.

Sold and distributed in the U.S.A. and Canada
by Kluwer Academic Publishers,
101 Philip Drive, Norwell, MA 02061, U.S.A.

In all other countries, sold and distributed
by Kluwer Academic Publishers Group,
P.O. Box 322, 3300 AH Dordrecht, The Netherlands.

Printed on acid-free paper

Contents

Preface

This book stems from teaching intensive, week-long workshops on twin methodology in Leuven, Belgium and Boulder, Colorado. The primary aim of these workshops was to teach students enough of the theory and practice of analyzing twin data that they could apply the methods to their own data in their own research institutions. The first two workshops were set up in Leuven in 1987 and 1989. Demand was so great that the 1989 workshop attendance was uncomfortably large even though many able students had been turned away. The following year an annual schedule was adopted with the Boulder workshop, which also was oversubscribed. Last year there were 55 students for each of two consecutive weeks, and still there were more students than available places on the course. Perhaps one of the reasons for this overwhelming popularity was the absence of any publication that could be considered a course text. Thus the only opportunities to learn were either to study with faculty at a very small number of places in the world, or to attend the workshop. We hope that this book will provide a third way in which undergraduate, graduate and postdoctoral students and faculty can learn how to analyze and interpret data collected from twin and family studies. This is not to say that those who have read this book will not be welcome at future workshops! We believe that there is no substitute for "hands-on" experience, and recommend that readers interleave their reading with active model fitting to get the most out of the text.

The lack of a course text was, in fact, immediately obvious during the first course, and a special issue of *Behavior Genetics* was published in 1989, featuring papers describing and applying some of the techniques. Although many of the models used in the special issue are featured in this book, there have been so many new developments and improvements to both the models and the software used to test them that there is relatively little redundancy. Furthermore, the examples given in this volume are completely different from those used for the special issue. Not all of the book is entirely new — parts of Chapter 6 appear in the LISREL manual, and some of the Figures and Tables in Chapters 16 and 17 appear in Hewitt *et al.*, 1992 and Cardon *et al.*, 1991.

Students for the workshops came from a broad range of disciplines including anthropology, biology, cardiology, genetics, physiology, psychology, psychiatry, sociology, nursing, mathematics, and statistics. For such a diverse group it was safest to assume that the audience 'knew nothing' and to try to provide a basic grounding in areas such as matrix algebra, statistics, linear modeling, and applied computing. Both feedback from the students and increasing demand for the workshops indicate that our approach was successful. We have adopted the same strategy in this volume, with background chapters on summarizing data, biometrical genetics, matrix algebra, path analysis, the LISREL model, and statistical power. As far as possible we have illustrated the methods with examples directly relevant to the analysis of genetically informative data. The real task of applied data analysis begins in Chapter 8 with univariate analysis of data from twins reared together. All subsequent chapters, except those on statistical power and the final chapter, describe a model or a class of models which is fitted to a real dataset. For the most part these applications focus on the models much more than on the background to the area, the details of the samples, the method of data collection, and the substantive interpretations of the results. We certainly do not believe that these latter issues are unimportant — on the contrary, they are crucial aspects of the scientific method. Our emphasis on the models reflects our concern that these methods should be thoroughly understood by the producers and consumers of research of human individual differences.

One of the striking features of the workshops was the strong coherence of the material, despite enormous variation in the lecturing styles, the subject matter taught, and the example datasets used. In this book, we have strived to preserve this logical coherence without destroying the variety. The net result, we hope, is a volume that will be useful for a large number of disciplines. There is no area of human science that could not benefit from the more fundamental understanding of individual differences offered by modeling genetically informative data. Though many may argue that their primary concern is 'the environment' we would counter that to study the environment properly it is necessary to control for the effects of genotype first. For example, suppose that high-school students whose parents are helpful and supportive about homework have higher grades than students without such assistance. Naively, one might conclude that the parents' treatment of their children causes improved academic performance. However, children and their parents are related genetically, and it is quite plausible that genes for good school performance lead to helpful and supportive parenting later in life. Without a genetically informative study, these radically different explanations of the same association are confounded. With designs such as MZ and DZ twins and their parents or biological and adopted children, the relative impact of genotypic and environmental effects may be estimated.

The study of variability is a relatively simple matter with animal populations, because (i) the environment can be directly controlled, and (ii) the genotype may be manipulated in breeding experiments. Among human populations, genetic control is unethical, and the same is true of a large number of environmental factors. In addition, experimental modification of the environment may be quite different from the occurence of the same events in a naturalistic setting. Thus, we are usually faced with an ethological approach to the study of human individual differences, and with statistical control of genetic effects. The methods described in this volume are a first step towards this control. While we have focused this introductory text largely on twin data, the models extend quite readily to many classes of relatives. One such extension is described in Chapter 17 in which data from MZ and DZ twins and their parents are used to test a model of mixed genetic and cultural transmission.

To model the genetic and environmental factors underlying human variation most effectively, we should apply certain basic principles of good mathematical modeling. These tenets include a good understanding of the biosocial problem in question, realistic mathematical representation of the salient features of the data, the ability to make quantitative predictions about related phenomena, and interpretation of the parameters of the model in terms of the biosocial problem. In this introductory text, we have limited our treatment to linear structural equation models which will no doubt prove to be inadequate for many applications. However, the advantage of a coherent framework for basic modeling of genetically informative data is clear. More complex mathematical models generally build on the principles involved in simple structural equation modeling, because both are driven by genetic theory. The mixture of genetics, statistics, and applied computing required to apply the methods is by itself an interdisciplinary exercise, and one that has potential to lead to advances in each of the component disciplines. But without data, these issues become largely dull and academic; the richest source of new knowledge comes from the interface of modeling with the endless array of variables that can be measured in man. It is only relatively recently that data have been collected in large quantities from genetically informative constellations of relatives. As this process continues, the data will drive the mathematical modeling in new directions. Likewise, methodological and computational advances will lead to more efficient and informative designs for the study of genetic and environmental effects.

The contributors to this volume have been supported by grants from a large number of sources. United States Public Health Service awards include: ADAMHA grants MH45268, AA08672, AG04945, MH43899, GM30250 MH31302, MH40828, DA05588, AA03539, AA07535, AA07728; and NICHD grants HD07289, HD18426, and HD10333. In Europe, funds were obtained from: the Interuniversitair Network for Fundamental Research; grants 3.0038.82 and 3.0038.90 from the Fund for Medical Scientific Research (Brussels, Belgium); Dutch Heart Foundation: 86.083 and 88.042; Dutch Praeventie Fonds: 28-1847.26 and 28-1847.29; Onderzoeksfonds K.U.Leuven OT/86/80; and Fonds voor Geneeskundig Wetenschappelijk Onderzoek 3.0098.91. In Australia, data collection was though the Australian Twin Registry which is supported by the National Health and Medical Research Council. Dr. Jöreskog was supported by Swedish Council for Research in the Humanities and Social Sciences under the program *Multivariate Statistical Analysis*. Private sponsors include the Carman Trust for Scientific Research, the Phillip Morris Group of Companies and Nationale Bank van Belgie. Specially important for this book were the grants to support the workshops: NATO 86/0823; Nationaal Fonds voor Wetenschappelijk Onderzoek 89/86 and 91/83; MH19392; Ministerie van Volksgezondheid and NATO ASI901115. The NATO Science Committee was particularly helpful. In anticipation of an award letter, we look forward to receiving MH19687 for funding two workshops during the next three years.

The plans for this book were originally hammered out at the end of the workshop in 1990. As is natural for a book on the study of individual differences, variation was everywhere. One or two contributors acted quickly, most took quite a long time, and a few were forever seeking deadline $n + 1$. For many, this deadline coincided with the NATO ASI in Leuven, 1991, and several chapters were drafted during the weekend between the introductory and advanced courses. Fortunately, none of the authors could be criticized for a short, choppy, writing style; unfortunately several seemed to aim to write in sentences long enough to pose a challenge to James Joyce! Thus certain sections required little editing, while others needed a lot of work. While we have tried to maintain consistent notation, style and assumed level of knowledge throughout, this has not been an easy task. We ask the reader to be patient with discrepancies and typographical errors where they occur, and to remember that camera-ready copy was supplied to the publisher with no copy-editing or proof-reading by their staff. Yes, the mistakes are all our own.

We are extremely grateful to Drs. R. Vlietinck, R. Derom, C. Derom and H. Maes from the Katholiek Universiteit in Leuven, Belgium for their superhuman efforts put in to organize the workshops. Similarly, we thank John DeFries for helping to arrange the Boulder workshop. We owe a great debt to the students of all the courses (a list of the participants of the 1991 NATO ASI may be found in Appendix A); their ready participation led to revisions of the course and reallocation of the proportions of time spent covering each topic. The structure and proportioning of this volume also reflects this process.

We are very grateful to Greg Porter for drawing almost all of the figures. Like so many authors, we owe Donald Knuth and Leslie Lamport for developing TℰX and LᴀTℰX for typesetting. Also significant is Trevor Darrell for writing Psfig, which allows postscript figures to be included in the text. We are very grateful to Daniel Pérusse for making helpful editorial comments on many aspects of the manuscript. At MCV we are fortunate to have superb support from Health Sciences Computing, and would like to thank John Fritz and Bob Langford for getting everything to work. Finally we thank our spouses and families for tolerating our absences and workaholic schedules!

List of Figures

List of Tables

CONTRIBUTING AUTHORS

Lindon J. Eaves
Department of Human Genetics
Medical College of Virginia

John K. Hewitt
Department of Human Genetics
Medical College of Virginia

Joanne M. Meyer
Department of Human Genetics
Medical College of Virginia

Michael C. Neale
Department of Human Genetics
Medical College of Virginia

Hermine H. M. Maes
Institute of Physical Education
Catholic University Leuven

Dorret I. Boomsma
Department of Experimental Psychology
Free University, Amsterdam

Conor V. Dolan
Department of Psychology
University of Amsterdam

Peter C. M. Molenaar
Department of Psychology
University of Amsterdam

Karl G. Jöreskog
Department of Statistics
University of Uppsala

Nicholas G. Martin
Queensland Institute of Medical
Research

Lon R. Cardon
Institute for Behavioral Genetics
University of Colorado

David W. Fulker
Institute for Behavioral Genetics
University of Colorado

Andrew C. Heath
Department of Psychiatry
Washington University School of Medicine

Chapter 1

The Scope of Genetic Analyses

1.1 Introduction and General Aims

This book has its origin in a week-long intensive course on methods of twin data analysis taught on several occasions over the last few years at the Katholieke Universiteit of Leuven in Belgium and the Institute for Behavioral Genetics, Boulder, in Colorado. Our principal aim here is to help those interested in the genetic analysis of individual differences to realize that there are more challenging questions than simply "Is trait X genetic?" or "What is the heritability of X?" and that there are more flexible and informative methods than those that have been popular for more than half a century. We shall achieve this goal primarily by considering those analyses of data on twins that can be conducted with the LISREL program. There are two main reasons for this restriction: 1) the basic structure and logic of the twin design is simple and yet can illustrate many of the conceptual and practical issues that need to be addressed in any genetic study of individual differences; 2) the LISREL program is well-documented, commercially available for personal computers and can be used to apply most of the basic ideas we shall discuss. These limitations not withstanding, however, we believe that the material to be presented will open many new horizons to investigators in a wide range of disciplines and provide them with the tools to begin to explore their own data more fruitfully.

This introductory chapter has four main aims:

1. to identify some of the scientific questions which have aroused the curiosity of investigators and led them to develop the approaches we describe

2. to trace part of the intellectual tradition that brings us to the approach we are to present in this text

1

3. to outline the overall logical structure of the approach

4. to accomplish all of these with the minimum of statistics and mathematics.

Before starting on what we are going to do, however, it is important to point out what we are not going to deal with, especially in the age of molecular genetics and linkage analysis. There will be almost nothing in this book about detecting the contribution of individual loci of large effect against the background of other genetic and environmental effects ("segregation analysis") nor about where such individual genes are situated on the genome, if such there be ("linkage analysis"). Our neglect of these issues is not because we think them unimportant. It is rather that they have been treated extensively elsewhere (see e.g., Ott, 1985) — often to the exclusion of issues that may still turn out to be equally important, such as those outlined in this chapter. When the history of genetic epidemiology is written, we believe that the approaches described here will be credited with revealing the naivete of many of the simple assumptions about the action of genes and environment that are usually made in the search for single loci of large effect. Our work may thus be seen in the context of exploring those parameters of the action of genes and environment which are frequently not considered in conventional segregation and linkage analysis.

1.2   Heredity and Variation

Genetic epidemiology is impelled by three basic questions:

1. Why isn't everyone the same?

2. Why are children like their parents?

3. Why aren't children from the same parents all alike?

These questions address variation within individuals and covariation between relatives. As we shall show, covariation between relatives can provide useful information about variation within individuals.

1.2.1   Variation

In this section we shall examine the ubiquity of variability, and its distinction from mean levels in populations and sub-populations.

Variation is Everywhere

Almost everything that can be measured or counted in humans shows variation around the mean value for the population. Figure 1.1 shows the pattern of variation for self-reported weight (lb.) in a U.S. sample. The observation that individuals differ is almost universal and covers the entire spectrum of measurable

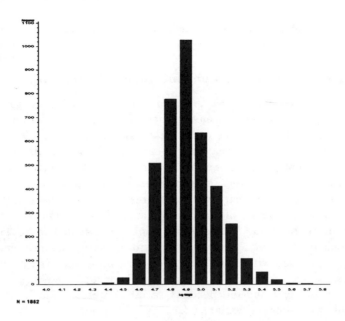

Figure 1.1: Variability in self reported weight in a sample of US twins.

traits, whether they be physical such as stature or weight, physiological such as heart rate and blood pressure, or psychological such as personality, abilities, or attitudes. The methods we shall describe are concerned with explaining why these differences occur.

Beyond the *a priori* Approach

As far as possible, the analyses we use are designed to be agnostic about the causes of variation in a particular variable. Unfortunately, the same absence of *a priori* bias is not always found among our scientific peers! A referee once wrote in a report on a manuscript describing a twin study:

> *It is probably alright to use the twin study to estimate the genetic contribution to variables which you know are genetic like stature and weight, and it's probably alright for things like blood pressure. But it certainly can't be used for behavioral traits which we know are environmental like social attitudes!*

Such a crass remark nevertheless serves a useful purpose because it illustrates an important principle which we should strive to satisfy, namely to find methods that are *trait-independent*; that is, they do not depend for their validity on investigators *a priori* beliefs about what causes variation in a particular trait. Such considerations may give weight to choosing one study design rather than another, but they cannot be used to decide whether we should believe our results when we have them.

Biometrical Genetical and Epidemiological Approaches

Approaches that use genetic manipulation, natural or artificial, to uncover latent (i.e. unmeasured) genetic and environmental causes of variation are sometimes called *biometrical genetical* (see e.g. Mather and Jinks, 1982). The methods may be contrasted to the more conventional ones used in individual differences, chiefly in the areas of psychology, sociology and epidemiology. The conventional approaches try to explain variation in one set of measures (the *dependent variables*) by references to differences in another set of measures (*dependent variables*) by references to differences in another set of measures (*independent variables*). For example, the risk for cardiovascular and lung diseases might be assumed to be dependent variables, and cigarette smoking, alcohol use, and life stress independent variables. A fundamental problem with this "epidemiological approach" is that its conclusions about causality can be seriously misleading. Erroneous inferences would be made if both the dependent and independent variables were caused by the same latent genetic and environmental variables (see e.g., Chapters 8 and 12).

Not Much Can Be Said About Means

It is vital to remember that almost every result in this book, and every conclusion that others obtain using these methods, relate to the causes of human differences, and may have almost nothing to do with the processes that account for the development of the mean expression of a trait in a particular population. We are necessarily concerned with what makes people vary around the mean of the population, race or species from which they are sampled. Suppose, for example, we were to find that differences in social attitudes had a very large genetic component of variation among U.S. citizens. What would that imply about the role of culture in the determination of social attitudes? It could imply several things. First, it might mean that culture is so uniform that only genetic effects are left to account for differences. Second, it might mean that cultural changes are adopted so rapidly that environmental effects are not apparent. A trivial example may make this clear. It is possible that understanding the genetic causes of variation in stature among humans may identify the genes responsible for the difference in stature between humans and chimpanzees, but it is by no means certain. Neither would a demonstration that all human variation in stature was due to the environment lead us to assume that the differences between humans and chimpanzees were not genetic. This point is stressed because, whatever subsequent genetic research on population and species differences might establish, there is no necessary connection between what is true of the typical human and what causes variation around the central tendency. For this reason, it is important to avoid such short-hand expressions as "height is genetic" when really we mean "individual differences in height are mainly genetic."

Variation and Modification

What has been said about means also extends to making claims about intervention. The causes of variation that emerge from twin and family studies relate to a particular population of genotypes at a specific time in its evolutionary and cultural history. Factors that change the gene frequencies, the expression of gene effects, or the frequencies of the different kinds of environment may all affect the outcome of our studies. Furthermore, if we show that genetic effects are important, the possibility that a rare but highly potent environmental agent is present cannot entirely be discounted. Similarly, a rare gene of major effect may hold the key to understanding cognitive development but, because of its rarity, accounts for relatively little of the total variation in cognitive ability. In either case, it would be foolhardy to claim too much for the power of genetic studies of human differences. This does not mean, however, that such studies are without value, as we shall show. Our task is to make clear what conclusions are justified on the basis of the data and what are not.

1.2.2 Graphing and Quantifying Familial Resemblance

Look at the two sets of data given in Figure 1.2. The first part of the figure is a scatterplot of measurements of weight in a large sample of non-identical (fraternal, dizygotic, DZ) twins. Each cross in the diagram represents a single twin pair. The second part of the figure is a scatterplot of pairs of completely unrelated people from the same population. Notice how the two parts of the figure differ. In the unrelated pairs the pattern of crosses gives the general impression of being circular; in general, if we pick a particular value on the X axis (first person's weight), it makes little difference to how heavy the second person is on average. This is what it means to say that measures are *uncorrelated* — knowing the score of the first member of a pair makes it no easier to predict the score of the second and *vice-versa*. By comparison, the scatterplot for the fraternal twins (who are related biologically to the same degree as brothers and sisters) looks somewhat different. The pattern of crosses is slightly elliptical and tilted upwards. This means that as we move from lighter first twins towards heavier first twins (increasing values on the X axis), there is also a general tendency for the average scores of the second twins (on the Y axis) to increase. It appears that the weights of twins are somewhat correlated. Of course, if we take any particular X value, the Y values are still very variable so the correlation is not perfect. The *correlation coefficient* (see Chapter 2) allows us to quantify the degree of relationship between the two sets of measures. In the unrelated individuals, the correlation turns out to be 0.02 which is well within the range expected simply by chance alone if the measures were really independent. For the fraternal twins, on the other hand, the correlation is 0.44 which is far

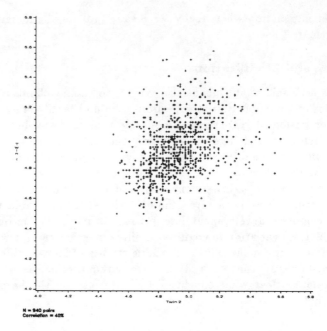

N = 940 pairs
Correlation = 40%

(a)

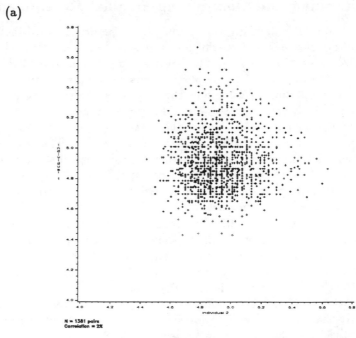

N = 1381 pairs
Correlation = 2%

(b)

Figure 1.2: Two scatterplots of measurements of weight: a) in a large sample of DZ twin pairs, and b) pairs of individuals matched at random.

greater than we would expect in so large a sample if the pairs of measures were truly independent.

The data on weight illustrate the important general point that relatives are usually much more alike than unrelated individuals from the same population. That is, although there are large individual differences for almost every trait than can be measured, we find that the trait values of family members are often quite similar. Figure 1.3 gives the correlations between relatives in large samples of nuclear families for stature, weight, and conservatism. One simple way of interpreting the correlation coefficient is to multiply it by 100 and treat it as a percentage. The correlation ($\times$ 100) is the "percentage of the total variation in a trait which is caused by factors shared by members of a pair." Thus, for example, our correlation of 0.44 for the weights of DZ twins implies that, of all the factors which create variation in weight, 44% are factors which members of DZ twin pair have in common. We can offer a similar interpretation for the other kinds of relationship. A problem becomes immediately apparent. Since the DZ twins, for example, have spent most of their lives together, we cannot know whether the 44% is due entirely to the fact that they shared the same environment *in utero*, lived with the same parents after birth, or simply have half their genes in common — and we shall never know until we can find another kind of relationship in which the degree of genetic similarity, or shared environmental similarity, is different.

Figure 1.4 gives a scattergram for the weights of a large sample of female identical (monozygotic, MZ) twins. Whereas DZ twins, like siblings, on average share only half their genes, MZ twins are genetically identical. The scatter of points is now much more clearly elliptical, and the 45° tilt of the major axis is especially obvious. The correlation in the weights in this sample of MZ twins is 0.77, almost twice that found for DZ's. The much greater resemblance of MZ twins, who are expected to have completely identical genes establishes a strong *prima facie* case for the contribution of genetic factors to differences in weight. One of the tasks to be addressed in this book is how to interpret such differential patterns of family resemblance in a more rigorous, quantitative, fashion.

1.2.3 Within Family Differences

At a purely anecdotal level, when parents hear about the possibility that genes create differences between people, they will sometimes respond "Well, that's pretty obvious. I've raised three sons and they've all turned out differently." At issue here is not whether their conclusions are soundly based on their data, so much as to indicate that not all variation is due to factors that family members share in common. No matter how much parents contribute genetically to their children and, it seems, no matter how much effort they put into parenting, a large part of the outcome appears beyond their immediate control. That is, there are large differences even within a family. Some of these differences are doubtless due to the environment since even identical twins are not perfectly alike. Figure 1.5 is a

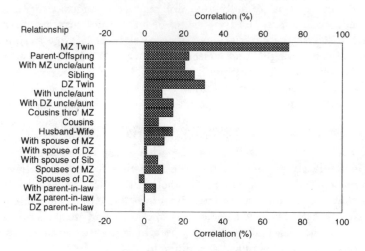

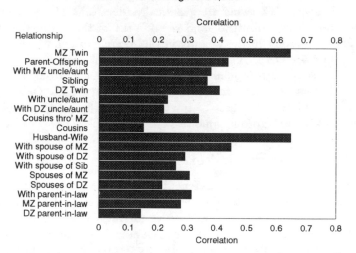

Figure 1.3: Correlations for body mass index (weight/height^2) and conservatism between relatives. Data were obtained from large samples of nuclear families ascertained through twins.

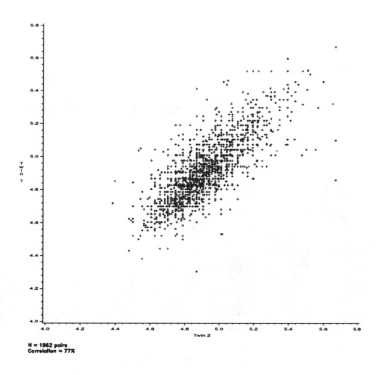

Figure 1.4: Scatterplot of weight in pounds of a large sample of MZ twins.

bar chart of the (absolute) weight differences within pairs of twins. The darker, left-hand column of each pair gives the percentage of the DZ sample falling in the indicated range of differences, and the lighter, right-hand column shows the corresponding percentages for MZ pairs. For MZ twins, these differences must be due to factors in the environment that differ even within pairs of genetically identical individuals raised in the same home. Obviously the differences within DZ pairs are much greater on average. The known mechanisms of Mendelian inheritance can account for this finding since, unlike MZ twins, DZ twins are not genetically identical although they are genetically related. DZ twins represent a separate sample from the genetic pool "cornered" by the parents. Thus, DZ twins will be correlated because their particular parents have their own particular selection of genes from the total gene pool in the population, but they will not be genetically identical because each DZ twin, like every other sibling in the same family, represents the result of separate, random, meioses[1] in the parental germlines.

---

[1] meiosis is the process of gametogenesis in which either sperm or ova are formed

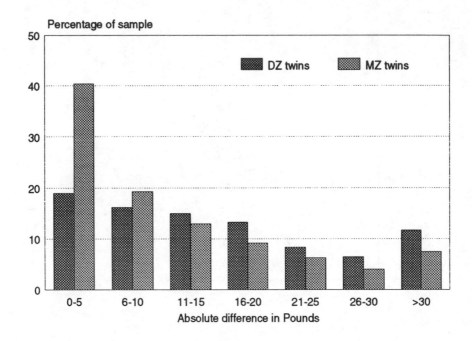

Figure 1.5: Bar chart of absolute differences in weight within 1826 pairs of identical twins, and within 927 pairs of fraternal twins.

1.3   Building and Fitting Models

As long as we study random samples of unrelated individuals, we shall limit our understanding of what causes the differences we see. The total population variation is simply an aggregate of all the various components of variance. One practical approach to the analysis of variation is to obtain several measures of it, each known to reflect a different proportion of genetic and environmental components of the differences. Then, if we have a model for how the effects of genes and environment contribute differentially to each distinct measure of variation, we can solve to obtain estimates of the separate components. Figure 1.6 shows the principal stages in this process. There are two aspects: *theory* and *data*. The *model* is a formal, in our case mathematical, statement which mediates between the logic of the theory and the reality of the data. Cnce a model is formulated consistently, the predictions implied for different sets of data can be derived by a series of elementary math-

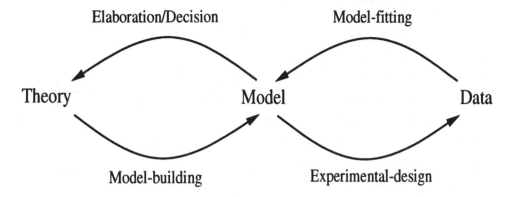

Elaboration/Decision   Model-fitting

Theory   Model   Data

Model-building   Experimental-design

Figure 1.6: Diagram of the interrelationship between theory, model and empirical observation.

ematical operations. *Model building* is the task of translating the ideas of theory into mathematical form. A large part of this book is devoted to a discussion of model building. Inspection of the model, sometimes aided by computer simulation (see Chapters 9 and 13), suggests appropriate study designs which may be used to generate critical data to test some or all parts of a current model. The statistical processes of *model fitting* allow us to compare the predictions of a particular model with the actual observations about a given population. If the model fails, then we are forced to revise all or some of our theory. If, on the other hand, the model fits then we cannot know it is "right" in some ultimate sense. However, we might now wish to base new testable conjectures on the theory in order to enlarge the scope of observations it can encompass.

1.4   The Elements of a Model: Causes of Variation

No model is built in isolation. Rather it is built upon a foundation of what is either already known or what might be a matter for fertile conjecture. Part of the difficulty, but also the intrinsic appeal, of genetic epidemiology is the fact that it seeks either to distinguish between major sets of theoretical propositions, or to integrate them into an overall framework. From biology, and especially through knowledge of genetics, we have a detailed understanding of the intricacies of gene expression. From the behavioral and social sciences we have strong proposals about the importance of the environment, especially the social environment, for the development of human differences. One view of our task may be that of giving a common conceptual and mathematical framework to both genetic and environmental theories so that we may decide which, if any, is more consistent with the facts in particular cases.

1.4.1 Genetic Effects

A complete understanding of genetic effects would need to answer a series of questions:

1. How important are genetic effects on human differences?

2. What kinds of action and interaction occur between gene products in the pathways between genotype and phenotype?

3. Are the genetic effects on a trait consistent across sexes?

4. Are there some genes that have particularly outstanding effects when compared to others?

5. Whereabouts on the human gene map are these genes located?

Questions 4 and 5 are clearly very important, but are not the immediate concern of this book. On the other hand, we shall have a lot to say about 1, 2, and 3. It is arguable that we shall not be able to understand 4 and 5 adequately, if we do not have a proper appreciation of these other issues.

The importance of genes is often expressed relative to all the causes of variation, both genetic and environmental. The proportion of variation associated with genetic effects is termed the *broad heritability*. However, the complete analysis of genetic factors does not end here because, as countless experiments in plant and animal genetics have shown (well in advance of modern molecular genetics; see e.g., Mather and Jinks, 1982), genes can act and interact in a variety of ways before their effects on the phenotype are measured.

Geneticists typically distinguish between *additive* and *non-additive* genetic effects (these terms will be defined more explicitly in Chapter 3). These influences have been studied in detail in many non-human species using selective breeding experiments, which directly alter the frequencies of particular genotypes. In such experiments, the bulk of genetic variation is usually explained by additive genetic effects. However, careful studies have shown two general types of non-additivity that may be important, especially in traits that have been subject to strong directional selection in the wild. The two main types of genetic non-additivity are *dominance* and *epistasis*.

The term dominance derives initially from Mendel's classical experiments in which it was shown that the progeny of a cross between two pure breeding lines often resembled one parent more than the other. That is, an individual who carries different alleles at a locus (the *heterozygote*) is not exactly intermediate in expression between individuals who are pure breeding (*homozygous*) for the two alleles. While dominance describes the interaction between alleles at the same locus, *epistasis* describes the interaction between alleles at different loci.

Epistasis is said to occur whenever the effects of one gene on individual differences depend on which genotype is expressed at another locus. For example, suppose that at locus A/a individuals may have genotype AA, Aa or aa, and at locus B/b genotype BB, Bb or bb[2]. If the difference between individuals having genotype AA and those with genotype aa depends on whether they are BB or bb, then there would be *additive* × *additive* epistatic interactions. Experimental studies have shown a rich variety of possible epistatic interactions depending on the number and effects of the interacting loci. However, their detailed resolution in humans is virtually impossible unless we are fortunate enough to identify a small handful of specific loci, so it is sufficient to acknowledge their conceptual importance. Failure to take non-additive genetic effects into account may be one of the main reasons studies of twins give different heritability estimates from studies of adoptees and nuclear families (Eaves *et al.*, 1992; Plomin *et al.*, 1991).

As studies in genetic epidemiology become larger and better designed, it is becoming increasingly clear that there are marked sex differences in gene expression. An important factor in establishing this view has been the incorporation of unlike-sex twin pairs in twin studies (Eaves *et al.*, 1990). However, comparison of statistics derived from any relationship of individuals of unlike sex with those of like sex would yield a similar conclusion (see Chapter 11). We shall make an important distinction between two types of *sex-limited gene expression*. In the simpler case, the same genes affect both males and females, but their effects are consistent across sexes and differ only by some constant multiple over all the loci involved. We shall refer to this type of effect as *scalar sex-limitation*. In other cases, however, we shall discover that genetic effects in one sex are not just a constant multiple of their effects in the other. Indeed, even though a trait may be measured in exactly the same way in males and females, it may turn out that quite different genes control its expression in the two sexes. A classic example would be the case of chest-girth since at least some of the variation expressed in females may be due to loci that, while still present in males, are only expressed in females. In this case we shall speak of *non-scalar sex-limitation*. None of us likes the term very much, but until someone suggests something better we shall continue to use it!

1.4.2 Environmental Effects

Paradoxically, one of the greatest benefits of studies that can detect and control for genetic effects is the information they can provide about the sources of environmental influence. We make an important distinction between deciding which are the best places to look for specific environmental agents and deciding what those specific agents are. For example, it may be possible to show that variation in diastolic blood pressure is influenced by environmental effects shared by family members long before it is possible to demonstrate that the salient environmental factor is the amount of sodium in the diet. We make a similar distinction between estimating the overall contribution of genetic effects and identifying specific loci that account for a significant fraction of the total genetic variation. Using

---

[2]This notation is described more fully in Chapter 3.

some of the methods we shall describe later in this book it may indeed be possible to estimate the contribution of specific factors to the environmental component of variation (see Chapter 12). However, using the *biometrical genetical* approach which relies only on the complex patters of family resemblance, it is possible to make some very important statements about the structure of the environment in advance of our ability to identify specific features of the environment which are most important. Although the full subtlety for analyzing the environment cannot be achieved with data on twins alone, much less on twins reared together, it is nevertheless possible to make some important preliminary statements about the major sources of environmental influence which can provide a basis for future studies.

We may conceive of the total environmental variation in a trait as arising from a number of sources. The first major distinction we make is between environmental factors which operate within families from those which create differences between families. Sometimes the environment within families is called the *unique environment* or the *specific environment* or the *random environment*. Different authors may refer to it as V_E, V_{SE}, E_1, E_W or e^2, but the important thing is to understand the concept behind the symbols. The within-family environment refers to all those environmental influences which are so random in their origin, and idiosyncratic in their effects, as to contribute to differences between members of the same family. They are captured by Hamlet's words from the famous 'to be or not to be' soliloquy:

...the slings and arrows of outrageous fortune.

The within-family environment will even contribute to differences between individuals of the same genotype reared in the same family. Thus, the single most direct measure of their impact is the variation within pairs of MZ twins reared together.

Obviously, if a large proportion of the total variation is due to environmental differences within families we might expect to look more closely at the different experiences of family members such as MZ twins in the hope of identifying particular environmental factors. However, we have to take account of a further important distinction, namely that between "long-term" and "short-term" environmental effects, even within families. If we only make a single measurement on every individual in a study of MZ twins, say, we cannot tell whether the observed phenotypic differences between members of an MZ twin pair are due to some lasting impact of an early environmental trauma, or due to much more transient differences that influence how the twins function on the particular occasion of measurement. Many of the latter kinds of influence are captured by the concept of "unreliability" variance in measurement theory. There is, of course, no hard and fast distinction between the two sources of variation because how far one investigator is prepared to treat short-term fluctuations as "unreliability" is largely a matter of his or her frame of reference. In depression, which is inherently episodic, short term fluctuations in behavior may point to quite specific environmental factors that trigger specific episodes (see, e.g., Kendler *et al.*, 1986). The main thing to realize is that what a single cross-sectional study assigns to the "within-family" environment may or may not be resolved into specific non-trivial environmental causes. How far to proceed with the analysis of "EW" is a matter for the judgement and ingenuity of the particular investigator, aided by such data on repeated measures as he or she may gather.

The between-family environment would seem to be the place that many of the conceptually important environmental effects might operate. Any environmental factors that are shared by family members will create differences between families and make family members relatively more similar. The environment between families is sometimes called the *shared environment,* the *common environment* or just the *family environment.* Sometimes it is represented by the symbols $E2$, EB, EC, CE, c^2 or V_{EC}. Again, all these symbols denote the same underlying processes.

In twin studies, the shared environment is expected to contribute to the correlation of both MZ and DZ twins as long as they are reared together. Just as we distinguish short-term and long-term effects of the within-family environment, so it is conceptually important to note that the effects of the shared environment may be more or less permanent and persist even if family members are separated later in life, or they may be relatively transient in that they are expressed as long as individuals are living together, perhaps as children with their parents, but are dissipated as soon as the source of shared environmental influence is removed. Such effects can be detected only by comparing the analyses of different age groups in a cross-sectional study, or by tracing changes in the contribution of the shared environment in a longitudinal genetic study (see Chapter 14).

It is a popular misconception that studies of twins reared together can offer no insight about the effects of the shared environment. As we shall see in the following chapters, this is far from the case. Large samples of twins reared together can provide a strong *prima facie* case for the importance of between-family environmental effects that account for a significant proportion of the total variance. The weakness of twin studies, however, is that the various sources of the shared environment cannot be discriminated. It is nevertheless essential for our understanding of what the twin study can achieve, to recognize some of the reasons why this design can never be a "one-shot," self-contained investigation and why investigators should be open to the possibility of significant extensions of the twin study (see Chapter 17).

The environmental similarity between twins may itself be due to several distinct sources whose resolution would require more extensive studies. First, we may identify the environmental impact of parents on their children. That is, part of the "EB" effect in twins, can be traced to the fact that children learn from their parents. Formally, this implies that some aspect of variation in the maternal or paternal phenotypes (or both) creates part of the environmental variation between pairs of children. An excellent starting point for exploring some of these effects is the extension of the classical twin study to include data on the parents of twins (see Chapter 17). In principle, we might find that parents do not contribute equally to the shared family environment. The effect of mothers on the environment of their offspring is usually called the "maternal effect" and the impact of fathers is called the "paternal effect." Although these effects can be resolved by parent-offspring data, they cannot be separated from each other as long as we only have twins in the sample.

Often, following the terms introduced by Cavalli-Sforza and Feldman (1981), the environmental effects of parent on child are called *vertical cultural transmission* to reflect the fact that non-genetic information is passed vertically down the family tree from parents to children. However, the precise effects of the parental environment on the pattern of family resemblance depend on which aspect of the parental phenotype is affecting the offspring's environment. The shared environment of the children may depend on the same trait in the parents that is being measured in the offspring. For example, the environment that makes offspring more or less conservative depends directly on the conservatism of their parents. In this case we normally speak of "phenotype-to-environment ('P to E')" transmission. It is quite possible, however, that part of the shared environment of the offspring is created by aspects of parental behavior that are different from those measured in the children, although the two may be somewhat correlated. Thus, for example, parental income may exercise a direct effect on offspring educational level through its effect on duration and quality of schooling. Another example would be the effect of parental warmth or protectiveness on the development of anxiety or depression in their children. In this case we have a case of *correlated variable transmission.* Haley, Jinks and Last (1981) make a similar distinction between the "one character" and "two character" models for maternal effects. The additional feature of the parental phenotype may or may not be measured in either parents or children. When such additional traits are measured in addition to the trait of primary interest we will require *multivariate genetic models* to perform the data analysis properly. Some simple examples of these methods will be described in later chapters. Two extreme examples of correlated variable transmission are where the variable causing the shared environment is:

1. an index purely of the environmental determinants of the phenotype — "environment-to- environment ('E to E')" transmission

2. purely genetic — "genotype-to- environment ('G to E')" transmission.

Although we can almost never claim to have a direct measure of the genotype for any quantitative trait, the latter conception recognizes that there may be a *genetic environment* (see e.g. Darlington, 1971), that is, genetic differences between some members of a population may be part of the environment of others. One consequence of the genetic environment is the seemingly paradoxical notion that *different genetic relationships also can be used to tease out certain important aspects of the environment.* For example, the children of identical twins can be used to provide a test of the environmental impact of the maternal genotype on the phenotypes of their children (see e.g., Nance and Corey, 1976). A concrete example of this phenomenon would be the demonstration that a mother's genes affect the birthweight of her children.

Although researchers in the behavioral sciences almost instinctively identify the parents as the most salient feature of the shared environment, we must recognize that there are other environmental factors shared by family members which do not depend directly on the parents. There are several factors that can create residual (non-parental) shared environmental effects. First, there may be factors that are shared between all types of offspring, twin or non-twin; these may be called *sibling shared environments*. Second, twins may share a more similar pre-and postnatal environment than siblings simply because they are conceived, born and develop at the same time. This additional correlation between the environments of twins is called the *special twin environment* and is expected to make both MZ and DZ twins more alike than siblings even in the absence of genetic effects. It is important to notice that even twins separated at birth share the same pre-natal environment so a comparison of twins reared together and apart is only able to provide a simple test of the post-natal shared environment[3].

A further type of environmental partition, the *special MZ twin environment* is sometimes postulated to explain the fact that MZ twins reared together are more correlated than DZ twins. This is the most usual environmental explanation offered as an alternative to genetic models for individual differences because the effects of the special MZ environment will tend to mimic those of genes in twins reared together. It is because of concern that genetic effects may be partly confounded with any special MZ twin environments that we stress the importance of thinking beyond the twin study to include other relationships. It becomes increasingly difficult to favor a purely non-genetic explanation of MZ twin similarity when the genetic model is able to predict the correlations for a rich variety of relationships from a few fairly simple principles. Since the special twin environment, however, would increase the correlation of MZ twins, its effects may often resemble those of non-additive genetic effects (dominance and epistasis) in models for family resemblance.

1.4.3   Genotype-Environment Effects

It has long been realized that the distinction we make for heuristic purposes between "genotype" and "environment" is an approximation which ignores several processes that might be important in human populations. Three factors defy the simple separation of genetic and environmental effects, but are likely to be of potential significance from what we know of the way genes operate in other species, and from the logical consequences of the grouping of humans into families of self-determining individuals who share both genes and environment in common.

The factors we need to consider are:

---

[3] Twins born serially by embryo implantation are currently far too rare for the purposes of statistical distinction between pre- and post-natal effects!

1. assortative mating

2. genotype-environment covariance (CovGE, or genotype-environment correlation, CorGE)

3. genotype × environment interaction (G×E).

Each of these will be discussed briefly.

Assortative Mating.

Any non-random pairing of mates on the basis of factors other than biological relatedness is subsumed under the general category of *assortative mating.* Mating based on relatedness is termed *inbreeding,* and will not be examined in this book. We discuss assortative mating under the general heading of genotype-environmental effects for two main reasons. First, when assortment is based on some aspect of the phenotype, it may be influenced by both genetic and environmental factors. Second, assortative mating may affect the transmission, magnitude, and correlation of both genetic and environmental effects.

In human populations, the first indication of assortative mating is often a correlation between the phenotypes of mates. Usually, such correlations are positive. Positive assortment is most marked for traits in the domains of education, religion, attitudes, and socioeconomic status. Somewhat smaller correlations are found in the physical and cognitive domains. Mating is effectively random, or only very slightly assortative, in the personality domain. We are not aware of any replicated finding of a significant negative husband-wife correlation, with the exception of gender!

Assortative mating may not be the sole source of similarity between husband and wife — social interaction is another plausible cause. *A priori,* we might expect social interaction to play a particularly important role in spousal resemblance for habits such as cigarette smoking and alcohol consumption. Two approaches are available for resolving spousal interaction from strict assortative mating. The first depends on tracing the change in spousal resemblance over time, and the second requires analyzing the resemblance between the spouses of biologically related individuals (see Heath, 1987). Although the usual treatment of assortative mating assumes that spouses choose one another on the basis of the trait being studied (*primary phenotypic assortment*), we should understand that this is only one model of a process that might be more complicated in reality. For example, mate selection is unlikely to be based on an actual psychological test score. Instead it is probably based on some related variable, which may or may not be measured directly. If the variable on which selection is based is something that we have also measured, we call it *correlated variable assortment.* If the correlated trait is not measured directly we have *latent variable assortment.* In the simplest case, the latent variable may simply be the *true value* of trait of which the actual measure is just a more or less unreliable index. We then speak of *phenotypic assortment with error.*

Once we begin to consider latent variable assortment, we recognize that the latent variable may be more or less genetic. If the latent variable is due entirely to the social environment we have one form of *social homogamy* (e.g., Rao *et al.*, 1974). We can conceive of a number of intriguing mechanisms of latent variable assortment according to the presumed causes of the latent variable on which mate selection is based. For example, mating may be based on one or more aspects of the phenotypes of relatives, such as parents' incomes, culinary skills, or siblings' reproductive history. In all these cases of correlated or latent variable assortment, mate selection may be based on variables that are more reliable indices of the genotype than the measured phenotype. This possibility was considered by Fisher (1918) in what is still the classical treatment of assortative mating.

Clearly, the resolution of these various mechanisms of assortment is beyond the scope of the conventional twin study, although multivariate studies that include the spouses of twins, or the parents and parents-in-law of twins may be capable of resolving some of these complex issues (see, e.g., Heath *et al.*, 1985).

Even though the classical twin study cannot resolve the complexities of mate selection, we have to keep the issue in mind all the time because of the *effects* of assortment on the correlations between relatives, including twins. When mates select partners like themselves phenotypically, they are also (indirectly) choosing people who resemble themselves genetically and culturally. As a result, positive phenotypic assortative mating increases the genetic and environmental correlations between relatives. Translating this principle into the context of the twin study, we will find that assortative mating tends to increase the similarity of DZ twins relative to MZ twins. As we shall see, in twins reared together, the genetic effects of assortative mating will artificially inflate estimates of the family environmental component. This means, in turn, that estimates of the genetic component based primarily on the difference between MZ correlations and DZ correlations will tend to be biased downwards in the presence of assortative mating.

Genotype-Environment Correlation.

Paradoxically, the factors that make humans difficult to study genetically are precisely those that make humans so interesting. The experimental geneticist can control matings and randomize the uncontrolled environment. In many human societies, for better or for worse, consciously or unconsciously, people likely decide for themselves on the genotype of the partner to whom they are prepared to commit the future of their genes. Furthermore, humans are more or less free living organisms who spend a lot of time with their relatives. If the problem of mate selection gives rise to fascination with the complexities of assortative mating, it is the fact that individuals create their own environment and spend so much time with their relatives that generates the intriguing puzzle of genotype-environment correlation.

As the term suggests, *genotype-environment correlation (CorGE)* refers to the fact that the environments which individuals experience may not be a random sample of the whole range of environments but may be caused by, or correlated with, their genes. Christopher Jencks (1972) spoke of the "double advantage" phenomenon in the context of ability and education. Individuals who begin life with the advantage of genes which increase their ability relative to the average may also be born into homes that provide them with more enriched environments, having more money to spend on books and education and being more committed to learning and teaching. This is an example of positive CorGE. Cattell (1963) raised the possibility of negative CorGE by formulating a principle of "cultural coercion to the biosocial norm." According to this principle, which has much in common with the notion of *stabilizing selection* in population genetics, individuals whose genotype predisposes them to extreme behavior in either direction will tend to evoke a social response which will "coerce" them back towards the mean. For example, educational programs that are designed specifically for the average student may increase achievement in below average students while attenuating it in talented pupils.

Many taxonomies have been proposed for CorGE. We prefer one that classifies CorGE according to specific detectable consequences for the pattern of variation in a population (see Eaves *et al.*, 1977). The first type of CorGE, *genotype-environment autocorrelation* arises because the individual creates or evokes environments which are functions of his or her genotype. This is the "smorgasbord" model which views a given culture as having a wide variety of environments from which the individual makes a selection on the basis of genetically determined preferences. Thus, an intellectually gifted individual would invest more time in mentally stimulating activities. An example of possible CorGE from a different context is provided by an ethological study of 32 month-old male twins published a number of years ago (Lytton, 1977). The study demonstrated that parent-initiated interactions with their twin children are more similar when the twins are MZ rather than DZ. Of course, like every other increased correlation in the environment of MZ twins, it may not be clear whether it is truly a result of a correlation between treatment and genotype rather than simply a matter of identical individuals being treated more similarly.

Insofar as the genotypes of individuals create or elicit environments, cross-sectional twin studies will not be able to distinguish the ensuing CorGE from any other effects of the genes. That is, positive CorGE will increase estimates of all the genetic components of variance and negative CorGE will decrease them. However, we will have no direct way of knowing which genetic effects act *directly* on the phenotype and which result from the action of environmental variation caused initially by genetic differences. In this latter case, the environment may be considered as part of the "extended phenotype" (see Dawkins, 1982). If the process we describe were to accumulate during behavioral development, positive CorGE would lead to an increase in the relative contribution of genetic factors with age, but a constant genetic correlation across ages (see Chapter 14). However, the fact that we find this pattern of developmental change does not necessarily imply that the actual mechanism of the change is specifically genotype-environment autocorrelation.

The second major type of CorGE is that which arises because the environment in which individuals develop is often provided by their biological relatives. Thus, one individual's environment is provided by the phenotype of someone who is genetically related. Typically, we think of the correlated genetic and environmental effects of parents on their children. For example, a child who inherits the genes that predispose to depression may also experience the pathogenic environment of rejection because the tendency of parents to reject their children may be caused by the same genes that increase risk to depression. As far as the offspring are concerned, therefore, a high genetic predisposition to depression is correlated with exposure to an adverse environment because both genes and environment derive originally from the parents. We should note (i) that this type of CorGE can occur only if there is evidence that parent-offspring transmission comprises both genetic factors and vertical cultural inheritance, and (ii) that the CorGE is broken in randomly adopted individuals since the biological parents no longer provide the salient environment. Adoption data thus provide one important test for the presence of this type of genotype-environment correlation.

Although most empirical studies have focused on the parental environment as that which is correlated with genotype, parents are not the only relatives who may be influential in the developmental process. Children are very often raised in the presence of one or more siblings. Obviously, this is always the case for twin pairs. In a world in which people did not interact socially, we would expect the presence or absence of a sibling, and the unique characteristics of that sibling, to have no impact on the outcome of development. However, if there is any kind of social interaction, the idiosyncrasies of siblings become salient features of one another's environment. Insofar as the effect of one sibling or twin on another depends on aspects of the phenotype that are under genetic control, we expect there to be a special kind of *genetic environment* which can be classified under the general category of *sibling effects*. When the trait being measured is partly genetic, and also responsible for creating the sibling effects, we have the possibility for a specific kind of CorGE. This CorGE arises because the genotype of one sibling, or twin, is genetically correlated with the phenotype of the other sibling which is providing part of the environment. When above average trait values in one twin tend to increase trait expression in the other, we speak of *cooperation* effects (Eaves, 1976b) or *imitation* effects (Carey, 1986b). An example of imitation effects would be any tendency of deceptive behavior in one twin to reinforce deception in the other. The alternative social interaction, in which a high trait value in one sibling tends to act on the opposite direction in the other, produces *competition* or *contrast* effects We might expect such effects to be especially marked in environments in which there is competition for limited resources. It has sometimes been argued that contrast effects are an important source of individual differences in extraversion (see Eaves *et al.*, 1989) with the more extraverted twin tending to engender introversion in his or her cotwin and vice-versa.

Sibling effects typically have two kinds of detectable consequence. First, they produce differences in trait mean and variance as a function of sibship size and density. One of the first indications of sibling effects may be differences in variance between twins and singletons. Second, the genotype-environment correlation created by sibling effects depends on the biological relationship between the socially interacting individuals. So, for example, the CorGE is greater in pairs of MZ twins because each twin is reared with an cotwin of identical genotype. If there are cooperation (imitation) effects we expect the CorGE to make the total variance of MZ twins significantly greater than that for DZ's, and the variance of both to exceed that for singletons (Eaves, 1976b). Competition (contrast) effects will tend to make the MZ variance less than that of DZ's. Other effects ensue for the covariances between relatives, as discussed in Chapter 10. Sibling effects may conceivably be reciprocal, if siblings influence each other, or non-reciprocal, if an elder sibling, for example, is a source of social influence on a younger sibling.

Genotype × Environment Interaction

The interaction of genotype and environment ("G × E") must always be distinguished carefully from CorGE. Genotype-environment correlation reflects a non-random distribution of environments among different genotypes. "Good" genotypes get more or less than their fair share of "good" environments. By contrast, G × E interaction has nothing to do with the distribution of genetic and environmental effects. Instead, it relates to the actual way genes and environment affect the phenotype. G × E refers to the genetic control of sensitivity to differences in the environment. The old adage "sauce for the goose is sauce for the gander" describes a world in which G × E is absent, because it implies that the same environmental treatment has the same positive or negative effect regardless of the genotype of the individual upon whom it is imposed.

An obvious example of G × E interaction is that of inherited disease resistance. Genetically susceptible individuals will be free of disease as long as the environment does not contain the pathogen. Resistant individuals will be free of the disease even in a pathogenic environment. That is, changing the environment by introducing the pathogen will have quite a different impact on the phenotype of susceptible individuals in comparison with resistant ones. More subtle examples may be the genetic control of sensitivity to the pathogenic effects of tobacco smoke or genetic differences in the effects of sodium intake on blood pressure.

The analysis of G × E in humans is extremely difficult in practice because of the difficulty of securing large enough samples to detect effects that may be small compared with the main effects of genes and environment. Studies of G × E in experimental organisms (see, e.g., Mather and Jinks, 1982) illustrate a number of issues which are also conceptually important in thinking about G×E in humans. We consider these briefly in turn.

The genes responsible for sensitivity to the environment are not always the same as those that control average trait values. For example, one set of genes may control overall liability to depression and a second set, quite distinct in their location and mode of action, may control whether individuals respond more or less to stressful environments. Another way of thinking about the issue is to consider measurements made in different environments as different traits which may or may not be controlled by the same genes. By analogy with our earlier discussion of sex-limitation, we distinguish between "scalar" and "non-scalar" G × E interaction. When the same genes are expressed consistently at all levels of a salient environmental variable so that only the amount of genetic variance changes between environments, we have "scalar genotype × environment interaction." If, instead of, or in addition to, changes in genetic variance, we also find that different genes are expressed in different environments we have "non-scalar G × E."

G × E interaction may involve environments that can be measured directly or whose effects can be inferred only from the correlations between relatives. Generally, our chances of detecting G × E are much greater when we can measure the relevant environments, such as diet, stress, or tobacco consumption. The simplest situation, which we shall discuss in Chapter 11, arises when each individual in a twin pair can be scored for the presence or absence of a particular environmental variable such as exposure to severe psychological stress. In this case, twin pairs can be divided into those who are concordant and discordant for environmental exposure and the data can be tested for different kinds of G × E using relatively simple methods.

One "measurable" feature of the environment may be the phenotype of an individual's parent. A problem frequently encountered, however, is the fact that many measurable aspects of the environment, such as smoking and alcohol consumption, themselves have a genetic component so that the problems of mathematical modelling and statistical analysis become formidable. If we are unable to measure the environment directly, our ability to detect and analyze G × E will depend on the same kinds of data that we use to analyze the main effects of genes and environment, namely the patterns of family resemblance and other, more complex, features of the distribution of trait values in families. Generally, the detection of any interaction between genetic effects and unmeasured aspects of the between-family environment will require adoption data, particularly separated MZ twins. Interaction between genes and the within-family environment will usually be detectable only if the genes controlling sensitivity are correlated with those controlling average expression of the trait (see, e.g., Jinks and Fulker, 1970).

1.5 Relationships between Variables

Many of the critics of the methods we are to describe argue that, for twin studies at least, the so-called traditional methods such as taking the difference between the MZ and DZ correlations and doubling it as a heritability estimate give much the same answer as the more sophisticated methods taught here. In the final analysis, it must be up to history and the consumer to decide, but in our experience there are several reasons for choosing to "do it our way." First, as we have already shown, the puzzle of human variation extends far beyond testing whether genes play any role in variation. The subtleties of the environment and the varieties of gene action call for methods that can integrate many more types of data and test more complex hypotheses than were envisioned fifty or a hundred years ago. Only a model building/model fitting strategy allows us to trace the implications of a theory across all kinds of data and to test systematically for the consistency of theory and observation. But even if the skeptic is left in doubt by the methods proposed for the interpretation of variables considered individually, we believe that the conventional approaches of fifty years ago pale utterly once we want to analyze the genetic and environmental causes of correlation between variables.

The genetic analysis of multiple variables will occupy many of the succeeding chapters, so here it is sufficient to preview the main issues. There are three kinds of "multivariate" questions which are generic issues in genetic epidemiology, although we shall address them in the context of the twin study. Each is outlined briefly.

1.5.1 The Contribution of Genes and Environment to the Correlation between Variables

The question of what causes variables to correlate is the usual entry point to multivariate genetic analysis. Students of genetics have long been familiar with the concept of pleiotropy, i.e., that one genetic factor can affect several different phenotypes. Obviously, we can imagine environmental advantages and insults that affect many traits in a similar way. Students of the psychology of individual differences, and especially of factor analysis, will be aware that Spearman introduced the concept of the "general intelligence factor" as a latent variable accounting for the pattern of correlations observed between multiple abilities. He also introduced an empirical test (the method of tetrad differences) of the consistency between his general factor theory and the empirical data on the correlations between abilities. Such factor models however, only operate at the descriptive phenotypic level. They aggregate into a single model genetic and environmental processes which might be quite separate and heterogeneous if only the genetic and environmental causes of inter-variable correlation could be analyzed separately. Cattell recognized this when he put forward the notion of "fluid" and "crystallized" intelligence. The former was dependent primarily on genetic processes and would tend to increase the correlation between measures that index genetic abilities. The latter was determined more by the content of the environment (an "environmental mold" trait) and would thus appear as loading more on traits that reflect the cultural environment. A recent analysis of multiple symptoms of anxiety and depression by Kendler *et al.* (1986) illustrates very nicely the point that the pattern of genetic and environmental effects on multiple measures may differ very markedly. They showed that twins' responses to a checklist of symptoms reflected a single underlying genetic dimension which influenced symptoms of both anxiety and depression. By contrast, the effects of the environment were organized along two dimensions ("group factors") — one affecting only symptoms of anxiety and the other symptoms of depression. More recently, this finding has been replicated with psychiatric diagnoses, which suggests that the liability to either disorder is due to a single common set of genes, while the specific expression of that liability as either anxiety or depression is a function of what kind of environmental event triggers the disorder in the vulnerable person. Such insights are impossible without methods that can analyze the correlations between multiple measures into their genetic and environmental components.

1.5.2 Analyzing the Direction of Causation

Students of elementary statistics have long been made to recite "correlation does not imply causation" and rightly so, because a premature assignment of causality to a mere statistical association could waste scientific resources and do actual harm if treatment were to be based upon it. However, one of the goals of science is to analyze complex systems into elementary processes which are thought to be *causal* or more *fundamental* and, when actual experimental intervention is difficult, it may be necessary to look to the nexus of intercorrelations among measures for clues about causality.

The claim that correlation does not imply causality comes from a fundamental indeterminacy of any general model for the correlation between a single pair of variables. Put simply, if we observe a correlation between A and B, it can arise from one or all of three processes: A causing B, B causing A, or latent variable C causing A and B. A general model for the correlation between A and B would need constants to account for the strength of the causal connections between A and B, B and A, C and A, C and B. Clearly, a single correlation cannot be used to determine four unknown parameters.

When we have more than two variables, however, matters may look a little different. It may now become possible to exclude some causal hypotheses as clearly inconsistent with the data. Whether or not this can be done will depend on the complexity of the causal nexus being analyzed. For example, a pattern of correlations of the form $r_{AC} = r_{AB} \times r_{BC}$ would support one or other of the causal sequences $A \longrightarrow B \longrightarrow C$ or $C \longrightarrow B \longrightarrow A$ in preference to orders that place A or C in the middle.

The fact that causality implies *temporal priority* has been used in some applications to advocate a longitudinal strategy for its analysis. One approach is the *cross-lagged panel study* in which the variables A and B are measured at two points in time, t_0 and t_1. If the correlation of A at t_0 with B at t_1 is greater than the correlation of B at t_0 with A at t_1, we might give some credence to the causal priority of A over B.

The cross-lagged approach, though strongly suggestive of causality in some circumstances, is not entirely foolproof. With this fact in view, researchers are always on the look-out for other approaches that can be used to test hypotheses about causality in correlational data. It has recently become clear that the cross-sectional twin study, in which multiple measures are made only on one occasion, may, under some circumstances, allow us to test hypotheses about direction of causality without the necessity of longitudinal data. The potential contribution of twin studies to resolving alternative models of causation will be discussed in Chapter 13. At this stage, however, it is sufficient to give a simple insight about one set of circumstances which might lead us to prefer one causal hypothesis over another.

Consider the ambiguous relationship between exercise and body weight. In free-living populations, there is a significant correlation between exercise and body weight. How much of that association is due to the fact that people who exercise use up more calories and how much to the fact that fat people don't like jogging? In the simplest possible case, suppose that we found variation in exercise to be purely environmental (i.e., having no genetic component) and variation in weight to be partly genetic. Then there is no way that the direction of causation can go from body weight to exercise because, if this were the case, some of the genetic effects on body weight would create genetic variation in exercise. In practice, things are seldom that simple. Data are nearly always more ambiguous and hypotheses more complex. But this simple example illustrates that the genetic studies, notably the twin study, may sometimes yield valuable insight about the causal relationships between multiple variables.

1.5.3   Analyzing Developmental Change

Any cross-sectional study is a slice at one time point across the continuing onto-genetic dialogue between the organism and the environment. While such studies help us understand outcomes, they may not tell us much about the process of "becoming". The longitudinal genetic study, for example repeated measures of twins, may be thought of as a multivariate genetic study in which the multiple occasions of measurement correspond to multiple traits in the conventional cross-sectional study. In the conventional multivariate study we ask such questions as "How much do genes create the correlation between different variables?", so in the longitudinal genetic study we ask "How far do genes (or environment) account for the developmental consistency of behavior?" and "How far are there specific genetic and environmental effects expressed at each point in time?". These are but two of a rich variety of questions which can be addressed with the methods we shall describe. One indication of the insight that can ensue from such an approach to longitudinal measures on twins comes from some of the data on cognitive growth obtained in the ground-breaking Louisville Twin Study. In a reanalysis by model fitting methods, Eaves *et al.* (1986) concluded that such data as had been published strongly suggested the involvement of a single common set of genes which were active from birth to adolescence and whose affects persisted and accumulated through time. By contrast, the shared environment kept changing during development. That is, parents who provided a better environment at one age did not necessarily do so at another, even though whatever they did had fairly persistent effects. The unique environment of the individual, however, was age-specific and very ephemeral in its effect. Such a model, based as it was on only that part of the data available in print, may not stand the test of more detailed scrutiny. Our aim here is not so much to defend a particular model for cognitive development as to indicate that a model fitting approach to longitudinal kinship data can lead to many important insights about the developmental process.

1.6 The Context of our Approach

Figure 1.7 summarizes the main streams of the intellectual tradition which converge to yield the ideas and methods we shall be discussing here. The streams divide and merge again at several places. The picture is not intended to be a comprehensive history of statistical or behavioral genetics, so a number of people whose work is extremely important to both disciplines are not mentioned. Rather, it tries to capture the main lines of thought and the "cast of characters" who have been especially influential in our own intellectual development. Not all of us would give the same weight to all the lines of descent.

1.6.1 19th Century Origins

Two geniuses of the last century provided the fundamental principles on which much of what we do today still depends. Francis Galton's boundless curiosity, ingenuity and passion for measurement were combined in seminal insights and contributions which established the foundations of the scientific study of individual differences. Karl Pearson's three-volume scientific biography of Galton is an enthralling testimony to Galton's fascination and skill in bringing a rich variety of intriguing problems under scientific scrutiny. His *Inquiry into the efficacy of prayer* reveals Galton to be a true "child of the Enlightenment" to whom nothing was sacred. To him we owe the first systematic studies of individual differences and family resemblance, the recognition that the difference between MZ and DZ twins provided a valuable point of departure for resolving the effects of genes and culture, the first mathematical model (albeit inadequate) for the similarity between relatives, and the development of the correlation coefficient as a measure of association between variables that did not depend on the units of measurement.

The specificity that Galton's theory of inheritance lacked was supplied by the classical experiments of Gregor Mendel on plant hybridization. Mendel's demonstration that the inheritance of model traits in carefully bred material agreed with a simple theory of particulate inheritance still remains one of the stunning examples of how the alliance of quantitative thinking and painstaking experimentation

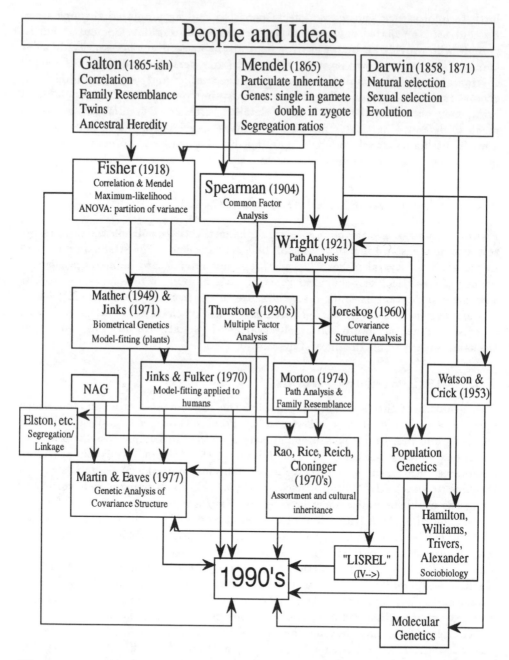

Figure 1.7: Diagram of the intellectual traditions leading to modern mathematical genetic methodology.

can predict, in advance of any observations of chromosome behavior or molecular science, the necessary properties of the elementary processes underlying such complex phenomena as heredity and variation.

1.6.2 Genetic, Factor, and Path Analysis

The conflict between those, like Karl Pearson, who followed a Galtonian model of inheritance and those, like Bateson, who adopted a Mendelian model, is well known to students of genetics. Although Pearson appeared to have some clues about how Galton's data might be explained on Mendelian principles, it fell to Ronald Fisher, in 1918, to provide the first coherent and general account of how the "correlations between relatives" could be explained "on the supposition of Mendelian inheritance." Fisher assumed what is now called the *polygenic model,* that is, he assumed the variation observed for a trait such as stature was caused by a large number of individual genes, each of which was inherited in strict conformity to Mendel's laws. By describing the effects of the environment, assortative mating, and non-additive gene action mathematically, Fisher was able to show remarkable consistency between Pearson's own correlations between relatives for stature and a strictly Mendelian mechanism of inheritance. Some of the ideas first expounded by Fisher will be the basis of our treatment of *biometrical genetics* (Chapter 3).

In the same general era we witness the seeds of two other strands of thought which continue to be influential today. Charles Spearman, adopting Galton's idea that a correlation between variables might reflect a common underlying causal factor, began to explore the pattern of correlations between multiple measures of ability. So began the tradition of multivariate analysis which was, for much of psychology at least, embodied chiefly in the method of factor analysis which sought the latent variables responsible for the observed patterns of correlation between multiple variables. The notion of multiple factors, introduced through the work of Thurstone, and the concept of factor rotation to *simple structure,* provided much of the early conceptual and mathematical foundation for the treatment of multivariate systems to be discussed in this book.

Sewall Wright, whose long and distinguished career spans all of the six decades which have seen the explosion of genetics into the most influential of the life sciences, was the founding father of American population genetics. His seminal paper on path analysis, published in 1921 established a parallel stream of thought to that created by Fisher in 1918. The emphasis of Fisher's work lay in the formulation of a mathematical theory which could reconcile observations on the correlation between relatives with a model of particulate inheritance. Wright, on the other hand, was less concerned with providing a theory which could integrate two views of genetic inheritance than he was with developing a method for exploring ways in which different causal hypotheses could be expressed in a simple, yet testable, form. It is not too gross an oversimplification to suggest that the contributions of Fisher and Wright were each stronger where the other was weaker. Thus, Fisher's

early paper established an explicit model for how the effects and interaction of
large numbers of individual genes could be resolved in the presence of a number of
different theories of mate selection. On the other hand, Fisher showed very little
interest in the environment, choosing rather to conceive of environmental effects as
a random variable uncorrelated between relatives. Fisher's environment is what we
have called the "within family" environment, which seems appropriate for the kinds
of anthropometric variables that Fisher and his predecessors chose to illustrate the
rules of quantitative inheritance. However, it seems a little less defensible, on *a
priori* grounds, as a model for the effects of environment on what Pearson (1904)
called "the mental and moral characteristics of man" or those habits and lifestyles
that might have a significant impact on risk for disease. By contrast, Wright's
approach virtually ignored the subtleties of gene action, considering only additive
genetic effects and treating them as a statistical aggregate which owed little to the
laws of Mendel beyond the fact that offspring received half their genes from their
mother and half from their father. On the other hand, Wright's strategy made it
much easier to specify familial environmental effects, especially those derived from
the social interaction of family members.

1.6.3   Integration of the Biometrical and Path-Analytic Approaches

These different strengths and weaknesses of the traditions derived from Fisher and
Wright persisted into the 1970's. The biometrical genetical approach, derived from
Fisher through the ground-breaking studies of Kenneth Mather and his student
John Jinks established what became known as the "Birmingham School." The emphasis of this tradition was on the detailed analysis of gene action through carefully
designed and properly randomized breeding studies in experimental organisms. Except where the environment could be manipulated genetically (e.g., in the study
of the environmental effects of the maternal genotype), the biometrical genetical
approach treated the environment as a random variable. Even though the environment might sometimes be correlated between families as a result of practical
limitations on randomization, it was independent of genotype. Thus, the Birmingham School's initial treatment of the environment in human studies allowed for
the partition of environmental components of variance into contributions within
families (EW) and between families (EB) but was very weak in its treatment of
genotype-environment correlation. Some attempt to remedy this deficiency was offered by Eaves (1976a; 1976b) in his treatment of vertical cultural transmission and
sibling interaction, but the value of these models was restricted by the assumption
of random mating.

The rediscovery of path analysis in a series of papers by Morton and his cowork-
ers in the early 70's showed how many of the more realistic notions of how environmental effects were transmitted, such as those suggested by Cavalli-Sforza and
Feldman (1981), could be captured much better in path models than they could by

the biometrical approach. However, these early path models assumed that assortative mating to be based on homogamy for the social determinants of the phenotype. Although the actual mechanism of assortment is a matter for empirical investigation, this strong assumption, being entirely different from the mechanisms proposed by Fisher, precluded an adequate fusion of the Fisher and Wright traditions.

A crucial step was achieved in 1978 and 1979 in a series of publications describing a more general path model by Cloninger, Rice, and Reich which integrated the path model for genetic and environmental effects with a Fisherian model for the consequences of assortment based on phenotype. Since then, the approach of path analysis has been accepted (even by the descendants of the Birmingham school) as a first strategy for analyzing family resemblance, and a number of different nuances of genetic and environmental transmission and mate selection have now been translated into path models. This does not mean that the method is without limitations in capturing non-additive effects of genes and environment, but it is virtually impossible today to conceive of a strategy for the analysis of a complex human trait that does not include path analysis among the battery of techniques to be considered.

1.6.4 Development of Statistical Methods

Underlying all of the later developments of the biometrical-genetical, path-analytic and factor-analytic research programs has been a concern for the statistical problems of estimation and hypothesis-testing. It is one thing to develop models; to attach the most efficient and reliable numerical values to the effects specified in a model, and to decide whether a particular model gives an adequate account of the empirical data, are completely different. All three traditions that we have identified as being relevant to our work rely heavily on the statistical concept of likelihood, introduced by Ronald Fisher as a basis for developing methods for parameter estimation and hypothesis testing. The approach of "maximum likelihood" to estimation in human quantitative genetics was first introduced in a landmark paper by Jinks and Fulker (1970) in which they first applied the theoretical and statistical methods of biometrical genetics to human behavioral data. Essential elements of their understanding were that:

1. complex models for human variation could be simplified under the assumption of polygenic inheritance

2. the goodness-of-fit of a model should be tested before waxing lyrical about the substantive importance of parameter estimates

3. the most precise estimates of parameters should be obtained

4. possibilities exist for specifying and analyzing gene action and genotype $\times$ environment interaction

It was the confluence of these notions in a systematic series of models and methods of data analysis which is mainly responsible for breaking the intellectual gridlock into which human behavioral genetics had driven itself by the end of the 1960's.

Essentially the same statistical concern was found among those who had followed the path analytic and factor analytic approaches. Rao, Morton, and Yee (1974) used an approach close to maximum likelihood for estimation of parameters in path models for the correlations between relatives, and earlier work on the analysis of covariance structures by Karl Jöreskog had provided some of the first workable computer algorithms for applying the method of maximum likelihood to parameter estimation and hypothesis-testing in factor analysis. Guided by Jöreskog's influence, the specification and testing of specific hypotheses about factor rotation became possible. Subsequently, with the collaboration of Dag Sörbom, the analysis of covariance structures became elaborated into the flexible model for Linear Structural Relations (LISREL) and the associated computer algorithms which, over two decades, have passed through a series of increasingly general versions.

The attempts to bring genetic methods to bear on psychological variables naturally led to a concern for how the psychometrician's interest in multiple variables could be reconciled with the geneticist's methods for separating genetic and environmental effects. For example, several investigators (Vandenberg, 1965; Loehlin and Vandenberg, 1968; Bock and Vandenberg, 1968) in the late 1960's began to ask whether the genes or the environment was mainly responsible for the general ability factor underlying correlated measures of cognitive ability. The approaches that were suggested, however, were relatively crude generalizations of the classical methods of univariate twin data analysis which were being superseded by the biometrical and path analytic methods. There was clearly a need to integrate the model fitting approach of biometrical genetics with the factor model which was still the conceptual framework of much multivariate analysis in psychology. In discussion with the late Owen White, it became clear that Jöreskog's analysis of covariance structures provided the necessary statistical formulation. In 1977, Martin and Eaves reanalyzed twin data on Thurstone's Primary Mental Abilities using their own FORTRAN program for a multi-group extension of Jöreskog's model to twin data and, for the first time, used the model fitting strategy of biometrical genetics to test hypotheses, however simple, about the genetic and environmental causes of covariation between multiple variables. The subsequent wide dissemination of a multi-group version of LISREL (LISREL III) generated a rash of demonstrations that what Martin and Eaves had achieved somewhat laboriously with their own program could be done much more easily with LISREL (Boomsma and Molenaar, 1986, Cantor, 1983; Fulker et al., 1983; Martin et al., 1982; McArdle et al, 1980).

In the past decade there were many significant new departures in the specification of multivariate genetic models for family resemblance. The main emphasis was on extending the path models, such as those of Cloninger et al., (1979a,b) to the multivariate case (Neale & Fulker, 1984; Vogler, 1985). Much of this work is described clearly and in detail by Fulker (1988) but requires designs and algorithms which are beyond the scope of this book. But all these later developments are cumulative and, although they set the research program for a significant part of the future, it may be a further ten years before the data are available on samples as large and diverse as those required to exploit all the theoretical developments now in hand.

The collection of large volumes of data in a rich variety of twin studies from around the world in the last ten years, coupled with the rocketing growth in the power of micro-computers, offer an unprecedented opportunity. What were once ground-breaking methods, available to those few who knew enough about statistics and computers to write their own programs, can now be placed in the hands of teachers and researchers alike.

Chapter 2

Data Summary

2.1 Introduction

By definition, the primary focus of the study of human individual differences is on variation. As we have seen, the covariation between family members can be especially informative about the causes of variation, so we now turn to the statistical techniques used to measure both variation within and covariation between family members. We start by reviewing the calculation of variances and covariances by hand, and then illustrate how one may use PRELIS to compute these summary statistics in a convenient form for use with LISREL. Our initial treatment assumes that we have well-behaved, normally-distributed variables for analysis. However, almost all studies involve some measures that are certainly not normal because they consist of a few ordered categories, which we call *ordinal* scales. In the second part of this Chapter, we deal with the summary of these cruder forms of measurement, and discuss the concepts of degrees of freedom and goodness-of-fit that arise in this context.

2.2 Continuous Data Analysis

Biometrical analyses of twin data normally make use of summary statistics that reflect differences, or variability, between and within members of twin pairs. Some early studies used mean squares and products, derived from an analysis of variance (Eaves et al., 1977; Martin and Eaves, 1977; Fulker et al., 1983; Boomsma and Molenaar, 1987; Molenaar and Boomsma, 1987), but recent work has embraced variance-covariance matrices as the summary statistics of choice. This approach, often called *covariance structure analysis*, provides greater flexibility in the treatment of some of the processes underlying individual differences, such as genotype $\times$ sex or genotype $\times$ environment interaction. In addition, variances and covariances are a more practical data summary for data that include the relatives of twins, such as parents or spouses (Heath et al., 1985). Because of the greater generality afforded by variances and covariances, we focus on these quantities rather than mean squares.

2.2.1 Calculating Summary Statistics by Hand

The variances and covariances used in twin analyses often are computed using a statistical package such as SPSS (SPSS, 1988) or SAS (SAS, 1988), or by PRELIS (Jöreskog and Sörbom, 1988), the preprocessor for LISREL (the usage of PRELIS is described below). Nevertheless, it is useful to examine how they are calculated in order to ensure a comprehensive understanding of one's observed data. In this Section we describe the calculation of means, variances, covariances, and correlations.

Some simulated measurements from 16 MZ and 16 DZ twin pairs are presented in Table 2.1. The observed values in the columns labelled *Twin 1* and *Twin 2* have

Table 2.1: Simulated Measurements from 16 MZ and 16 DZ Twin Pairs.

MZ		DZ	
Twin 1	*Twin 2*	*Twin 1*	*Twin 2*
3	2	0	1
3	3	2	3
2	1	1	2
1	2	4	3
0	0	3	1
2	2	2	2
2	2	2	2
3	2	1	3
3	3	3	4
2	3	1	0
1	1	1	1
1	1	2	1
4	4	3	3
2	3	3	2
2	1	2	2
1	2	2	2

been selected to illustrate some elementary principles of variation in twins[1].

---

[1] These data are for illustration *only*; they would normally be treated as ordinal, not continuous,

In order to obtain the summary statistics of variances and covariances for genetic analysis, it is first necessary to compute the average value for a set of measurements, called the *mean*. The mean is typically denoted by a bar over the variable name for a group of observations, for example $\overline{X}$ or $\overline{Twin1}$ or $\overline{Twin2}$. The formula for calculation of the mean is:

$$\overline{X} = \frac{X_1 + X_2 + \cdots + X_n}{n}$$

$$= \frac{\sum_{i=1}^{n} X_i}{n}, \tag{2.1}$$

in which X_i represents the ith observation and n is the total number of observations. In the twin data of Table 2.1, the mean of the measurements on Twin 1 of the MZ pairs is

$$\overline{Twin1} = \frac{3 + 3 + 2 + \cdots + 2 + 2 + 1}{16}$$

$$= 32/16$$

$$= 2.0$$

The mean for the second MZ twin ($\overline{Twin2}$) also is 2.0, as are the means for both DZ twins.

The *variance* of the observations represents a measure of dispersion around the mean; that is, how much, on average, observations differ from the mean. The variance formula for a sample of measurements, often represented as s^2 or V_{MZ} or V_{DZ}, is

$$s^2 = \frac{(X_1 - \overline{X})^2 + (X_2 - \overline{X})^2 + \cdots + (X_n - \overline{X})^2}{n - 1}$$

$$= \frac{\sum_{i=1}^{n} (X_i - \overline{X})^2}{n - 1} \tag{2.2}$$

We note two things: first, the difference between each observation and the mean is squared. In principle, absolute differences from the mean could be used as a measure of variation, but absolute differences have a greater variance than squared differences (Fisher, 1920), and are therefore less efficient for use as a summary statistic. Likewise, higher powers (e.g. $\sum_{i=1}^{n}(X_i - \overline{X})^4$) also have greater variance. In fact, Fisher showed that the square of the difference is the most informative measure of variance, i.e., it is a *sufficient statistic*. Second, the sum of the squared

---

and would be summarized differently, as described in Section 2.3. Note also that we do not need to have equal numbers of pairs in the two groups.

deviations is divided by $n-1$ rather than n. The denominator is $n-1$ in order to compensate for an underestimate in the sample variance which would be obtained if s^2 were divided by n. (This arises from the fact that we have already used one parameter — the mean — to describe the data; see Mood & Graybill, 1963 for a discussion of bias in sample variance). Again using the twin data in Table 2.1 as an example, the variance of MZ Twin 1 is

$$
\begin{aligned}
V_{MZT1} &= \frac{(3-2)^2 + (3-2)^2 + \cdots + (2-2)^2 + (1-2)^2}{15} \\
&= \frac{1+1+0+\cdots+0+0+1}{15} \\
&= 16/15
\end{aligned}
$$

The variances of data from the second MZ twin, DZ Twin 1, and DZ Twin 2 also equal 16/15.

Covariances are computationally similar to variances, but represent mean deviations which are shared by two sets of observations. In the twin example, covariances are useful because they indicate the extent to which deviations from the mean by Twin 1 are similar to the second twin's deviations from the mean. Thus, the covariance between observations of Twin 1 and Twin 2 represents a scale-dependent measure of twin similarity. Covariances are often denoted by $s_{x,y}$ or Cov_{MZ} or Cov_{DZ}, and are calculated as

$$
\begin{aligned}
s_{x,y} &= \frac{(X_1-\overline{X})(Y_1-\overline{Y}) + (X_2-\overline{X})(Y_2-\overline{Y}) + \cdots + (X_n-\overline{X})(Y_n-\overline{Y})}{n-1} \\
&= \frac{\displaystyle\sum_{i=1}^{n}(X_i-\overline{X})(Y_i-\overline{Y})}{n-1}
\end{aligned}
\tag{2.3}
$$

Note that the variance formula shown in Eq. 2.2 is just a special case of the covariance when $Y_i = X_i$. In other words, the variance is simply the covariance between a variable and itself.

For the twin data in Table 2.1, the covariance between MZ twins is

$$
\begin{aligned}
\text{Cov}_{MZ} &= \frac{(3-2)(2-2) + (3-2)(3-2) + \cdots + (1-2)(2-2)}{15} \\
&= \frac{0+1+0+0+\cdots+4+0+0+0}{15} \\
&= 12/15
\end{aligned}
$$

The covariance between DZ pairs may be calculated similarly to give 8/15.

The *correlation coefficient* is closely related to the covariance between two sets of observations. Correlations may be interpreted in a similar manner as covariances, but are rescaled to give a lower bound of -1.0 and an upper bound of 1.0.

The correlation coefficient, r, may be calculated using the covariance between two measures and the square root of the variance (the *standard deviation*) of each measure:

$$r = \frac{\text{Cov}_{x,y}}{\sqrt{V_x V_y}} \qquad (2.4)$$

For the simulated MZ twin data, the correlation between twins is

$$
\begin{aligned}
r_{MZ} &= \frac{12/15}{\sqrt{(16/15)(16/15)}} \\
&= 12/16 = .75,
\end{aligned}
$$

and the DZ twin correlation is

$$
\begin{aligned}
r_{DZ} &= \frac{8/15}{\sqrt{(16/15)(16/15)}} \\
&= 8/16 = .50
\end{aligned}
$$

Although variances and covariances typically define the observed information for biometrical analyses of twin data, correlations are useful for comparing resemblances between twins as a function of genetic relatedness. In the simulated twin data, the MZ twin correlation ($r = .75$) is greater than that of the DZ twins ($r = .50$). This greater similarity of MZ twins may be due to several sources of variation (discussed in subsequent chapters), but at the least is suggestive of a heritable basis for the trait, as increased MZ similarity could result from the fact that MZ twins are genetically identical, whereas DZ twins share only 1/2 of their genes on average.

2.2.2   Using PRELIS to Summarize Continuous Data

Here we apply PRELIS to the simulated MZ twin data, and briefly discuss some of the further features of the software. In practice, data on MZ and DZ twins may be placed in separate files, often with one or more lines of data per twin pair[2]. It is easy to use PRELIS to generate summary statistics such as means and covariances for structural equation model fitting.

PRELIS

Suppose that the MZ twin data in Table 2.1 are stored in a file called MZ.RAW in the following way:

```
3   2
3   3
```

---

[2]It is possible to use data files that contain both types of twins and some code to discriminate between them, but it is less efficient.

```
  .    .
  .    .
  .    .
  2    1
  1    2
```

We can use "free format" to read these data. Free format means that there is at least one space or end-of-line character between consecutive data items. These data could be entered using any simple text editor such as the Norton Editor. If a wordprocessor such as Wordperfect or Microsoft Word were used, it would be necessary to save the file as a DOS or ASCII text file. Next, we would prepare an ASCII file containing the PRELIS commands to read these data and compute the means and covariances. We refer to files containing PRELIS or LISREL commands as 'scripts'; the PRELIS script in this case might look like this:

```
Simple prelis example to compute MZ covariances
DA NI=2 NO=0
LA
Twin1 Twin2
COntinuous Twin1 Twin2
RAw FIle=MZ.RAW
OU SM=MZ.COV MA=CM
```

The first line is simply a title. PRELIS will treat all lines as part of the title until a line beginning with DA is encountered. The DA line is used to specify basic features of the input (raw) data such as the number of input variables (NI) and the number of observations. Here we have specified the number of observations as zero (NO=0), which asks PRELIS to count the number of cases for us. The next two lines of the script supply labels (LA) for the variables; these are optional but highly recommended when more than a few variables are to be read. Next, we define the variables Twin1 and Twin2 as *continuous*. By default, PRELIS 2 will treat any variable with less than 15 categories as ordinal. Although this is a reasonable statistical approach, it is not what we want for the purposes of this example. The next line in the script (beginning RA) tells PRELIS where to find the data, and the last line signifies the end of the script, and requests the covariances (MA=CM) to be saved in the file MZ.COV. This output file is created by PRELIS — it is also ASCII format and looks like this:

```
(6D13.6)
 .106667D+01   .800000D+00   .106667D+01
```

The first line of the file contains a FORTRAN format for reading the data. The reader is referred to almost any text on FORTRAN, including User's Guides, for a detailed description of formats. The format used here is D format, for double precision. The 3 characters after the D give the power of 10 by which the printed number should be multiplied, so our .106667D+01 is really $.106667 \times 10^1 = 1.06667$. This number is part of the *lower triangle* of the covariance matrix. Since covariance matrices are always symmetric, only the lower triangle is needed. The file may in turn be read by LISREL for the purposes of structural equation model fitting using syntax such as

```
CM FIle=MZ.COV
```

within a LISREL script — LISREL by default expects only the lower triangle of covariance matrices to be supplied.

Suppose that, instead of just two variables, we had a data file with 20 variables per subject, with two lines for a twin pair. Also suppose that one of the variables identifies the zygosity of the pair, we wish to select only those pairs where zygosity is 1, and we only want the covariance of four of the variables. We could read these data into PRELIS using a FORTRAN format statement explicitly given in the PRELIS script. The script might look like this:

```
PRELIS script to select MZ's and compute covariances of 4
        variables
DA NI=40 NO=0
LA
Zygosity Twin1P1 Twin1P2 Twin2P1 Twin2P2
RAw FIle=MZ.RAW FO
(3X,F1.0,2x,F5.0,12X,F5.0/6X,F5.0,12X,F5.0)
SD Zygosity=1
OU SM=MZ.COV MA=CM
```

The SD command selects cases where zygosity is 1, and deletes zygosity from the list of variables to be analyzed. Note that the FORTRAN format implicitly skips all the irrelevant variables, retaining only five (as specified by the F1.0 and F5.0 fields). Although we could have started with a more complete list of variables, read them in with an appropriate FORMAT, and used the PRELIS command SD to delete those we didn't want, it is more efficient to save the program the trouble of reading these data by adjusting our NI and format statement. On the other hand, if the data file is not large or if a powerful computer is available, it may be better to use SD to save user time spent modifying the script.

2.3   Ordinal Data Analysis

Suppose that instead of making measurements on a continuous scale, we are able to discriminate only a few ordered categories with our measuring instrument. This situation is commonly encountered when assessing the presence or absence of disease, or responses to a single item on a questionnaire. Although it is possible to calculate a covariance matrix from these data, *the correlations usually will be biased*. The degree of bias depends on factors such as the number of categories and

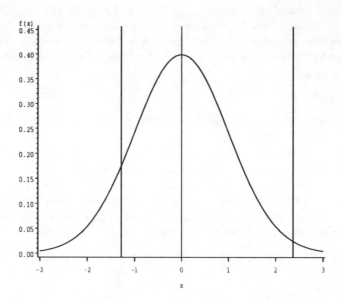

Figure 2.1: Univariate normal distribution with thresholds distinguishing ordered response categories.

the number of observations in each category, and usually results in an underestimate of the true liability correlation in the population. In this section we describe methods of summarizing ordinal data.

2.3.1   Univariate Normal Distribution of Liability

One approach to the analysis of ordinal data is to assume that the ordered categories reflect imprecise measurement of an underlying normal distribution of liability. A second assumption is that the liability distribution has one or more threshold values that discriminate between the categories (see Figure 2.1). This model has been used widely in genetic applications (Falconer, 1960; Neale *et al.*, 1986; Neale, 1988; Heath *et al* 1989a). As long as we consider one variable at a time, it is always possible to place the thresholds so that the proportion of the distribution lying between adjacent thresholds *exactly* matches the observed proportion of the sample that is found in each category. For example, suppose we had an item with four possible responses: 'none', 'a little', 'quite a lot', and 'a great deal'. In a sample of 200 subjects, 20 say 'none', 80 say 'a little', 98 say 'quite a lot' and 2 say 'a great deal'. If our assumed underlying normal distribution has mean 0 and variance 1, then placing thresholds at z-values of -1.282, 0.0 and 2.326 would partition the normal distribution as required. In mathematical terms, let the number of categories be p, so there are $p-1$ thresholds needed to divide the distribution. The expected proportion lying in category i is

$$\int_{t_{i-1}}^{t_i} \phi(x)\, dx$$

where $t_0 = -\infty$, $t_p = \infty$, and $\phi(x)$ is the normal probability density function, given by

$$\phi(x) = \frac{e^{-.5x^2}}{\sqrt{2\pi}}$$

2.3.2 Bivariate Normal Distribution of Liability

When we have only one variable, there is no goodness-of-fit test for the liability model because it always gives a perfect fit. However, this is not necessarily so when we move to the multivariate case. Consider first, the example where we have two variables, each measured as a simple 'yes/no' binary response. Data collected from a sample of subjects could be summarized as a contingency table:

	Item 1	
Item 2	No	Yes
Yes	13	55
No	32	15

It is at this point that we encounter the crucial statistical concept of degrees of freedom (df). Fortunately, though important, calculating the number of df for a model is usually very easy; it is simply the difference between the number of observed statistics and the number of parameters in the model. In the present case we have a 2×2 contingency table in which there are four observed frequencies. However, if we take the total sample size as given and work with the proportion of the sample observed in each cell, we only need three proportions to describe the table completely, because the total of the cell proportions is 1 and the last cell proportion always can be obtained by subtraction. Thus in general for a table with r rows and c columns we can describe the data as rc frequencies or as $rc - 1$ proportions and the total sample size. The next question is, how many parameters does our model contain?

The natural extension of the univariate liability model described above is to assume that there is a continuous, bivariate normal distribution underlying the distribution of our observations. Given this model, we can compute the expected proportions for the four cells of the contingency table[3]. The model is illustrated graphically as contour and 3-D plots in Figure 2.2. The figures contrast the uncorrelated case ($r = 0$) with a high correlation in liability ($r = .9$) and are dramatically

---

[3]Mathematically these expected proportions can be written as double integrals. We do not explicitly define them here, but return to the subject in context of ascertainment discussed in Chapter 18

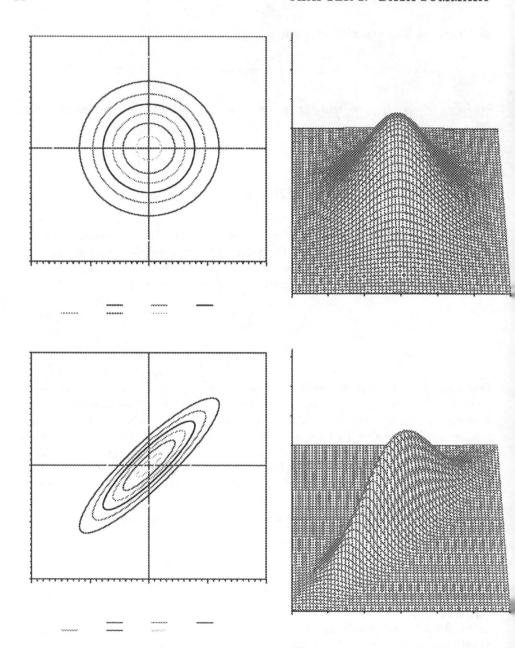

Figure 2.2: Contour and 3-D plots of the bivariate normal distribution with thresholds distinguishing two response categories. Contour plot in top left shows zero correlation in liability and plot in bottom left shows correlation of .9; the panels on the right shows the same data as 3-D plots.

similar to the scatterplots of data from unrelated persons and from MZ twins, shown in Figures 1.3 and 1.4 on pages 8 and 9. By adjusting the correlation in liability and the two thresholds, the model can predict any combination of proportions in the four cells. Because we use 3 parameters to predict the 3 observed proportions, there are no degrees of freedom to test the goodness of fit of the model. This can be seen when we consider an arbitrary non-normal distribution created by mixing two normal distributions, one with $r = +.9$ and the second with $r = -.9$, as shown in Figure 2.3. With thresholds imposed as shown, equal proportions are expected in each cell, corresponding to a zero correlation and zero thresholds, not an unreasonable result *but with just two categories we have no knowledge at all that our distribution is such a bizarre non-normal example.* The case of a 2×2 contingency table is really a 'worst case scenario' for no degrees of freedom associated with a model, since absolutely any pattern of observed frequencies could be accounted for with the liability model. Effectively, all the model does is to transform the data; it cannot be *falsified.*

2.3.3   Testing the Normal Distribution Assumption

The problem of having no degrees of freedom to test the goodness of fit of the bivariate normal distribution to two binary variables is solved when we have at least three categories in one variable and at least two in the other. To illustrate this point, compare the contour plots shown in Figure 2.4 in which two thresholds have been specified for the two variables. With the bivariate normal distribution, there is a very strong pattern imposed on the relative magnitudes of the cells on the diagonal and elsewhere. There is a similar set of constraints with the mixture of normals, but quite different predictions are made about the off-diagonal cells; all four corner cells would have an appreciable frequency given a sufficient sample size, and probably in excess of that in each of the four cells in the middle of each side [e.g., (1,2)]. The bivariate normal distribution could never be adjusted to perfectly predict the cell proportions obtained from the mixture of distributions.

This intuitive idea of *opportunities for failure* translates directly into the concept of degrees of freedom. When we use a bivariate normal liability model to predict the proportions in a contingency table with r rows and c columns, we use $r - 1$ thresholds for the rows, $c - 1$ thresholds for the columns, and one parameter for the correlation in liability, giving $r + c - 1$ in total. The table itself contains $rc - 1$ proportions, neglecting the total sample size as above. Therefore we have degrees of freedom equal to:

$$\text{d.f.} = rc - 1 - (r + c - 1) \text{d.f.} = rc - r - c \qquad (2.5)$$

The discrepancy between the frequencies predicted by the model and those actually observed in the data can be measured using the χ^2 statistic given by:

$$\chi^2 = \sum_{i=1}^{r} \sum_{j=1}^{c} \frac{(O_{ij} - E_{ij})^2}{E_{ij}}$$

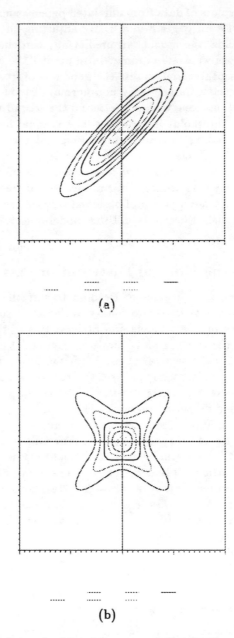

(a)

(b)

Figure 2.3: Contour plots of a bivariate normal distribution with correlation .9 (top); and of a mixture of bivariate normal distributions (bottom), one with .9 correlation and the other with -.9 correlation. One threshold in each dimension is shown.

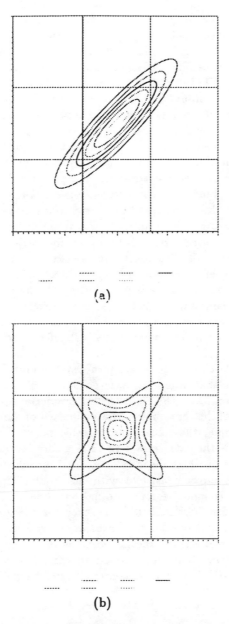

Figure 2.4: Contour plots of a bivariate normal distribution with correlation .9 (top) and a mixture of bivariate normal distributions, one with .9 correlation and the other with -.9 correlation (bottom). Two thresholds in each dimension are shown.

Given a large enough sample, the model's failure to predict the observed data would be reflected in a significant χ^2 for the goodness of fit.

In principle, models could be fitted by maximum likelihood directly to contingency tables, employing the observed and expected cell proportions. This approach is general and flexible, especially for the multigroup case — the programs LISCOMP (Muthen, 1987) and Mx (Neale, 1991) use the method — but it is currently limited by computational considerations. When we move from two variables to larger examples involving many variables, integration of the multivariate normal distribution (which has to be done numerically) becomes extremely time-consuming, perhaps increasing by a factor of ten or so for each additional variable. To circumvent this problem, we use advanced numerical methods available in PRELIS 2 to compute each correlation in a pairwise fashion, and to compute a weight matrix. The weight matrix is an estimate of the variances and covariances of the correlations. The variances of the correlations certainly have some intuitive appeal, being a measure of how precisely a correlation is estimated. However, the idea of a correlation correlating with another correlation may seem strange to a newcomer to the field. Yet this covariation between correlations is precisely what we need in order to represent how much *additional* information the second correlation supplies over and above that provided by the first correlation. Armed with these two types of summary statistics — the correlation matrix and the covariances of the correlations — we may fit models using a structural equation modeling package such as LISREL, and make statistical inferences from the goodness of fit of the model.

It is also possible to use the bivariate normal liability distribution to infer the patterns of statistics that would be observed if an ordinal and continuous variables were correlated. Essentially, there are specific predictions made about the expected mean and variance of the continuous variable in each of the categories of the ordinal variable. For example, the continuous variable means are predicted to increase monotonically across the categories if there is a correlation between the liabilities. An observed pattern of a high mean in category 1, low in category 2 and high again in category 3 would not be consistent with the model. The number of parameters used to describe this model for an ordinal variable with r categories is $r + 2$, since we use $r - 1$ for the thresholds, one each for the mean and variance of the continuous variable, and one for the covariance between the two variables. The observed statistics involved are the proportions in the cells (less one because the final proportion may be obtained by subtraction from 1) and the mean and variance of the continuous variable in each category. Therefore we have:

$$\begin{aligned}
\text{d.f.}_{\text{oc}} &= (r-1) + 2r - (r+2) \qquad\qquad (2.6)\\
&= 2r - 3
\end{aligned}$$

So the number of degrees of freedom for such a test is $2r - 3$ where r is the number of categories.

Table 2.2: Classification of correlations according to their observed distribution.

Measurement	Two Categories	Three or more Categories	Continuous
Two	Tetrachoric	Polychoric	Biserial
Three +	Polychoric	Polychoric	Polyserial
Continuous	Biserial	Polyserial	Product Moment

2.3.4 Terminology for Types of Correlation

One of the difficulties encountered by the newcomer to statistics is the use of a wide variety of terms for correlation coefficients. There are many measures of association between variables; here we confine ourselves to the parametric statistics computed by PRELIS. These statistics correspond most naturally to our genetic theory, in which we assume that a large number of independent genetic and environmental factors give rise to variation — "multifactorial inheritance"[4].

Table 2.2 shows the name given to the correlation coefficient calculated under normal distribution theory, according to whether each variable has: two categories (dichotomous); several categories (polychotomous); or an infinite number of categories (continuous). If both variables are dichotomous, then the correlation is called a tetrachoric correlation *as long as it is calculated using the bivariate normal integration approach described in Section 2.3 above.* If we simply use the Pearson product moment formula (described in Section 2.2.1 above) then we have computed a phi-coefficient which will probably underestimate the population correlation in liability. Because the tetrachoric and polychoric are calculated with the same method, some authors refer to the tetrachoric as a polychoric, and the same is true of the use of polyserial instead of biserial. As we shall see, the theory behind all these statistics is essentially the same.

2.3.5 Using PRELIS with Ordinal Data

Here we give a PRELIS script to read only two from a long list of psychiatric diagnoses, coded as 1 or 0 in these data.

```
Diagnoses and age MZ twins: VARIABLES ARE:
 DEPLN4 DEPLN2 DEPLN1 DEPLB4 DEPLB2 DEPLB1 GADLN6 GADLN1
 GADLB6 GADLB1 GAD88B GAD88N PANN PANB PHON PHOB ETOHN
 ETOHB ANON ANOB BULN BULB DEPLN4T2 DEPLN2T2 DEPLN1T2
```

---

[4]In fact quite a small number of genetic factors may give rise to a distribution which is for almost all practical purposes indistinguishable from a normal distribution (Kendler and Kidd, 1986).

```
DEPLB4T2 DEPLB2T2 DEPLB1T2 GADLN6T2 GADLN1T2 GADLB6T2
GADLB1T2 GAD88BT2 GAD88NT2 PANNT2 PANBT2 PHONT2 PHOBT2
ETOHNT2 ETOHBT2 ANONT2 ANOBT2 BULNT2 BULBT2/
FORMAT IN FULL IS:
(2X, F8.2,F1.0, 43(1X,F1.0)
```

```
Diagnoses and age MZ twins
DA NI=3 NO=0
LA; DOB DEPLN4 DEPLN4T2
RA FI=DIAGMZ.DAT FO
(2X, F8.2,F1.0, 43x,F1.0)
OR DEPLN4-DEPLN4T2
OU MA=PM SM=DEPLN4MZ.COR SA=DEPLN4MZ.ASY PA
```

```
Diagnoses and age DZ twins
DA NI=3 NO=0
LA; DOB DEPLN4 DEPLN4T2
RA FI=DIAGdZ.DAT FO
(2X, F8.2,F1.0, 43x,F1.0)
OR DEPLN4-DEPLN4T2
OU MA=PM SM=DEPLN4dZ.COR SA=DEPLN4dZ.ASY PA
```

Note that again we have used the FORTRAN format to control which variables
are read. One key difference from the continuous case is the use of MA=PM, which
requests calculation of a matrix of polychoric, polyserial and product moment correlations. The program uses product moment correlations when both variables
are continuous, a polyserial (or biserial) when one is ordinal and the other continuous, and a polychoric (or tetrachoric) when both are ordinal. Running the
script produces four output files DEPLN4MZ.COR, DEPLN4MZ.ASY, DEPLN4DZ.COR and
DEPLN4DZ.ASY which may be read directly into LISREL using PM and AC commands.
Notice that we have 'stacked' two scripts in one file, one to read and compute statistics from the MZ data file (FI=DIAGMZ.DAT) and a second to do the same thing for
the DZ data. Also notice that the SM command is used to output the correlation
matrix and SA is to save the asymptotic weight matrix. In fact, PRELIS saves
the weight matrix multiplied by the sample size which is what LISREL expects
to receive when the AC command is used. The PA command requests that the
asymptotic weight matrix itself be printed in the output.

Output from running the PRELIS script has several notable features, particularly PRELIS 2, which is in beta test version at the time of writing. The authors
hope that PRELIS 2 will be generally available in the near future, because weight
matrices calculated in PRELIS 1 are inaccurate (Rigdon & Ferguson, 1991). So,
in the PRELIS 2 output, there are a number of summary statistics for continuous variables (means and standard deviations, and histograms) and frequency
distributions with bar graphs, for the ordinal variables. To provide the user with

some guide to the origin of statistics describing the covariance between variables, PRELIS prints means and standard deviations of continuous variables separately for each category of each pair of ordinal variable, and contingency tables between each ordinal variables. Towards the end of the output there is a table printed with the following format:

```
                                TEST OF MODEL
                CORRELATION   CHI-SQU.  D.F.  P-VALUE

                -----------   --------  ----  -------

DEPLN4 VS.    DOB  -.233 (PS)   5.067     1    .024
DEPLN4T2 VS.  DOB   .010 (PS)   6.703     1    .010
```

There are two quite different chi-squared tests printed on the output. The first, under TEST OF MODEL is a test of the goodness of fit of the bivariate normal distribution model to the data. In the case of two ordinal variables with r and c categories in each, there are $rc - r - c$ d.f. as described in expression 2.5 above. Likewise there will be $2r - 3$ d.f. for the continuous by ordinal statistics, as described in expression 2.6. If the p-value reported by PRELIS is low (e.g. $< .05$), then concern arises about whether the bivariate normal distribution model is appropriate for these data. For a polyserial correlation (correlations between ordinal and continuous variables), it may simply be that the continuous variable is not normally distributed, or that the association between the variables does not follow a bivariate normal distribution. For polychoric correlations, there is no univariate test of normality involved, so failure of the model would imply that the latent liability distributions do not follow a bivariate normal. Remember however that significance levels for these tests are not often the reported p-value, because we are performing multiple tests. If the tests were independent, then with n such tests the α significance level would not be the reported p-value but $1 - (1 - p)^n$. Therefore concern would arise only if p was very small and a large number of tests had been performed. In our case, the tests are not independent because, for example, the correlation of A and B is not independent of the correlation of A and C, so the attenuation of the α level of significance is not so extreme as the $1 - (1 - p)^n$ formula predicts. The amount of attenuation will be application specific, but would often be closer to $1 - (1 - p)^n$ than simply to p.

The second chi-squared statistic printed by PRELIS (not shown in the above sample of output) tests whether the correlation is significantly different from zero. A similar result should be obtained if the summary statistics are supplied to LISREL, and a chi-squared difference test (see Chapter 6) is performed between a model which allows the correlation to be a free parameter, and one in which the correlation is set to zero.

The use of weight matrices as input to LISREL is described elsewhere in this book. Here we have described the generation of a weight matrix for a correlation matrix, but it is also possible to use weight matrices for covariance matrices[5]. Both methods are part of the asymptotically distribution free (ADF) methods pioneered by Browne (1984). It is not yet clear whether maximum likelihood or ADF methods are generally better for coping with data that are not multinormally distributed; further simulation studies are required. The ADF methods require more numerical effort and become cumbersome to use with large numbers of variables. This is so because the size of the weight matrix rapidly increases with number of variables. The number of elements on and below the diagonal of a matrix is a *triangular number* given by $k(k+1)/2$. The number of elements in this weight matrix is a triangular number of a triangular number, or

$$\frac{k^4 + 2k^3 + 3k^2 + 2k}{8}$$

In the case of correlation matrices, the number of elements is somewhat less, but still increases as a quartic function:

$$\frac{k^4 - 2k^3 + 3k^2 - 2k}{8}$$

As a compromise when the number of variables is large, Jöreskog and Sörbom suggest the use of diagonal weights, i.e. just the variances of the correlations and not their covariances. However, tests of significance are likely to be inaccurate with this method and estimates of anything other than the full or true model would be biased.

2.4   Summary

We have described in detail the statistical operations involved in, and the use of PRELIS for, the measurement of variation and covariation. When we have continuous measures, the calculations are quite simple and can be done by hand, but for ordinal data the process is more complex. We obtain estimates of polychoric and polyserial correlations by using software that numerically integrates the bivariate normal distribution. In the process, we are effectively fitting a model of continuous multivariate normal liability with abrupt thresholds to the contingency table. This model cannot be rejected when there are only two categories for each measure, but may fail as the number of cells in the table increases.

While ordinal data are far more common than continuous measures in the behavioral sciences, we note that as the number of categories gets large (e.g., more than 15) the difference between the continuous and the ordinal treatments gets

---

[5] The number of elements in a weight matrix for a covariance matrix is greater than that for a correlation matrix. For this reason, it is necessary to specify MA=PM on the DA line of a LISREL job that is to read a weight matrix.

small. In general, the researcher should try to obtain continuous measures if possible, since considerable statistical power can be lost when only a few response categories are used, as we shall show in Chapter 9.

Chapter 3

Biometrical Genetics

3.1 Introduction and Description of Terminology

The principles of biometrical and quantitative genetics lie at the heart of virtually all of the statistical models examined in this book. Thus, an understanding of biometrical genetics is fundamental to our statistical approach to twin and family data. Biometrical models relate the "latent," or unobserved, variables of our structural models to the functional effects of genes. It is these effects, based on the principles of Mendelian genetics, that give our structural models a degree of validity quite unusual in the social sciences. The purpose of this chapter is to provide a brief introduction to biometrical models. Extensive treatments of the subject have been provided by Mather and Jinks (1982) and Falconer (1990). Here we employ the notation of Mather and Jinks.

Before we begin our discussion of biometrical genetics, we must describe some of the terms that are encountered frequently in biometrical and classical genetic discourse. For the present purposes, we use the term *gene* in reference to a "unit factor of inheritance" that influences an observable trait or traits, following the earlier usage by Fuller and Thompson (1978). Observable characteristics are referred to as *phenotypes*. The site of a gene on a chromosome is known as the *locus*. *Alleles* are alternative forms of a gene that occupy the same locus on a chromosome. They often are symbolized as A and a or B and b or A_1 and A_2. The simplest system for a segregating locus involves only two alleles (A and a), but there also may be a large number of alleles in a system. For example, the HLA locus on chromosome 6 is known to have 18 alleles at the A locus, 41 alleles at the B locus, 8 at C, about 20 at DR, 3 at DQ, and 6 at DP (Bodmer 1987). Nevertheless, if one or two alleles are much more frequent than the others, a two-allele system provides a useful approximation and leads to an accurate account for the phenotypic variation and covariation with which we are concerned. The *genotype* is the chromosomal complement of alleles for an individual. At a single locus (with two alleles) the

55

genotype may be symbolized AA, Aa, or aa; if we consider multiple loci the genotype of an individual may be written as $AABB$, $AABb$, $AAbb$, $AaBB$, $AaBb$, $Aabb$,
$aaBB$, $aaBb$, or $aabb$, in the case of two loci, for example. *Homozygosity* refers to
a state of identical alleles at corresponding loci on homologous chromosomes; for
example, AA or aa for one locus, or $AABB$, $aabb$, $AAbb$, or $aaBB$ for two loci. In
contrast, *heterozygosity* refers to a state of unlike alleles at corresponding loci, Aa
or $AaBb$, for example. When numeric or symbolic values are assigned to specific
genotypes they are called *genotypic values*. The *additive value* of a gene is the
sum of the average effects of the individual alleles. *Dominance deviations* refer to
the extent to which genotypes differ from the additive genetic value. A system in
which multiple loci are involved in the expression of a single trait is called *polygenic*
("many genes"). A *pleiotropic* system ("many growths") is one in which the same
gene or genes influence more than one trait.

Biometrical models are based on the measurable effects of different genotypes
that arise at a segregating locus, which are summed across all of the loci that contribute to a continuously varying trait. The number of loci generally is not known,
but it is usual to assume that a relatively large number of genes of equivalent effect are at work. In this way, the categories of Mendelian genetics that lead to
binomial distributions for traits in the population tend toward continuous distributions such as the normal curve. Thus, the statistical parameters that describe
this model are those of continuous distributions, including the first moment, or the
mean; second moments, or variances, covariances, and correlation coefficients; and
higher moments such as measures of skewness where these are appropriate. This
polygenic model was originally developed by Sir Ronald Fisher in his classic paper
"*The correlation between relatives on the supposition of Mendelian inheritance*"
(Fisher, 1918), in which he reconciled Galtonian biometrics with Mendelian genetics. One interesting feature of the polygenic biometrical model is that it predicts
normal distributions for traits when very many loci are involved and their effects
are combined with a multitude of environmental influences. Since the vast majority
of biological and behavioral traits approximate the normal distribution, it is an inherently plausible model for the geneticist to adopt. We might note, however, that
although the normality expected for a polygenic system is statistically convenient
as well as empirically appropriate, none of the biometrical expectations with which
we shall be concerned depend on how many or how few genes are involved. The
expectations are equally valid if there are are only one or two genes, or indeed no
genes at all.

In the simplest two–allele system (A and a) there are two parameters that define
the measurable effects of the three possible genotypes, AA, Aa, and aa. These
parameters are d, which is twice the measured difference between the homozygotes
AA and aa, and h, which defines the measured effect of the heterozygote Aa, insofar
as it does not fall exactly between the homozygotes. The point between the two
homozygotes is m, the mean effect of homozygous genotypes. We refer to the
parameters d and h as *genotypic effects*. The scaling of the three genotypes is

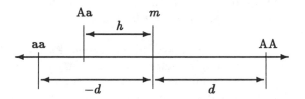

Figure 3.1: The d and h increments of the gene difference $A - a$. Aa may lie on either side of m and the sign of h will vary accordingly; in the case illustrated h would be negative. (Adapted from Mather and Jinks, 1977, p. 32).

shown in Figure 3.1.

To make the simple two–allele model concrete, let us imagine that we are talking about genes that influence adult stature. Let us assume that the normal range of height for males is from 4 feet 10 inches to 6 feet 8 inches; that is, about 22 inches[1]. And let us assume that each somatic chromosome has one gene of roughly equivalent effect. Then, roughly speaking, we are thinking in terms of loci for which the homozygotes contribute $+\frac{1}{2}$ inch (from the midpoint), depending on whether they are AA, the increasing homozygote, or aa, the decreasing homozygotes. In reality, although some loci may contribute greater effects than this, others will almost certainly contribute less; thus we are talking about the kind of model in which any particular polygene is having an effect that would be difficult to detect by the methods of classical genetics. Similarly, while the methods of linkage analysis may be appropriate for a number of quantitative loci, it seems unlikely that the majority of causes of genetic variation would be detectable by these means. The biometrical approach, being founded upon an assumption that inheritance may be polygenic, is designed to elucidate sources of genetic variation is these types of systems.

3.2   Breeding Experiments: Gametic Crosses

The methods of biometrical genetics are best understood through controlled breeding experiments with inbred strains, in which the results are simple and intuitively

---

[1]Note: 1 inch = 2.54cm; 1 foot = 12 inches.

obvious. Of course, in the present context we are dealing with continuous variation in humans, where inbred strains do not exist and controlled breeding experiments are impossible. However, the simple results from inbred strains of animals apply directly, albeit in more complex form, to those of free mating organisms such as humans. We feel an appreciation of the simple results from controlled breeding experiments provides insight and lends credibility to the application of the models to human beings.

Let us consider a cross between two inbred parental strains, P_1 and P_2, with genotypes AA and aa, respectively. Since individuals in the P_1 strain can produce gametes with only the A allele, and P_2 individuals can produce only a gametes, all of the offspring of such a mating will be heterozygotes, Aa, forming what Gregor Mendel referred to as the "first filial," or F_1 generation. A cross between two F_1 individuals generates what he referred to as the "second filial" generation, or F_2, and it may be shown that this generation comprises $\frac{1}{4}$ individuals of genotype AA, $\frac{1}{4}$ aa, and $\frac{1}{2}$ Aa. Mendel's first law, the *law of segregation*, states that parents with genotype Aa will produce the gametes A and a in equal proportions. The pioneer Mendelian geneticist Reginald Punnett developed a device known as the *Punnett square*, which he found useful in teaching Mendelian genetics to Cambridge undergraduates, that gives the proportions of genotypes that will arise when these gametes unite at random. (Random unions of gametes occur under the condition of random mating among individuals). The result of other matings such as $P_1 \times F_1$, the first backcross, B_1, and more complex combinations may be elucidated in a similar manner. A simple usage of the Punnett square is shown in Table 3.1 for the mating of two heterozygous parents in a two–allele system. The gamete frequencies in Table 3.1 (shown outside the box) are known as *gene or allelic frequencies*, and they give rise to the *genotypic frequencies* by a simple product of independent probabilities. It is this assumption of independence based on random mating that makes the biometrical model straightforward and tractable in more complex situations, such as random mating in populations where the gene frequencies are unequal. It also forms a simple basis for considering the more complex effects of non-random mating, or assortative mating, which are known to be important in human populations.

In the simple case of equal gene frequencies as we have in an F_2 population, it is easily shown that random mating over successive generations changes neither the gene nor genotype frequencies of the population. Male and female gametes of the type A and a from an F_2 population are produced in equal proportions so that random mating may be represented by the same Punnett square as given in Table 3.1, which simply reproduces a population with identical structure to the F_2 from which we started. This remarkable result is known as *Hardy–Weinberg equilibrium* and is the cornerstone of quantitative and population genetics. From this result, the effects of non-random mating and other forces that change populations, such as natural selection, migration, and mutation, may be deduced. Hardy-Weinberg equilibrium is achieved in one generation and applies whether or

Table 3.1: Punnett square for mating between two heterozygous parents.

	Male Gametes	
	$\frac{1}{2}A$	$\frac{1}{2}a$
Female Gametes $\frac{1}{2}A$	$\frac{1}{4}AA$	$\frac{1}{4}Aa$
$\frac{1}{2}a$	$\frac{1}{4}Aa$	$\frac{1}{4}aa$

not the gene frequencies are equal and whether or not there are more than two alleles. It also holds among polygenic loci, linked or unlinked, although in these cases joint equilibrium depends on a number of generations of random mating.

For our purposes the genotypic frequencies from the Punnett square are important because they allow us to calculate the simple first and second moments of the phenotypic distribution that result from genetic effects; namely, the mean and variance of the phenotypic trait. The genotypes, frequencies, and genotypic effects of the biometrical model in Table 3.1 are shown below, and from these we can calculate the mean and variance.

Genotype (i)	AA	Aa	aa
Frequency (f)	$\frac{1}{4}$	$\frac{1}{2}$	$\frac{1}{4}$
Genotypic effect (x)	d	h	$-d$

The mean effect of the A locus is obtained by summing the products of the frequencies and genotypic effects in the following manner:

$$
\begin{aligned}
\mu_A &= \sum f_i x_i \\
&= \frac{1}{4}d + \frac{1}{2}h - \frac{1}{4}d \\
&= \frac{1}{2}h
\end{aligned}
\tag{3.1}
$$

The variance of the genetic effects is given by the sum of the products of the genotypic frequencies and their squared deviations from the mean[2]:

$$
\sigma_A^2 = \sum f_i (x_i - \mu_A)^2
$$

---

[2]This is an application of the method described in Section 2.2.1. It looks a bit more intimidating here because of (a) the multiplication by the frequency, and (b) the use of letters not numbers. To gain confidence in this method, the reader may wish to choose values for d and h and work through an example.

$$= \frac{1}{4}(d - \frac{1}{2}h)^2 + \frac{1}{2}(h - \frac{1}{2}h)^2 + \frac{1}{4}(-d - \frac{1}{2}h)^2$$

$$= \frac{1}{4}d^2 - \frac{1}{4}dh + \frac{1}{16}h^2 + \frac{1}{8}h^2 + \frac{1}{4}d^2 + \frac{1}{4}dh + \frac{1}{16}h^2$$

$$= \frac{1}{2}d^2 + \frac{1}{4}h^2 \tag{3.2}$$

For this single locus with equal gene frequencies, $\frac{1}{2}d^2$ is known as the additive genetic variance, or V_A, and $\frac{1}{4}h^2$ is known as the dominance variance, V_D. When more than one locus is involved, perhaps many loci as we envisage in the polygenic model, Mendel's *law of independent assortment* permits the simple summation of the individual effects of separate loci in both the mean and the variance. Thus, for (k) multiple loci,

$$\mu = \frac{1}{2} \sum_{i=1}^{k} h_i , \tag{3.3}$$

and

$$\sigma^2 = \frac{1}{2} \sum_{i=1}^{k} d_i^2 + \frac{1}{4} \sum_{i=1}^{k} h_i^2$$

$$= V_A + V_D . \tag{3.4}$$

It is the parameters V_A and V_D that we estimate using the LISREL structural equations in this book.

In order to see how this biometrical model and the LISREL equations estimate V_A and V_D, we need to consider the joint effect of genes in related individuals. That is, we need to derive expectations for MZ and DZ covariances in terms of the genotypic frequencies and the effects of d and h.

3.3 Derivation of Expected Twin Covariances

3.3.1 Equal Gene Frequencies

Twin correlations may be derived in a number of different ways, but the most direct method is to list all possible twin-pair genotypes (taken as deviations from the population mean) and the frequency with which they arise in a random-mating population. Then, the expected covariance may be obtained by multiplying the genotypic effects for each pair, weighting them by the frequency of occurrence, and summing across all possible pairs. By this method the covariance among pairs is calculated directly. The overall mean for such pairs is, of course, simply the population mean, $\frac{1}{2}h$, in the case of equal gene frequencies, as shown in the previous section. There are shorter methods for obtaining the same result, but these are less direct and less intuitively obvious.

The covariance calculations are laid out in Table 3.2 for MZ, DZ, and Unrelated pairs of siblings, the latter being included in order to demonstrate the expected zero covariance for genetically unrelated individuals. The nine possible combinations of genotypes are shown in column 1, with their genotypic effects, x_{1i} and x_{2i}, in columns 2 and 3. From these values the mean of all pairs, $\frac{1}{2}h$, is subtracted in columns 4 and 5. Column 6 shows the products of these mean deviations. The final three columns show the frequency with which each of the genotype pairs occurs for the three kinds of relationship. For MZ twins, the genotypes must be identical, so there are only three possibilities and these occur with the population frequency of each of the possible genotypes. For unrelated pairs, the population frequencies of the three genotypes are simply multiplied within each pair of siblings since genotypes are paired at random. The frequencies for DZ twins, which are the same as for ordinary siblings, are more difficult to obtain. All possible parental types and the proportion of paired genotypes they can produce must be enumerated, and these categories collected up across all possible parental types. These frequencies and the method by which they are obtained may be found in standard texts (e.g., Crow and Kimura, 1970, pp. 136-137; Falconer, 1960, pp. 152-157; Mather and Jinks, 1971, pp. 214-215).

The products in column 6, weighted by the frequencies for the three sibling types, yield the degree of genetic resemblance between siblings. In the case of MZ twins, the covariance equals

$$\text{Cov(MZ)} = d^2(\frac{1}{4} + \frac{1}{4}) + dh(-\frac{1}{4} + \frac{1}{4}) + \frac{1}{4}h^2(\frac{1}{4} + \frac{2}{4} + \frac{1}{4})$$

$$= \frac{1}{2}d^2 + \frac{1}{4}h^2 , \tag{3.5}$$

which is simply expression 3.2, the total genetic variance in the population. If we sum over loci, as we did in expression 3.4, we obtain $V_A + V_D$, the additive and dominance variance, as we would intuitively expect since identical twins share all genetic variance. The calculation for DZ twins, with terms in d^2, dh, and h^2 initially separated for convenience, and collected together at the end, is

$$\begin{aligned}
\text{Cov(DZ)} &= d^2(\frac{9}{64} - \frac{1}{64} - \frac{1}{64} + \frac{9}{64}) \\
&+ dh(-\frac{9}{64} + \frac{3}{64} + \frac{3}{64} - \frac{3}{64} - \frac{3}{64} + \frac{9}{64}) \\
&+ \frac{1}{4}h^2(\frac{9}{64} - \frac{6}{64} + \frac{1}{64} - \frac{6}{64} + \frac{20}{64} - \frac{6}{64} + \frac{1}{64} - \frac{6}{64} + \frac{9}{64}) \\
&= \frac{1}{4}d^2 + \frac{1}{16}h^2 \tag{3.6}
\end{aligned}$$

When summed over all loci, this expression gives $\frac{1}{2}V_A + \frac{1}{4}V_D$. The calculation for unrelated pairs of individuals yields a zero value as expected, since, on average,

Table 3.2: Genetic covariance components for MZ, DZ, and Unrelated siblings with equal gene frequencies at a single locus ($u = v = \frac{1}{2}$).

Genotype Pair	Effect		$x_{1i} - \mu_1$	$x_{2i} - \mu_2$	$(x_{1i} - \mu_1)(x_{2i} - \mu_2)$	Frequency		
	x_{1i}	x_{2i}				MZ	DZ	U
AA, AA	d	d	$d - \frac{1}{2}h$	$d - \frac{1}{2}h$	$d^2 - dh + \frac{1}{4}h^2$	$\frac{1}{4}$	$\frac{9}{64}$	$\frac{1}{16}$
AA, Aa	d	h	$d - \frac{1}{2}h$	$\frac{1}{2}h$	$\frac{1}{2}dh - \frac{1}{4}h^2$	-	$\frac{3}{32}$	$\frac{1}{8}$
AA, aa	d	$-d$	$d - \frac{1}{2}h$	$-d - \frac{1}{2}h$	$-d^2 + \frac{1}{4}h^2$	-	$\frac{1}{64}$	$\frac{1}{16}$
Aa, AA	h	d	$\frac{1}{2}h$	$d - \frac{1}{2}h$	$\frac{1}{2}dh - \frac{1}{4}h^2$	-	$\frac{3}{32}$	$\frac{1}{8}$
Aa, Aa	h	h	$\frac{1}{2}h$	$\frac{1}{2}h$	$\frac{1}{4}h^2$	$\frac{1}{2}$	$\frac{5}{16}$	$\frac{1}{4}$
Aa, aa	h	$-d$	$\frac{1}{2}h$	$-d - \frac{1}{2}h$	$-\frac{1}{2}dh - \frac{1}{4}h^2$	-	$\frac{3}{32}$	$\frac{1}{8}$
aa, AA	$-d$	d	$-d - \frac{1}{2}h$	$d - \frac{1}{2}h$	$-d^2 + \frac{1}{4}h^2$	-	$\frac{1}{64}$	$\frac{1}{16}$
aa, Aa	$-d$	h	$-d - \frac{1}{2}h$	$\frac{1}{2}h$	$-\frac{1}{2}dh - \frac{1}{4}h^2$	-	$\frac{3}{32}$	$\frac{1}{8}$
aa, aa	$-d$	$-d$	$-d - \frac{1}{2}h$	$-d - \frac{1}{2}h$	$d^2 + dh + \frac{1}{4}h^2$	$\frac{1}{4}$	$\frac{9}{64}$	$\frac{1}{16}$

$\mu_{x_1} = \mu_{x_2} = \frac{1}{2}h$ in all cases; genetic covariance $= \sum_i f_i(x_{1i} - \mu_1)(x_{2i} - \mu_2)$

unrelated siblings have no genetic variation in common at all:

$$
\begin{aligned}
\text{Cov(U)} &= d^2(\frac{1}{16} - \frac{1}{16} - \frac{1}{16} + \frac{1}{16}) \\
&= dh(-\frac{1}{16} + \frac{1}{16} + \frac{1}{16} - \frac{1}{16} - \frac{1}{16} + \frac{1}{16}) \\
&= \frac{1}{4}h^2(\frac{1}{16} - \frac{2}{16} + \frac{1}{16} - \frac{2}{16} + \frac{4}{16} - \frac{2}{16} + \frac{1}{16} - \frac{2}{16} + \frac{1}{16}) \\
&= 0
\end{aligned}
\tag{3.7}
$$

It is the fixed coefficients in front of V_A and V_D, 1.0 and 1.0 in the case of MZ twins and $\frac{1}{2}$ and $\frac{1}{4}$, respectively, for DZ twins that allow us to specify the LISREL model and estimate V_A and V_D, as will be explained in subsequent chapters. These coefficients are the correlations between additive and dominance deviations for the specified twin types. This may be seen easily in the case where we assume that dominance is absent. Then, MZ and DZ genetic covariances are simply V_A and $\frac{1}{2}V_A$, respectively. The variance of twin 1 and twin 2 in each case, however, is the population variance, V_A. For example, the DZ genetic correlation is derived as

$$
r_{DZ} = \frac{\text{Cov(DZ)}}{\sqrt{V_{T1}V_{T2}}} = \frac{\frac{1}{2}V_A}{\sqrt{V_A V_A}} = \frac{1}{2}
$$

3.3.2 Unequal Gene Frequencies

The simple results for equal gene frequencies described in the previous section were appreciated by a number of biometricians shortly after the rediscovery of Mendel's work (Castle, 1903; Pearson, 1904; Yule, 1902). However, it was not until Fisher's remarkable 1918 paper that the full generality of the biometrical model was elucidated. Gene frequencies do not have to be equal, nor do they have to be the same for the various polygenic loci involved in the phenotype for the simple fractions, 1, $\frac{1}{2}$, $\frac{1}{4}$, and 0 to hold, providing we define V_A and V_D appropriately. The algebra is considerably more complicated with unequal gene frequencies and it is necessary to define carefully what we mean by V_A and V_D. However, the end result is extremely simple, which is perhaps somewhat surprising. We give the flavor of the approach in this section, and refer the interested reader to the classic texts in this field for further information (Crow and Kimura, 1970; Falconer, 1990; Kempthorne, 1960; Mather and Jinks, 1982). We note that the elaboration of this biometrical model and its power and elegance has been largely responsible for the tremendous strides in inexpensive plant and animal food production throughout the world, placing these activities on a firm scientific basis.

Consider the three genotypes, AA, Aa, and aa, with genotypic frequencies P, Q, R:

Genotypes	AA	Aa	aa
Frequency	P	Q	R

The proportion of alleles, or gene frequency, is given by

$$\text{gene frequency } (A) \quad = \quad P + \frac{Q}{2} = u$$

$$(a) \quad = \quad R + \frac{Q}{2} = v . \tag{3.8}$$

These expressions derive from the simple fact that the AA genotype contributes only A alleles and the heterozygote, Aa, contributes $\frac{1}{2}$ A and $\frac{1}{2}$ a alleles. A Punnett square showing the allelic form of gametes uniting at random gives the genotypic frequencies in terms of the gene frequencies:

| | | Male Gametes | |
		u A	v a
Female Gametes	u A	$u^2 AA$	$uv Aa$
	v a	$uv Aa$	$v^2 aa$

which yields an alternative representation of the genotypic frequencies

Genotypes	AA	Aa	aa
Frequency	u^2	$2uv$	v^2

That these genotypic frequencies are in Hardy-Weinberg equilibrium may be shown by using them to calculate gene frequencies in the new generation, showing them to be the same, and then reapplying the Punnett square. Using expression 3.8, substituting u^2, $2uv$, and v^2, for P, Q, and R, and noting that the sum of gene frequencies is 1 $(u+v = 1.0)$, we can see that the new gene frequencies are the same as the old, and that genotypic frequencies will not change in subsequent generations

$$u_1 \quad = \quad u^2 + \frac{1}{2} 2uv = u^2 + uv = u(u + v) = u$$

$$v_1 \quad = \quad v^2 + \frac{1}{2} 2uv = v^2 + uv = v(u + v) = v . \tag{3.9}$$

The biometrical model is developed in terms of these equilibrium frequencies and genotypic effects as

Genotypes	AA	Aa	aa
Frequency	u^2	$2uv$	v^2
Genotypic effect	d	h	$-d$

(3.10)

The mean and variance of a population with this composition is obtained in analogous manner to that in 3.1. The mean is

$$\mu = u^2 d + 2uvh - v^2 d = (u - v)d + 2uvh \tag{3.11}$$

Because the mean is a reasonably complex expression, it is not convenient to sum weighted deviations to express the variance as in 3.2, instead, we rearrange the variance formula

$$\begin{aligned}
\sigma^2 &= \sum f_i(x_i - \mu)^2 \\
&= \sum f_i(x_i^2 - 2x_i\mu + \mu^2) \\
&= \sum f_i x_i^2 - 2\mu \sum f_i x_i + \mu^2 \\
&= \sum f_i x_i^2 - 2\mu^2 + \mu^2 \\
&= \sum f_i x_i^2 - \mu^2
\end{aligned} \tag{3.12}$$

Applying this formula to the genotypic effects and their frequencies given in 3.10 above, we obtain

$$\begin{aligned}
\sigma^2 &= u^2 d^2 + 2uvh^2 + v^2 d^2 - [(u-v)d + 2uvh]^2 \\
&= u^2 d^2 + 2uvh^2 + v^2 d^2 - [(u-v)^2 d^2 + 4uvdh(u-v) + 4u^2 v^2 h^2] \\
&= u^2 d^2 + 2uvh^2 + v^2 d^2 - [(u^2 - 2uv - v^2)d^2 + 4uvdh(u-v) + 4u^2 v^2 h^2] \\
&= 2uv[d^2 + 2(v-u)dh + (1 - 2uv)h^2] \\
&= 2uv[d^2 + 2(v-u)dh + (v-u)h^2 + 2uvh^2] \\
&= 2uv[d + (v-u)h]^2 + 4u^2 v^2 h^2 .
\end{aligned} \tag{3.13}$$

When the variance is arranged in this form, the first term $(2uv[d+(v-u)h]^2)$ defines the additive genetic variance, V_A, and the second term $(4u^2 v^2 h^2)$ the dominance variance, V_D. Why this particular arrangement is used to define V_A and V_D rather than some other may be seen if we introduce the notion of gene dose and the regression of genotypic effects on this variable, which essentially is how Fisher proceeded to develop the concepts of V_A and V_D.

If A is the increasing allele, then we can consider the three genotypes, AA, Aa, aa, as containing 2, 1, and 0 doses of the A allele, respectively. The regression of genotypic effects on these gene doses is shown in Figure 3.2. The values that enter into the calculation of the slope of this line are

Genotype	AA	Aa	aa
Genotypic effect (y)	d	h	$-d$
Frequency (f)	u^2	$2uv$	v^2
Dose (x)	2	1	0

From these values the slope of the regression line of y on x in Figure 3.2 is given by $\beta_{y,x} = \sigma_{x,y}/\sigma_x^2$. In order to calculate σ_x^2 we need μ_x, which is

$$\begin{aligned}
\mu_x &= 2u^2 + 2uv \\
&= 2u(u+v) \\
&= 2u .
\end{aligned} \tag{3.14}$$

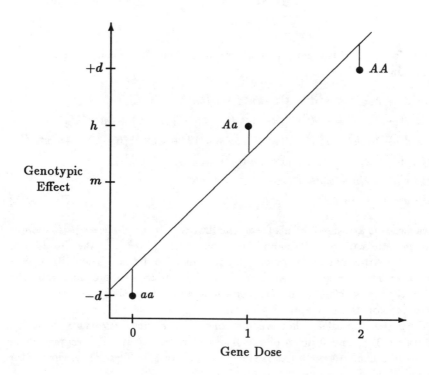

Figure 3.2: Regression of genotypic effects on gene dosage showing additive and dominance effects under random mating. The figure is drawn to scale for $u = v = \frac{1}{2}$, $d = 1$, and $h = \frac{1}{2}$.

Then, σ_x^2 is

$$
\begin{aligned}
\sigma_x^2 &= 2^2 u^2 + 1^2 2uv - 2^2 u^2 \\
&= 4u^2 + 2uv - 4u^2 \\
&= 2uv
\end{aligned}
$$

using the variance formula in 3.12. In order to calculate $\sigma_{x,y}$ we need to employ the covariance formula

$$
\sigma_{x,y} = \sum f_i x_i y_i - \mu_x \mu_y , \tag{3.15}
$$

where μ_y and μ_x are defined as in 3.11 and 3.14, respectively. Then,

$$
\begin{aligned}
\sigma_{xy} &= 2u^2 d + 2uvh - 2u[(u - v)d + 2uvh] \\
&= 2u^2 d + 2uvh - 2u^2 d + 2uvd - 4u^2 vh \\
&= 2uvd + h(2uv - 4u^2 v) \\
&= 2uvd + 2uvh(1 - 2u) \\
&= 2uvd + 2uvh(1 - u - u) \\
&= 2uvd + 2uvh(v - u) \\
&= 2uv[d + (v - u)h] . \tag{3.16}
\end{aligned}
$$

Therefore, the slope is

$$
\begin{aligned}
\beta_{y,x} &= \frac{\sigma_{xy}}{\sigma_x^2} \\
&= 2uv[d + (v - u)h]/2uv \\
&= d + (v - u)h . \tag{3.17}
\end{aligned}
$$

Following standard procedures in regression analysis, we can partition σ_y^2 into the variance due to the regression and the variance due to residual. The former is equivalent to the variance of the expected y; that is, the variance of the hypothetical points on the line in Figure 3.2, and the latter is the variance of the difference between observed y and the expected values.

The variance due to regression is

$$
\begin{aligned}
\beta \sigma_{xy} &= 2uv[d + (v - u)h][d + (v - u)h] \\
&= 2uv[d + (v - u)h]^2 \\
&= V_A \tag{3.18}
\end{aligned}
$$

and we may obtain the residual variance simply by subtracting the variance due to regression from the total variance of y. The variance of genotypic effects (σ_y^2) was given in 3.13, and when we subtract the expression obtained for the variance due to regression 3.18, we obtain the residual variances:

$$
\begin{aligned}
\sigma_y^2 - \beta \sigma_{x,y} &= 4u^2 v^2 h^2 \\
&= V_D . \tag{3.19}
\end{aligned}
$$

In this representation, genotypic effects are defined in terms of the regression line and are known as genotypic values. They are related to d and h, the genotypic effects we defined in Figure 3.1, but now reflect the population mean and gene frequencies of our random mating population. Defined in this way, the genotypic value (G) is $G = A + D$, the additive (A) and dominance (D) deviations of the individual.

G	$=$	A	$+$	D	frequency
G_{AA}	$=$	$2v[d + h(v - u)]$	$-$	$2v^2h$	u^2
G_{Aa}	$=$	$(v - u)[d + h(v - u)]$	$+$	$2uvh$	$2uv$
G_{aa}	$=$	$-2u[d + h(v - u)]$	$-$	$2u^2h$	v^2

In the case of $u = v = \frac{1}{2}$, this table becomes

G	$=$	A	$+$	D	frequency
G_{AA}	$=$	d	$-$	$\frac{1}{2}h$	$\frac{1}{4}$
G_{Aa}	$=$			$\frac{1}{2}h$	$\frac{1}{2}$
G_{aa}	$=$	$-d$	$-$	$\frac{1}{2}h$	$\frac{1}{4}$

from which it can be seen that the weighted sum of all G's is zero $(\sum f_i G_i = 0)$. In this case the additive effect is the same as the genotypic effect as originally scaled, and the dominance effect is measured around a mean of $\frac{1}{2}h$. This representation of genotypic value accurately conveys the extreme nature of unusual genotypes. Let $d = h = 1$, an example of complete dominance. In that case, $G_{AA} = G_{Aa} = \frac{1}{2}$ and $G_{aa} = -1\frac{1}{2}$ on our scale. Thus, aa genotypes, which form only $\frac{1}{4}$ of the population, fall far below the mean of 0, while the remaining $\frac{3}{4}$ of the population genotypes fall only slightly above the mean of 0. Thus, the bulk of the population appears relatively normal, whereas aa genotypes appear abnormal or unusual. When dominance is absent $(h = 0)$, Aa genotypes, which form $\frac{1}{2}$ of the population, have a mean of 0 and the less frequent genotypes AA and aa appear deviant. This situation is accentuated as the gene frequencies depart from $\frac{1}{2}$. For example, with $u = \frac{3}{4}$, $v = \frac{1}{4}$, and $h = d = 1$, then AA and Aa combined form $\frac{15}{16}$ of the population with a genotypic value of $\frac{1}{8}$, just slightly above the mean of 0, whereas the aa genotype has a value of $-1\frac{7}{8}$. In the limiting case of a very rare allele, AA and Aa tend to 0, the population mean, while only aa genotypes take an extreme value. These values intuitively correspond to our notion of a rare disorder of extreme effect, such as untreated phenylketonuria (PKU).

The genotypic values A and D that we employ in the LISREL model have precisely the expectations given above in 3.18 and 3.19, but are summed over all polygenic loci contributing to the trait. Thus, the biometrical model gives a precise definition to the latent variables employed in LISREL for the analysis of twin data.

Table 3.3: Genetic covariance components for MZ, DZ, and Unrelated Siblings with unequal gene frequencies at a single locus.

Genotype Pair	Effect x_{1i}	x_{2i}	MZ	Frequency DZ	U
AA, AA	d	d	u^2	$u^4 + u^3v + \frac{1}{4}u^2v^2$	u^4
AA, Aa	d	h	–	$u^3v + \frac{1}{2}u^2v^2$	$2u^3v$
AA, aa	d	$-d$	—	$\frac{1}{4}u^2v^2$	u^2v^2
Aa, AA	h	d	—	$u^3v + \frac{1}{2}u^2v^2$	$2u^3v$
Aa, Aa	h	h	$2uv$	$u^3v + 3u^2v^2 + uv^3$	$4u^2v^2$
Aa, aa	h	$-d$	—	$\frac{1}{2}u^2v^2 + uv^3$	$2uv^3$
aa, AA	$-d$	d	—	$\frac{1}{4}u^2v^2$	u^2v^2
aa, Aa	$-d$	h	—	$\frac{1}{2}u^2v^2 + uv^3$	$2uv^3$
aa, aa	$-d$	$-d$	u^4	$\frac{1}{4}u^2v^2 + uv^3 + v^4$	v^4

3.4 Summary

Table 3.3 replicates Table 3.2 employing genotypic frequencies appropriate to random mating and unequal gene frequencies. Using the table to calculate covariances among sibling pairs of the three types, MZ twins, DZ twins, and unrelated siblings, gives

$$
\begin{aligned}
\text{Cov(MZ)} &= 2uv[d + (v - u)h]^2 + 4u^2v^2h^2 &= V_A + V_D \\
\text{Cov(DZ)} &= uv[d + (v - u)h]^2 + u^2v^2h^2 &= \tfrac{1}{2}V_A + \tfrac{1}{4}V_D \\
\text{Cov(U)} &= 0 &= 0
\end{aligned}
$$

By similar calculations, the expectations for half-siblings and for parents and their offspring may be shown to be $\frac{1}{4}V_A$ and $\frac{1}{2}V_A$, respectively. That is, these relationships do not reflect dominance effects. The MZ and DZ resemblances are the primary focus of this text, but all five relationships we have just discussed may be analyzed in the extended LISREL approaches we discuss in Chapter 17.

With more extensive genetical data, we can assess the effects of *epistasis*, or non-allelic interaction, since the biometrical model may be extended easily to include such genetic effects. Another important problem we have not considered is that of assortative mating, which one might have thought would introduce insuperable problems for the model. However, once we are working with genotypic values such as A and D, the effects of assortment can be readily accommodated in the model by means of reverse path analysis (Wright, 1968) and the Pearson–Aitken treatment of selected variables (Aitken, 1934). Fulker (1988) describes this approach in the context of Fisher's (1918) model of assortment.

In this chapter, we have given a brief introduction to the biometrical model that underlies the LISREL approach employed in this book, and we have indicated how additional genetic complexities may be accommodated in the model. However, in addition to genetic influences, we must consider the effects of the environment in any phenotype. These may be easily accommodated by defining environmental influences that are common to sib pairs and those that are unique to the individual. If these environmental effects are unrelated to the genotype, then the variances due to these influences simply add to the genetic variances we have just described. If they are not independent of genotype, as in the case of sibling interactions and cultural transmission, both of which are likely to occur in some behavioral phenotypes, then the LISREL model may be suitably modified to account for these complexities, as we describe in Chapters 10 and 17.

Chapter 4

Matrix Algebra

4.1 Matrix Notation

Many people regard journal articles and books that contain matrix algebra as prohibitively complicated and ignore them or shelve them indefinitely. This is a sad state of affairs because learning matrix algebra is not difficult and can reap enormous benefits. Science in general, and genetics in particular, is becoming increasingly quantitative. Matrix algebra provides a very economical language to describe our data and our models; it is essential for understanding LISREL and other data analysis packages. In common with most languages, the way to make it "stick" is to *use* it. Those unfamiliar with, or out of practice at, using matrices will benefit from doing the worked examples in the text. Readers with a strong mathematics background may skim this chapter, or skip it entirely, using it for reference only. We do not give an exhaustive treatment of matrix algebra and operations but limit ourselves to the bare essentials needed for structural equation modeling. There are many excellent texts for those wishing to extend their knowledge; we recommend Searle (1982) and Graybill (1969).

Although matrices and certain matrix operations were used as long ago as 2000 BC in ancient China, it is only relatively recently that a comprehensive matrix algebra has been developed. During the 1850's, Cayley worked on general algebraic systems (Boyer, 1985 p. 627) and developed the basis of matrix algebra as it is used today. The concept of a matrix is a very simple one, being just a table of numbers or symbols laid out in *rows* and *columns*,

$$\text{e.g.,} \quad \begin{pmatrix} 1 & 4 \\ 2 & 5 \\ 3 & 6 \end{pmatrix} \quad \text{or} \quad \begin{pmatrix} \alpha_{11} & \alpha_{12} & \alpha_{13} \\ \alpha_{21} & \alpha_{22} & \alpha_{23} \\ \alpha_{31} & \alpha_{32} & \alpha_{33} \end{pmatrix}$$

In most texts, the table is enclosed in brackets, either: curved, (); square, [ ]; or curly, {}.

It is conventional to specify the configuration of the matrix in terms of Rows ×
Columns and these are its *dimensions* or *order*. Thus the first matrix above is of
order 3 by 2 and the second is a 3 × 3 matrix.

A common occurrence of matrices in behavioral sciences is the *data matrix*
where the *rows are subjects* and the *columns are measures*, e.g.,

	Weight	*Height*
S_1	50	20
S_2	100	40
S_3	150	60
S_4	200	80

It is convenient to let a single letter symbolize a matrix. This is written in UP-
PERCASE **boldface**. Thus we might say that our data matrix is **A**, which in
handwriting we would underline with either a straight or a wavy line. Sometimes a
matrix is written $_4\mathbf{A}_2$ to specify its dimensions. The economy of using matrices is
immediately apparent: we can represent a whole table by a single symbol, whether
it contains just one row and one column, or a billion rows and a billion columns!
There are several special terms for matrices with one row or one column or both.
When a matrix consists of a single number, it is called a *scalar*; when it consists of
single column (row) of numbers it is called a column (row) *vector*. Scalars are usually represented as lower case, non-bold letters. Vectors are normally represented
as a **bold** lowercase letter. Thus, the weight measurements of our four subjects are

$$
\begin{bmatrix} 50 \\ 100 \\ 150 \\ 200 \end{bmatrix} = \mathbf{a}
$$

We can refer to the specific elements of matrix **A** as a_{ij} where i indicates the row
number and j indicates the column number.

Certain special forms of matrices exist. We have already defined scalars and
row and column vectors. A matrix full of zeroes is called a *null* matrix and a matrix
full of ones is called a *unit matrix*. Matrices in which the number of rows is equal
to the number of columns are called *square* matrices. Among square matrices,
diagonal matrices have at least one non-zero diagonal element, with every off-
diagonal element zero. By diagonal, we mean the 'leading diagonal' from the top
left element of the matrix to the bottom right element. A special form of the
diagonal matrix is the *identity matrix*, **I**, which has every diagonal element one
and every non-diagonal element zero. The identity matrix functions much like the
number one in ordinary algebra.

4.2 Matrix Algebra Operations

Matrix algebra defines a set of operations that may be performed on matrices. These operations include addition, subtraction, multiplication, inversion (multiplication by the inverse is similar to division) and transposition. We may separate the operations into two mutually exclusive categories: *unary* and *binary*. Unary operations are performed on a single matrix, and binary operations combine two matrices to obtain a single matrix result. Binary operations will be described first.

4.2.1 Binary Operations

Addition and subtraction

Matrices may be *added* if and only if they have the *same dimension*. They are then said to be *conformable for addition*. Each element in the first matrix is added to the corresponding element in the second matrix to form the same element in the solution.

$$\text{e.g.} \begin{pmatrix} 1 & 4 \\ 2 & 5 \\ 3 & 6 \end{pmatrix} + \begin{pmatrix} 8 & 11 \\ 9 & 12 \\ 10 & 13 \end{pmatrix} = \begin{pmatrix} 9 & 15 \\ 11 & 17 \\ 13 & 19 \end{pmatrix}$$

or symbolically,

$$\mathbf{A} + \mathbf{B} = \mathbf{C}.$$

One *cannot add*

$$\begin{pmatrix} 1 & 4 \\ 2 & 5 \\ 3 & 6 \end{pmatrix} + \begin{pmatrix} 8 & 10 \\ 9 & 11 \end{pmatrix}$$

because they have a different number of rows. Subtraction works in the same way as addition, e.g.

$$\begin{pmatrix} 1 & 4 \\ 2 & 5 \\ 3 & 6 \end{pmatrix} - \begin{pmatrix} 2 & 5 \\ 2 & 5 \\ 2 & 5 \end{pmatrix} = \begin{pmatrix} -1 & -1 \\ 0 & 0 \\ 1 & 1 \end{pmatrix}$$

which is written

$$\mathbf{A} - \mathbf{B} = \mathbf{C}.$$

Matrix multiplication

Matrices are *conformable for multiplication* if and only if the number of columns in the first matrix equals the number of rows in the second matrix. This means that *adjacent columns and rows must be of the same order*. For example, the matrix product $_3\mathbf{A}_2 \times {_2}\mathbf{B}_1$ may be calculated; the result is a 3×1 matrix. In general, if we multiply two matrices $_i\mathbf{A}_j \times {_j}\mathbf{B}_k$, the result will be of order $i \times k$.

Matrix multiplication involves calculating a *sum of cross products* among *rows of the first matrix* and *columns of the second matrix* in all possible combinations.

$$\text{e.g.} \begin{pmatrix} 1 & 4 \\ 2 & 5 \\ 3 & 6 \end{pmatrix} \begin{pmatrix} 1 & 3 \\ 2 & 4 \end{pmatrix} = \begin{pmatrix} 1 \times 1 + 4 \times 2 & 1 \times 3 + 4 \times 4 \\ 2 \times 1 + 5 \times 2 & 2 \times 3 + 5 \times 4 \\ 3 \times 1 + 6 \times 2 & 3 \times 3 + 6 \times 4 \end{pmatrix}$$

$$= \begin{pmatrix} 9 & 19 \\ 12 & 26 \\ 15 & 33 \end{pmatrix}$$

This is written

$$\mathbf{AB} = \mathbf{C}$$

The only exception to the above rule is multiplication by a *single number* called a scalar[1]. Thus, for example,

$$2 \begin{pmatrix} 1 & 4 \\ 2 & 5 \\ 3 & 6 \end{pmatrix} = \begin{pmatrix} 2 & 8 \\ 4 & 10 \\ 6 & 12 \end{pmatrix}$$

by convention this is often written as

$$2\mathbf{A} = \mathbf{C}.$$

Although convenient and often found in the literature, we do not recommend this style of matrix formulation, but prefer use of the kronecker product.

The simplest example of matrix multiplication is to multiply a vector by itself. If we premultiply a column vector ($n \times 1$) by its transpose[2], the result is a scalar called the *inner product*. For example, if

$$\mathbf{a}' = \begin{pmatrix} 1 & 2 & 3 \end{pmatrix}$$

then the inner product is

$$\mathbf{a}'\mathbf{a} = \begin{pmatrix} 1 & 2 & 3 \end{pmatrix} \begin{pmatrix} 1 \\ 2 \\ 3 \end{pmatrix} = 1^2 + 2^2 + 3^2 = 14$$

which is the sum of the squares of the elements of the vector **a**. This has a simple graphical representation when **a** is of dimension 2×1 (see Figure 4.1).

---

[1] Such an operation also may be expressed as a kronecker product, symbolized $\otimes$, in which every element of the matrix is multiplied by the scalar.

[2] Transposition is defined in Section 4.2.2 below. Essentially the rows become columns and *vice versa*.

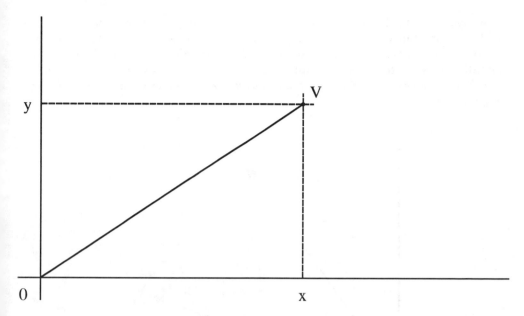

Figure 4.1: Graphical representation of the inner product $\mathbf{a}'\mathbf{a}$ of a (2×1) vector $\mathbf{a}$, with $\mathbf{a}' = (xy)$. By Pythagoras' theorem, the distance of the point V from the origin O is $\sqrt{x^2 + y^2}$, which is the square root of the inner product of the vector.

4.2.2 Unary Operations

Transposition

A matrix is transposed when the rows are written as columns and the columns are written as rows. This operation is denoted by writing $\mathbf{A}'$ or $\mathbf{A}^T$. For our example data matrix on page 72,

$$\mathbf{A}' = \begin{pmatrix} 50 & 100 & 150 & 200 \\ 20 & 40 & 60 & 80 \end{pmatrix}$$

a row vector is usually written

$$\mathbf{a}' = \begin{pmatrix} 50 & 100 & 150 & 200 \end{pmatrix}$$

Clearly, $(\mathbf{A}')' = \mathbf{A}$.

Determinant of a matrix

For a square matrix $\mathbf{A}$ we may calculate a scalar called the *determinant* which we write as $|\mathbf{A}|$. In the case of a 2×2 matrix, this quantity is calculated as

$$|\mathbf{A}| = a_{11}a_{22} - a_{12}a_{21}$$

. We shall be giving numerical examples of calculating the determinant when we address matrix inversion. The determinant has an interesting geometric representation. For example, consider two standardized variables that correlate r. This situation may be represented graphically by drawing two vectors, each of length 1.0, having the same origin and an angle a, whose cosine is r, between them (see Figure 4.2).

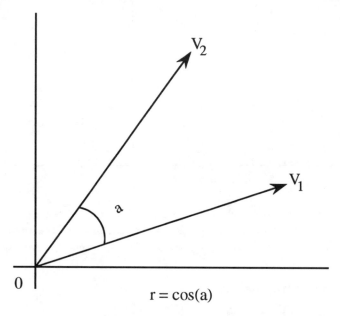

$$r = \cos(a)$$

Figure 4.2: Geometric representation of the determinant of a matrix. The angle between the vectors is the cosine of correlation between two variables, so the determinant is given by twice the area of the triangle OV_1V_2.

It can be shown (the proof involves symmetric square root decomposition of matrices) that the area of the triangle OV_1V_2 is $.5\sqrt{|\mathbf{A}|}$. Thus as the correlation r increases, the angle between the lines decreases, the area decreases, and *the determinant decreases*. For two variables that correlate perfectly, the determinant of the correlation (or covariance) matrix is zero. Conversely, the determinant is at a maximum when $r = 0$; the angle between the vectors is 90°, and we say that the variables are *orthogonal*. For larger numbers of variables, the determinant is a function of the hypervolume in n-space; if any single pair of variables correlates perfectly then the determinant is zero. In addition, if one of the variables is a linear combination of the others, the determinant will be zero. For a set of variables with given variances, the determinant is maximized when all the variables are orthogonal, i.e., all the off-diagonal elements are zero.

Many software packages [e.g., Mx (Neale, 1991); SAS, 1985] and numerical libraries (e.g., IMSL, 1987; NAG, 1990) have algorithms for finding the determinant and inverse of a matrix. But it is useful to know how matrices can be inverted by hand, so we present a method for use with paper and pencil. To calculate the determinant of larger matrices, we employ the concept of a *cofactor*. If we delete row i and column j from an $n \times n$ matrix, then the determinant of the remaining matrix is called the *minor* of element a_{ij}. The cofactor, written A_{ij} is simply:

$$A_{ij} = (-1)^{i+j} \text{minor } a_{ij}$$

The determinant of the matrix $\mathbf{A}$ may be calculated as

$$|\mathbf{A}| = \sum_{i=1}^{n} a_{ij} A_{ij}$$

where n is the order of $\mathbf{A}$.

The determinant of a matrix is related to the concept of *definiteness* of a matrix. In general, for a null column vector $\mathbf{x}$, the quadratic form $\mathbf{x}'\mathbf{A}\mathbf{x}$ is always zero. For some matrices, this quadratic is zero *only* if $\mathbf{x}$ is the null vector. If $\mathbf{x}'\mathbf{A}\mathbf{x} > 0$ for all non-null vectors $\mathbf{x}$ then we say that the matrix is *positive definite*. Conversely, if $\mathbf{x}'\mathbf{A}\mathbf{x} < 0$ for all non-null $\mathbf{x}$, we say that the matrix is *negative definite*. However, if we can find some non-null $\mathbf{x}$ such that $\mathbf{x}'\mathbf{A}\mathbf{x} = 0$ then the matrix is said to be *singular*, and its determinant is zero. As long as no two variables are perfectly correlated, and there are more subjects than measures, a covariance matrix calculated from data on random variables will be *positive definite*. LISREL will complain (and rightly so!) if it is given a covariance matrix that is not positive definite. The determinant of the covariance matrix can be helpful when there are problems with model-fitting that seem to originate with the data. However, it is possible to have a matrix with a positive determinant yet which is negative definite (consider $-\mathbf{I}$ with an even number of rows), so the determinant is not an adequate diagnostic. Instead we note that all the eigenvalues of a positive definite matrix are greater than zero. Eigenvalues and eigenvectors may be obtained from software packages and the numerical libraries listed above[3].

Trace of a matrix

The trace of a matrix is simply the sum of its diagonal elements. Thus the trace of the matrix

$$\begin{pmatrix} 1 & 2 & 3 \\ 4 & 5 & 6 \\ 7 & 8 & 9 \end{pmatrix} = 1 + 5 + 9$$
$$= 15$$

---

[3]Those readers wishing to know more about the uses of eigenvalues and eigenvectors may consult Searle (1982) or any general text on matrix algebra.

Inverse of a matrix

In ordinary algebra the division operation $a \div b$ is equivalent to multiplication of the reciprocal $a \times \frac{1}{b}$. Thus one binary operation, division, has been replaced by two operations, one binary (multiplication) and one unary (forming $\frac{1}{b}$). In matrix algebra we make an equivalent substitution of operations, and we call the unary operation *inversion*. We write the inverse of the matrix $\mathbf{A}$ as $\mathbf{A}^{-1}$, and calculate it so that

$$\mathbf{A}\mathbf{A}^{-1} = \mathbf{I}$$

and

$$\mathbf{A}^{-1}\mathbf{A} = \mathbf{I}\,,$$

where $\mathbf{I}$ is the identity matrix. In general the inverse of a matrix is not simply formed by finding the reciprocal of each element (this holds only for scalars and diagonal matrices[4]), but is a more complicated operation involving the determinant.

There are many computer programs available for inverting matrices. Some routines are general, but there are often faster routines available if the program is given some information about the matrix, for example, whether it is symmetric, positive definite, triangular, or diagonal. Here we describe one general method that is useful for matrix inversion; we recommend undertaking this hand calculation at least once for at least a 3×3 matrix in order to fully understand the concept of a matrix inverse.

Procedure: In order to invert a matrix, the following four steps can be used:

1. Find the determinant

2. Set up the matrix of cofactors

3. Transpose the matrix of cofactors

4. Divide (3) by the determinant

For example, the matrix

$$\mathbf{A} = \begin{pmatrix} 1 & 2 \\ 1 & 5 \end{pmatrix}$$

can be inverted by:

1.

$$|\mathbf{A}| = (1 \times 5) - (2 \times 1) = 3$$

---

[4]N.B. For a diagonal matrix one takes the reciprocal of only the diagonal elements!

2.

$$A_{ij} = \begin{bmatrix} (-1)^2 \times 5 & (-1)^3 \times 1 \\ (-1)^3 \times 2 & (-1)^4 \times 1 \end{bmatrix}$$
$$= \begin{pmatrix} 5 & -1 \\ -2 & 1 \end{pmatrix}$$

3.

$$A'_{ij} = \begin{pmatrix} 5 & -2 \\ -1 & 1 \end{pmatrix}$$

4.

$$A^{-1} = \frac{1}{3} \begin{pmatrix} 5 & -2 \\ -1 & 1 \end{pmatrix} = \begin{pmatrix} \frac{5}{3} & -\frac{2}{3} \\ -\frac{1}{3} & \frac{1}{3} \end{pmatrix}$$

To verify this, we can multiply $\mathbf{A}\mathbf{A}^{-1}$ to obtain the identity matrix:

$$\frac{1}{3} \begin{pmatrix} 5 & -2 \\ -1 & 1 \end{pmatrix} \begin{pmatrix} 1 & 2 \\ 1 & 5 \end{pmatrix} = \frac{1}{3} \begin{pmatrix} 3 & 0 \\ 0 & 3 \end{pmatrix} = \begin{pmatrix} 1 & 0 \\ 0 & 1 \end{pmatrix}$$

The result that $\mathbf{A}\mathbf{A}^{-1} = \mathbf{I}$ may be used to solve the pair of simultaneous equations:

$$\begin{aligned} x_1 + 2x_2 &= 8 \\ x_1 + 5x_2 &= 17 \end{aligned}$$

which may be written

$$\begin{pmatrix} 1 & 2 \\ 1 & 5 \end{pmatrix} \begin{pmatrix} x_1 \\ x_2 \end{pmatrix} = \begin{pmatrix} 8 \\ 17 \end{pmatrix}$$

i.e.,

$$\mathbf{A}\mathbf{x} = \mathbf{y}$$

premultiplying both sides by the inverse of $\mathbf{A}$, we have

$$\begin{aligned} \mathbf{A}^{-1}\mathbf{A}\mathbf{x} &= \mathbf{A}^{-1}\mathbf{y} \\ \mathbf{x} &= \mathbf{A}^{-1}\mathbf{y} \\ &= \frac{1}{3} \begin{pmatrix} 5 & -2 \\ -1 & 1 \end{pmatrix} \begin{pmatrix} 8 \\ 17 \end{pmatrix} \\ &= \frac{1}{3} \begin{pmatrix} 6 \\ 9 \end{pmatrix} \\ &= \begin{pmatrix} 2 \\ 3 \end{pmatrix} \end{aligned}$$

which may be verified by substitution.

For a larger matrix it is more tedious to compute the inverse. Let us consider the matrix

$$\mathbf{A} = \begin{pmatrix} 1 & 1 & 0 \\ 1 & 0 & 1 \\ 1 & -1 & 0 \end{pmatrix}$$

1. The determinant is

$$\begin{aligned} |\mathbf{A}| &= +1 \begin{vmatrix} 0 & 1 \\ -1 & 0 \end{vmatrix} - 1 \begin{vmatrix} 1 & 1 \\ 1 & 0 \end{vmatrix} + 0 \begin{vmatrix} 1 & 0 \\ 1 & -1 \end{vmatrix} \\ &= +1 + 1 + 0 \\ &= 2 \end{aligned}$$

2. The matrix of cofactors is:

$$A_{ij} = \begin{bmatrix} + \begin{vmatrix} 0 & 1 \\ -1 & 0 \end{vmatrix} & - \begin{vmatrix} 1 & 1 \\ 1 & 0 \end{vmatrix} & + \begin{vmatrix} 1 & 0 \\ 1 & -1 \end{vmatrix} \\ - \begin{vmatrix} 1 & 0 \\ -1 & 0 \end{vmatrix} & + \begin{vmatrix} 1 & 0 \\ 1 & 0 \end{vmatrix} & - \begin{vmatrix} 1 & 1 \\ 1 & -1 \end{vmatrix} \\ + \begin{vmatrix} 1 & 0 \\ 0 & 1 \end{vmatrix} & - \begin{vmatrix} 1 & 0 \\ 1 & 1 \end{vmatrix} & + \begin{vmatrix} 1 & 1 \\ 1 & 0 \end{vmatrix} \end{bmatrix}$$

$$= \begin{pmatrix} 1 & 1 & -1 \\ 0 & 0 & 2 \\ 1 & -1 & -1 \end{pmatrix}$$

3. The transpose is

$$A'_{ij} = \begin{pmatrix} 1 & 0 & 1 \\ 1 & 0 & -1 \\ -1 & 2 & -1 \end{pmatrix}$$

4. Dividing by the determinant, we have

$$\mathbf{A}^{-1} = \frac{1}{2} \begin{pmatrix} 1 & 0 & 1 \\ 1 & 0 & -1 \\ -1 & 2 & -1 \end{pmatrix} = \begin{pmatrix} .5 & 0 & .5 \\ .5 & 0 & -.5 \\ -.5 & 1 & -.5 \end{pmatrix}$$

which may be verified by multiplication with **A** to obtain the identity matrix.

4.3   Equations in Matrix Algebra

Matrix algebra provides a very convenient short hand for writing sets of equations. For example, the pair of *simultaneous equations*

$$y_1 = 2x_1 + 3x_2$$

$$y_2 \quad = \quad x_1 + x_2$$

may be written

$$y \quad = \quad \mathbf{Ax}$$

i.e.,

$$\begin{pmatrix} y_1 \\ y_2 \end{pmatrix} = \begin{pmatrix} 2 & 3 \\ 1 & 1 \end{pmatrix} \begin{pmatrix} x_1 \\ x_2 \end{pmatrix}$$

Also if we have the following pair of equations:

$$\mathbf{y} = \mathbf{Ax}$$

$$\mathbf{x} = \mathbf{Bz} \, ,$$

then

$$\begin{aligned} \mathbf{y} \quad &= \quad \mathbf{A(Bz)} \\ &= \quad \mathbf{ABz} \\ &= \quad \mathbf{Cz} \end{aligned}$$

where $\mathbf{C} = \mathbf{AB}$. This is very convenient notation compared with direct substitution. The LISREL structural equations are written in this general form, i.e.,

Real variables (y) = Matrix × hypothetical variables.

To show the simplicity of the matrix notation, consider the following equations:

$$\begin{aligned} y_1 \quad &= \quad 2x_1 + 3x_2 \\ y_2 \quad &= \quad x_1 + x_2 \\ x_1 \quad &= \quad z_1 + z_2 \\ x_2 \quad &= \quad z_1 - z_2 \end{aligned}$$

Then we have

$$\begin{aligned} y_1 \quad &= \quad 2(z_1 + z_2) + 3(z_1 - z_2) \\ &= \quad 5z_1 - z_2 \\ y_2 \quad &= \quad (z_1 + z_2) + (z_1 - z_2) \\ &= \quad 2z_1 + 0 \end{aligned}$$

Similarly, in matrix notation, we have $\mathbf{y} = \mathbf{ABz}$, where

$$\mathbf{A} = \begin{pmatrix} 2 & 3 \\ 1 & 1 \end{pmatrix}, \mathbf{B} = \begin{pmatrix} 1 & 1 \\ 1 & -1 \end{pmatrix}$$

and

$$\mathbf{AB} = \begin{pmatrix} 5 & -1 \\ 2 & 0 \end{pmatrix},$$

or

$$y_1 = 5z_1 - z_2$$
$$y_2 = 2z_2$$

4.4 Applications of Matrix Algebra

Matrix algebra is used extensively throughout multivariate statistics (see e.g., Graybill, 1969; Mardia *et al.*, 1979; Maxwell, 1977; Searle, 1982). Here we do not propose to discuss statistical methods, but simply to show two examples of the utility of matrices in expressing general formulae applicable to any number of variables or subjects.

4.4.1 Calculation of Covariance Matrix from Data Matrix

Suppose we have a data matrix $\mathbf{A}$ with rows corresponding to subjects and columns corresponding to variables. We can calculate a mean for each variable and replace the data matrix with a matrix of *deviations from the mean*. That is, each element a_{ij} is replaced by $a_{ij} - \mu_j$ where μ_j is the mean of the jth variable. Let us call the new matrix $\mathbf{Z}$. The covariance matrix is then simply calculated as

$$\frac{1}{N-1}\mathbf{Z}'\mathbf{Z}$$

where N is the number of subjects.

For example, suppose we have the following data:

X	Y	$X - \overline{X}$	$Y - \overline{Y}$
1	2	-2	-4
2	8	-1	2
3	6	0	0
4	4	1	-2
5	10	2	4

So the matrix of deviations from the mean is

$$\mathbf{Z} = \begin{pmatrix} -2 & -4 \\ -1 & 2 \\ 0 & 0 \\ 1 & -2 \\ 2 & 4 \end{pmatrix}$$

and therefore the covariance matrix of the observations is

$$\frac{1}{N-1}\mathbf{Z}'\mathbf{Z} = \frac{1}{4}\begin{pmatrix} -2 & -1 & 0 & 1 & 2 \\ -4 & 2 & 0 & -2 & 4 \end{pmatrix}\begin{pmatrix} -2 & -4 \\ -1 & 2 \\ 0 & 0 \\ 1 & -2 \\ 2 & 4 \end{pmatrix}$$

$$= \frac{1}{4}\begin{pmatrix} 10 & 12 \\ 12 & 40 \end{pmatrix}$$

$$= \begin{pmatrix} 2.5 & 3.0 \\ 3.0 & 10.0 \end{pmatrix} = \begin{pmatrix} S_x^2 & S_{xy} \\ S_{xy} & S_y^2 \end{pmatrix}$$

The diagonal elements of this matrix are the variances of the variables, and the off-diagonal elements are the covariances between the variables. The *standard deviation* is the square root of the variance (see Chapter 2).

The correlation is

$$\frac{S_{xy}}{\sqrt{S_x^2 S_y^2}} = \frac{S_{xy}}{S_x S_y}$$

In general, a correlation matrix may be calculated from a covariance matrix by pre- and post-multiplying the covariance matrix by a diagonal matrix $\mathbf{D}$ in which each diagonal element d_{ii} is $\frac{1}{S_i}$, i.e., the reciprocal of the standard deviation for that variable. Thus, in our two variable example, we have:

$$\begin{pmatrix} \frac{1}{S_x} & 0 \\ 0 & \frac{1}{S_y} \end{pmatrix}\begin{pmatrix} S_x^2 & S_{xy} \\ S_{xy} & S_y^2 \end{pmatrix}\begin{pmatrix} \frac{1}{S_x} & 0 \\ 0 & \frac{1}{S_y} \end{pmatrix} = \begin{pmatrix} 1.0 & R_{xy} \\ R_{xy} & 1.0 \end{pmatrix}$$

4.4.2 Transformations of Data Matrices

Matrix algebra provides a natural notation for *transformations*. If we premultiply the matrix $_j\mathbf{B}_j$ by another, say $_k\mathbf{T}_i$, then the rows of $\mathbf{T}$ describe linear combinations of the rows of $\mathbf{B}$. The resulting matrix will therefore consist of k rows corresponding to the linear transformations of the rows of $\mathbf{B}$ described by the rows of $\mathbf{T}$. A very simple example of this is premultiplication by the identity matrix, $\mathbf{I}$, which, as noted earlier, merely has 1's on the leading diagonal and zeroes everywhere else.

Thus, the transformation described by the first row may be written as 'multiply the first row by 1 and add zero times the other rows.' In the second row, we have 'multiply the second row by 1 and add zero times the other rows,' and so the identity matrix transforms the matrix **B** into the same matrix. For a less trivial example, let our data matrix be **X**, then

$$\mathbf{X}' = \begin{pmatrix} -2 & -1 & 0 & 1 & 2 \\ -4 & 2 & 0 & -2 & 4 \end{pmatrix}$$

and let

$$\mathbf{T} = \begin{pmatrix} 1 & 1 \\ 1 & -1 \end{pmatrix}$$

then

$$\begin{aligned} \mathbf{Y}' &= \mathbf{T}\mathbf{X}' \\ &= \begin{pmatrix} -6 & 1 & 0 & -1 & 6 \\ 2 & -3 & 0 & 3 & -2 \end{pmatrix}. \end{aligned}$$

In this case, the transformation matrix specifies two transformations of the data: the first row defines the sum of the two variates, and the second row defines the difference (row 1 − row 2). In the above, we have applied the transformation to the raw data, but for these linear transformations it is easy to apply the transformation to the covariance matrix. The covariance matrix of the transformed variates is

$$\begin{aligned} \frac{1}{N-1}\mathbf{Y}'\mathbf{Y} &= \frac{1}{N-1}(\mathbf{T}\mathbf{X}')(\mathbf{T}\mathbf{X}')' \\ &= \frac{1}{N-1}\mathbf{T}\mathbf{X}'\mathbf{X}\mathbf{T}' \\ &= \mathbf{T}(\mathbf{V_x})\mathbf{T}' \end{aligned}$$

which is a useful result, meaning that linear transformations may be applied directly to the covariance matrix, instead of going to the trouble of transforming all the raw data and recalculating the covariance matrix.

4.4.3 Further Operations and Applications

There exists a great variety of matrix operations and functions with much broader scope than the limited selection given in this chapter. For example, there are two other forms of matrix multiplication in common use, direct or kronecker products, and dot products. Similar extensions to addition and subtraction exist, and numerous matrix functions beyond determinant and trace can be defined. One place to study further operations is Searle (1982); applications and some definitions can be found in Neale (1991). We hope that the outline provided here will make understanding structural equation modeling of twin data much easier, and provide a starting point for those who wish to study the subject in more detail.

4.5   Exercises

If you find these exercises insufficient practice, more may be found in almost any text on matrix algebra. Further practice may be obtained by computing the expected covariance matrix of almost any model in this book, selecting a set of trial values for the parameters. The exercise can be extended by computing fit functions (Chapter 7) for the model and parameter values selected. For the purposes of general introduction, however, the few given in this section should suffice.

4.5.1   Binary operations

Let
$$\mathbf{A} = \begin{pmatrix} 3 & 6 \\ 2 & 1 \end{pmatrix}, \mathbf{B} = \begin{pmatrix} 1 & 0 & 3 & 2 \\ 0 & -1 & -1 & 1 \end{pmatrix}$$

1. Form **AB**.

2. Form **BA**. (Careful, this might be a trick question!)

Let
$$\mathbf{C} = \begin{pmatrix} 3 & 6 \\ 2 & 1 \end{pmatrix}, \mathbf{D} = \begin{pmatrix} 1 & 2 \\ 3 & 4 \end{pmatrix}$$

1. Form **CD**.

2. Form **DC**.

3. In ordinary algebra, multiplication is *commutative*, i.e. $xy = yx$. In general, is matrix multiplication commutative?

Let
$$\mathbf{E'} = \begin{pmatrix} 1 & 0 & 3 \\ 1 & 2 & 1 \end{pmatrix}$$

1. Form $\mathbf{E}(\mathbf{C} + \mathbf{D})$.

2. Form $\mathbf{EC} + \mathbf{ED}$.

3. In ordinary algebra, multiplication is *distributive over addition*, i.e. $x(y+z) = xy+xz$. In general, is matrix multiplication distributive over matrix addition? Is matrix multiplication distributive over matrix subtraction?

4.5.2   Unary operations

1. Show for two (preferably non-trivial) matrices conformable for multiplication that

$$(\mathbf{AB})' = \mathbf{B}'\mathbf{A}'$$

2. If $\mathbf{C}$ is

$$\begin{pmatrix} 2 & 6 \\ .5 & 4 \end{pmatrix},$$

   find the determinant of $\mathbf{C}$.

3. What is the inverse of matrix $\mathbf{C}$?

4. If $\mathbf{D}$ is

$$\begin{pmatrix} .2 & .3 \\ .4 & .6 \end{pmatrix},$$

   find the determinant of $\mathbf{D}$.

5. What is the inverse of $\mathbf{D}$?

6. If $tr(\mathbf{A})$ means the trace of $\mathbf{A}$, what is $tr(\mathbf{C}) + tr(\mathbf{D})$?

Chapter 5

Path Analysis and Structural Equations

5.1 Introduction

Path analysis was invented by the geneticist Sewall Wright (1921a, 1934, 1960, 1968), and has been widely applied to problems in genetics and the behavioral sciences. It is a technique which allows us to represent, in diagrammatic form, linear 'structural' models and hence derive predictions for the variances and covariances (the *covariance structure*) of our variables under that model. The books by Kenny (1979), Li (1975), or Wright (1968) supply good introductory treatments of path analysis, and general descriptions of structural equation modeling can be found in Bollen (1989) and Loehlin (1987). In this chapter we provide only the basic background necessary to understand models used in the genetic analyses presented in this text.

A path diagram is a useful heuristic tool to graphically display causal and correlational relations or the paths between variables. Used correctly, it is one of several mathematically complete descriptions of a linear model, which include less visually immediate forms such as (i) structural equations and (ii) expected covariances derived in terms of the parameters of the model. Since all three forms are mathematically complete, it is possible to translate from one to another for such purposes as applying it to data, increasing understanding of the model, verifying its identification, or presenting results.

The advantage of the path method is that it goes beyond measuring the degree of association by the correlation coefficient or determining the best prediction by the regression coefficient. Instead, the user makes explicit hypotheses about relationships between the variables which are quantified by path coefficients. Better still, the model's predictions may be statistically compared with the observed data,

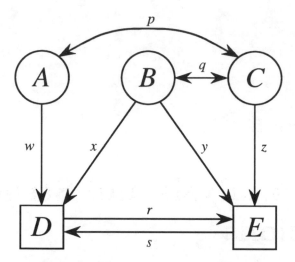

Figure 5.1: Path diagram for three latent (A, B and C) and two observed (D and E) variables, illustrating correlations (p and q) and path coefficients (r, s, w, x, y and z).

as we shall go on to discuss in Chapters 6 and 7. Path models are in fact extremely general, subsuming a large number of multivariate methods, including (but not limited to) multiple regression, principle component or factor analysis, canonical correlation, discriminant analysis and multivariate analysis of variance and covariance. Therefore those that take exception to 'path analysis' in its broadest sense, should be aware that they dismiss a vast array of multivariate statistical methods.

We begin by considering the conventions used to draw and read a path diagram, and explain the difference between correlational paths and causal paths (Section 5.2). In Sections 5.3 and 5.4 we briefly describe assumptions of the method and tracing rules for path diagrams. Then, to illustrate their use, we present simple linear regression models familiar to most readers. We define these both as path diagrams and as structural equations — some individuals handle path diagrams more easily, others respond better to equations! Finally we apply the method to two basic representations of a simple genetic model for covariation in twins, with special reference to the identity between the matrix specification of a model and its graphical representation.

5.2   Conventions Used in Path Analysis

A path diagram usually consists of boxes and circles, which are connected by arrows. Consider the diagram in Figure 5.1 for example. Squares or rectangles are used to enclose *observed* (manifest or measured) variables, and circles or ellipses surround *latent* (unmeasured) variables.

Single-headed arrows ('paths') are used to define causal relationships in the model, with the variable at the tail of the arrow causing the variable at the head. Omission of a path from one variable to another implies that there is no direct causal influence of the former variable on the latter. In the path diagram in (Figure 5.1) D is determined by A and B, while E is determined by B and C. When two variables cause each other, we say that there is a feedback-loop, or 'reciprocal causation' between them. Such a feedback-loop is shown between variables D and E in our example.

Double-headed arrows are used to represent a covariance between two variables, which might arise through a common cause or their reciprocal causation or both. In many treatments of path analysis, double-headed arrows may be placed *only* between variables that do not have causal arrows pointing at them. This convention allows us to discriminate between *dependent/endogenous* variables and *independent/ultimate/exogenous* variables.

Dependent variables are those variables we are trying to predict (in a regression model) or whose intercorrelations we are trying to explain (in a factor model). Dependent variables may be determined or caused by either independent variables or other dependent variables or both. In Figure 5.1, D and E are the dependent variables. *Independent* variables are the variables that explain the intercorrelations between the dependent variables or, in the case of the simplest regression models, predict the dependent variables. The causes of independent variables are not represented in the model. A, B and C are the independent variables in Figure 5.1.

Omission of a double-headed arrow reflects the hypothesis that two independent variables are uncorrelated. In Figure 5.1 the independent variables B and C correlate, C also correlates with A, but A does not correlate with B. This illustrates (i) that two variables which correlate with a third do not necessarily correlate with each other, and (ii) that when two factors cause the same dependent variable, it does not imply that they correlate. In some treatments of path analysis, a double-headed arrow from an independent variable to itself is used to represent its variance, but this is often omitted if the variable is standardized to unit variance.

By convention, lower-case letters (or numeric values, if these can be specified) are used to represent the values of paths or double-headed arrows, in contrast to the use of upper-case for variables. We call the values corresponding to causal paths *path coefficients,* and those of the double-headed arrows simply *correlation coefficients* (see Figure 5.1 for examples). In some applications, subscripts identify the origin and destination of a path. The first subscript refers to the variable being caused, and the second subscript tells which variable is doing the causing. In most genetic applications we assume that the variables are scaled as deviations from the means, in which case the constant intercept terms in equations will be zero and can be omitted from the structural equations.

Each dependent variable usually has a *residual*, unless it is fixed to zero *ex-hypothesi*. The residual variable does not correlate with any other determinants of its dependent variable, and will usually (but not always) be uncorrelated with other independent variables.

In summary therefore, the conventions used in path analysis:

- Observed variables are enclosed in squares or rectangles. Latent variables are enclosed in circles or ellipses. Error variables are included in the path diagram, and may be enclosed by circles or ellipses or (occasionally) not enclosed at all.

- Upper-case letters are used to denote observed or latent variables, and lower-case letters or numeric values represent the values of paths or two-way arrows, respectively called path coefficients and correlation coefficients.

- A one-way arrow between two variables indicates a postulated direct influence of one variable on another. A two-way arrow between two variables indicates that these variables may be correlated without any assumed direct relationship.

- There is a fundamental distinction between independent variables and dependent variables. Independent variables are not caused by any other variables in the system.

- Coefficients may have two subscripts, the first indicating the variable to which arrow points, the second showing its origin.

5.3 Assumptions of Path Analysis

Sewall Wright (Wright, 1968, p. 299) described path diagrams in the following manner:

> "[In path analysis] *every included variable, measured or hypothetical, is represented by arrows as either completely determined by certain others* (the dependent variables), *which may in turn be represented as similarly determined, or as an ultimate variable* (our independent variables). *Each ultimate factor in the diagram must be connected by lines with arrowheads at both ends with each of the other ultimate factors, to indicate possible correlations through still more remote, unrepresented factors, except in cases in which it can safely be assumed that there is no correlation .... the strict validity of the method depends on the properties of formally complete linear systems of unitary variables.*"

Some assumptions of the method, implicit or explicit in Wright's description, are:

- Linearity: All relationships between variables are linear. The assumption of a linear model seems valid as a wide variety of non-linear functions are well approximated by linear ones particularly within a limited range. (Sometimes non-linearity can be removed by appropriate transformation of the data prior to statistical analysis; but some models are inherently non-linear).

- Causal closure: All direct influences of one variable on another must be included in the path diagram. Hence the non-existence of an arrow between two variables means that it is assumed that these two variables are not directly related. The formal completeness of the diagram requires the introduction of residual variables if they are not represented as one of the ultimate variables, unless there is reason to assume complete additivity and determination by the specified factors.

- Unitary Variables: Variables may not be composed of components that behave in different ways with different variables in the system, but they should vary as a whole. For example, if we have three variables, A, B, and C, but A is really a composite of A1 and A2, and A1 is positively correlated with B and C, but A2 is positively correlated with B but negatively correlated with C, we have a potential for disaster!

5.4 Tracing Rules of Path Analysis

One of the greatest advantages of path diagrams is their foundation upon standard rules for reading paths, called "tracing rules," which yield the expected variances and covariances among the variables in the diagram.

In this section we first describe the tracing rules for standardized variables, following Wright's (1934, 1968) development of the method, and then outline the rules for unstandardized variables. Although nearly all path diagrams may be traced using rules for unstandardized variables,[1] we present path derivations for standardized and unstandardized variables separately because the former are much easier to trace than the latter, and because rules for unstandardized variables are fairly simple generalizations of the principles used in tracing paths between standardized variables. An excellent resource for learning tracing rules is the program RAMPATH (McArdle and Boker, 1990), which has a 'draw_bridges' command that illustrates the rules for any model.

5.4.1 Tracing Rules for Standardized Variables

The basic principle of tracing rules is described by Sewall Wright (1934) with the following words:

---

[1] Multivariate path diagrams, including delta path (van Eerdewegh, 1982), copath (Cloninger, 1980), and conditional path diagrams (Carey, 1986a) employ slightly different rules, but are outside the scope of this book. See Vogler (1985) for a general description.

> *"Any correlation between variables in a network of sequential relations
> can be analyzed into contributions from all the paths (direct or through
> common factors) by which the two variables are connected, such that the
> value of each contribution is the product of the coefficients pertaining to
> the elementary paths. If residual correlations are present (represented by
> bidirectional arrows) one (but never more than one) of the coefficients
> thus multiplied together to give the contribution of the connecting path,
> may be a correlation coefficient. The others are all path coefficients."*

In general, the expected correlation between two variables in a path diagram of
standardized variables may be derived by tracing all connecting routes (or "chains")
between the variables, while adhering to the following conditions. One may:

1. Trace backward along an arrow and then forward, or simply forwards from
   one variable to the other but *never forward and then back*

2. Pass through each variable only once in each chain of paths

3. Trace through at most one two-way arrow in each chain of paths

A corollary of the first rule is that one may *never pass through adjacent arrowheads*.
   The contribution of each chain traced between two variables to their expected
correlation is the *product* of its standardized coefficients. The expected correlation
between two variables is the sum of the contributions of all legitimate routes between those two variables. Note that these rules assume that there are no feedback
loops; i.e., that the model is 'recursive'.

5.4.2   Tracing Rules for Unstandardized Variables

If we are working with unstandardized variables, the tracing rules of the previous
section are insufficient to derive expected correlations. However, in the absence of
paths from dependent variables to other dependent variables, expected *covariances*,
rather than correlations, may be derived with only slight modifications to the
tracing rules (see Heise, 1975):

1. At any change of direction in a tracing route which is not a two-way arrow connecting different variables in the chain, the expected variance of the
   variable at the point of change is included in the product of path coefficients;
   thus, any path from an dependent variable to an independent variable will include the double-headed arrow from the independent variable to itself, unless
   it also includes a double-headed arrow connecting that variable to another independent variable (since this would violate the rule against passing through
   adjacent arrowheads)

2. In deriving variances, the path from an dependent variable to an independent
   variable and back to itself is only counted once

Perhaps a simpler approach to unstandardized path analysis is to make certain that all residual variances are included explicitly in the diagram with double-headed arrows pointing to the variable itself. Then the chains between two variables are formed simply if we

1. Trace backwards, change direction at a two-headed arrow, then trace forwards.

As before, the expected covariance is computed by multiplying all the coefficients in a chain and summing over all possible chains. We consider chains to be different if either a) they don't have the same coefficients, or b) the coefficients are in a different order. For a clear and thorough mathematical treatment, see the RAMPATH manual (McArdle and Boker, 1990).

5.5 Path Models for Linear Regression

In this Section we attempt to clarify the conventions, the assumptions and the tracing rules of path analysis by applying them to regression models. The path diagram in Figure 5.2a represents a linear regression model, such as might be used, for example, to predict systolic blood pressure [SBP], η_1 ('eta1'), from sodium intake, ξ_1 ('ksi1') [2]. The model asserts that high sodium intake is a *cause*, or *direct effect*, of high blood pressure (i.e., sodium intake $\to$ blood pressure), but that blood pressure also is influenced by other, unmeasured ('residual'), factors. The regression equation represented in Figure 5.2a is

$$\eta_1 = \alpha_1 + \gamma_{1,1}\xi_1 + \zeta_1, \tag{5.1}$$

where α is a constant intercept term, $\gamma_{1,1}$ the regression or 'structural' coefficient, and ζ_1 ('zeta1') the residual error term or disturbance term, which is uncorrelated with ξ_1. This is indicated by the absence of a double-headed arrow between ξ_1 and ζ_1 or an indirect common cause between them [$\mathrm{Cov}(\xi_1,\zeta_1) = 0$]. The double-headed arrow from ξ_1 to itself represents the variance of this variable: $\mathrm{Var}(\xi) = \phi_{1,1}$; the variance of ζ_1 is $\mathrm{Var}(\zeta) = \psi_{1,1}$. In this example systolic BP is the dependent variable and sodium intake is the independent variable.

We can extend the model by adding more independent variables or more dependent variables or both. The path diagram in Figure 5.2b represents a multiple regression model, such as might be used if we were trying to predict blood pressure (η_1) from sodium intake (ξ_1), exercise (ξ_2), and body mass index [BMI] (ξ_3), allowing once again for the influence of other residual factors (ζ_1) on blood pressure. The double-headed arrows between the three independent variables indicate that correlations are allowed between sodium intake and exercise ($\phi_{2,1}$), sodium intake and BMI ($\phi_{3,1}$), and BMI and exercise ($\phi_{3,2}$). For example, a negative covariance

---

[2] This usage of Greek variables corresponds to the LISREL model, to be discussed in greater detail in the next chapter. The Greek alphabet is presented in Appendix B.

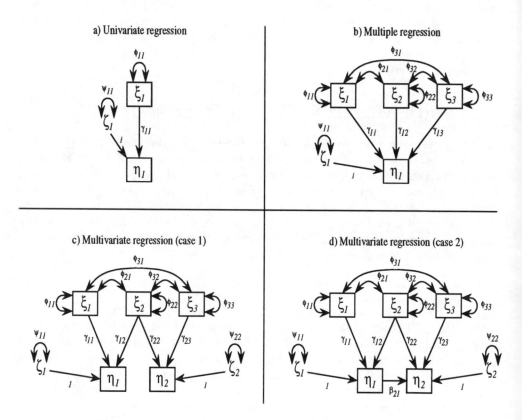

Figure 5.2: Regression models with manifest variables.

between exercise and sodium intake might arise if the health-conscious exercised more and ingested less sodium; positive covariance between sodium intake and BMI could occur if obese individuals ate more (and therefore ingested more sodium); and a negative covariance between BMI and exercise could exist if overweight people were less inclined to exercise. In this case the regression equation is

$$\eta_1 = \alpha_1 + \gamma_{1,1}\xi_1 + \gamma_{1,2}\xi_2 + \gamma_{1,3}\xi_3 + \zeta_1. \tag{5.2}$$

Note that the estimated values for α_1, $\gamma_{1,1}$ and ζ_1 will not usually be the same as in equation 5.1 due to the inclusion of additional independent variables in the multiple regression equation 5.2. Similarly, the only difference between Figures 5.2a and 5.2b is that we have multiple independent or predictor variables in Figure 5.2b.

Figure 5.2c represents a multivariate regression model, where we now have two dependent variables (blood pressure, η_1, and a measure of coronary artery disease [CAD], η_2), as well as the same set of independent variables (case 1). The model postulates that there are direct influences of sodium intake and exercise on blood pressure, and of exercise and BMI on CAD, but no direct influence of sodium intake on CAD, nor of BMI on blood pressure. Because the ξ_2 variable, exercise, causes both blood pressure, η_1, and coronary artery disease, η_2, it is termed a *common cause* of these dependent variables. The regression equations are

$$\eta_1 = \alpha_1 + \gamma_{1,1}\xi_1 + \gamma_{1,2}\xi_2 + \zeta_1$$

and

$$\eta_2 = \alpha_2 + \gamma_{2,2}\xi_2 + \gamma_{2,3}\xi_3 + \zeta_2. \tag{5.3}$$

Here α_1 and ζ_1 are the intercept term and error term, respectively, and $\gamma_{1,1}$ and $\gamma_{1,2}$ the regression coefficients for predicting blood pressure, and α_2, ζ_2, $\gamma_{2,2}$, and $\gamma_{2,3}$ the corresponding coefficients for predicting coronary artery disease. We can rewrite equation 5.3 using matrices (see Chapter 4 on matrix algebra),

$$\begin{pmatrix} \eta_1 \\ \eta_2 \end{pmatrix} = \begin{pmatrix} \alpha_1 \\ \alpha_2 \end{pmatrix} + \begin{pmatrix} \gamma_{1,1} & \gamma_{1,2} & 0 \\ 0 & \gamma_{2,2} & \gamma_{2,3} \end{pmatrix} \begin{pmatrix} \xi_1 \\ \xi_2 \\ \xi_3 \end{pmatrix} + \begin{pmatrix} \zeta_1 \\ \zeta_2 \end{pmatrix}$$

or, using matrix notation,

$$\eta = \alpha + \Gamma\xi + \zeta,$$

where η, α, ξ, and ζ are column vectors and Γ is a matrix of regression coefficients. Note that each variable in the path diagram which has an arrow pointing to it appears exactly one time on the left side of the matrix expression.

Figure 5.2d differs from Figure 5.2c only by the addition of a causal path $(\beta_{1,2})$ from blood pressure to coronary artery disease, implying the hypothesis that high blood pressure increases CAD (case 2). The presence of this path also provides a link between η_2 and ξ_1 ($\eta_2 \leftarrow \eta_1 \leftarrow \xi_1$); this type of process with multiple intervening variables is typically called an *indirect effect* (of ξ_1 on η_2). Thus we see that dependent variables can be influenced by other dependent variables, as well as by independent variables. Figure 5.3 adds an additional causal path from CAD to blood pressure ($\beta_{2,1}$), thus creating a 'feedback-loop' (hereafter designated as $\Longleftrightarrow$) between CAD and blood pressure. If both β parameters are positive, the interpretation of the model would be that high SBP increases CAD and increased CAD in turn increases SBP. Such reciprocal causation of variables requires special treatment and is discussed further in Chapters 10 and 13. Figure 5.3 implies the structural equations

$$\eta_1 = \alpha_1 + \beta_{1,2}\eta_2 + \gamma_{1,1}\xi_1 + \gamma_{1,2}\xi_2 + \zeta_1$$

and

$$\eta_2 = \alpha_2 + \beta_{2,1}\eta_1 + \gamma_{2,2}\xi_2 + \gamma_{2,3}\xi_3 + \zeta_2 \tag{5.4}$$

In matrix form, we may write these equations as

$$\begin{pmatrix} \eta_1 \\ \eta_2 \end{pmatrix} = \begin{pmatrix} \alpha_1 \\ \alpha_2 \end{pmatrix} + \begin{pmatrix} 0 & \beta_{1,2} \\ \beta_{2,1} & 0 \end{pmatrix} \begin{pmatrix} \eta_1 \\ \eta_2 \end{pmatrix} + \begin{pmatrix} \gamma_{1,1} & \gamma_{1,2} & 0 \\ 0 & \gamma_{2,2} & \gamma_{2,3} \end{pmatrix} \begin{pmatrix} \xi_1 \\ \xi_2 \\ \xi_3 \end{pmatrix}$$
$$+ \begin{pmatrix} \zeta_1 \\ \zeta_2 \end{pmatrix}$$

i.e.,

$$\boldsymbol{\eta} = \boldsymbol{\alpha} + \boldsymbol{B}\boldsymbol{\eta} + \boldsymbol{\Gamma}\boldsymbol{\xi} + \boldsymbol{\zeta}$$

Now that some examples of regression models have been described both in the form of path diagrams and structural equations, we can apply the tracing rules of path analysis to derive the expected variances and covariances under the models. The regression models presented in this chapter are all examples of unstandardized variables. We illustrate the derivation of the expected variance or covariance between some variables by applying the tracing rules for unstandardized variables in Figures 5.2a, 5.2b and 5.2c. As an exercise, the reader may wish to trace some of the other paths.

In the case of Figure 5.2a, to derive the expected covariance between ξ_1 and η_1, we need trace only the path:

$$\text{(i)} \qquad \xi_1 \xleftrightarrow{\phi_{1,1}} \xi_1 \xrightarrow{\gamma_{1,1}} \eta_1$$

yielding an expected covariance of ($\phi_{1,1}\gamma_{1,1}$). Two paths contribute to the expected variance of η_1,

$$\text{(i)} \qquad \eta_1 \xleftarrow{\gamma_{1,1}} \xi_1 \xleftrightarrow{\phi_{1,1}} \xi_1 \xrightarrow{\gamma_{1,1}} \eta_1,$$
$$\text{(ii)} \qquad \eta_1 \xleftarrow{1} \zeta_1 \xleftrightarrow{\psi_{1,1}} \zeta_1 \xrightarrow{1} \eta_1;$$

yielding an expected variance of η_1 of ($\gamma_{1,1}^2\phi_{1,1} + \psi_{1,1}$).

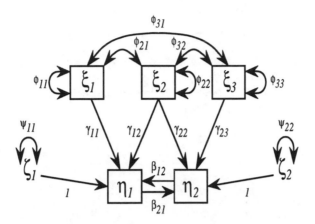

Figure 5.3: Non-recursive model: Multivariate regression model with reciprocal causation.

In the case of Figure 5.2b, to derive the expected covariance of ξ_1 and η_1, we can trace paths:

$$
\begin{array}{ll}
\text{(i)} & \eta_1 \xleftarrow{\gamma_{1,1}} \xi_1 \xleftrightarrow{\phi_{1,1}} \xi_1, \\[4pt]
\text{(ii)} & \eta_1 \xleftarrow{\gamma_{1,2}} \xi_2 \xleftrightarrow{\phi_{2,1}} \xi_1, \\[4pt]
\text{(iii)} & \eta_1 \xleftarrow{\gamma_{1,3}} \xi_3 \xleftrightarrow{\phi_{3,1}} \xi_1,
\end{array}
$$

to obtain an expected covariance of $(\gamma_{1,1}\phi_{1,1} + \gamma_{1,2}\phi_{2,1} + \gamma_{1,3}\phi_{3,1})$. To derive the expected variance of η_1, we can trace paths:

$$
\begin{array}{ll}
\text{(i)} & \eta_1 \xleftarrow{\gamma_{1,1}} \xi_1 \xleftrightarrow{\phi_{1,1}} \xi_1 \xrightarrow{\gamma_{1,1}} \eta_1, \\[4pt]
\text{(ii)} & \eta_1 \xleftarrow{\gamma_{1,2}} \xi_2 \xleftrightarrow{\phi_{2,2}} \xi_2 \xrightarrow{\gamma_{1,2}} \eta_1, \\[4pt]
\text{(iii)} & \eta_1 \xleftarrow{\gamma_{1,3}} \xi_3 \xleftrightarrow{\phi_{3,3}} \xi_3 \xrightarrow{\gamma_{1,3}} \eta_1, \\[4pt]
\text{(iv)} & \eta_1 \xleftarrow{1} \zeta_1 \xleftrightarrow{\psi_{1,1}} \zeta_1 \xrightarrow{1} \eta_1, \\[4pt]
\text{(v)} & \eta_1 \xleftarrow{\gamma_{1,1}} \xi_1 \xleftrightarrow{\phi_{2,1}} \xi_2 \xrightarrow{\gamma_{1,2}} \eta_1, \\[4pt]
\text{(vi)} & \eta_1 \xleftarrow{\gamma_{1,2}} \xi_2 \xleftrightarrow{\phi_{2,1}} \xi_1 \xrightarrow{\gamma_{1,1}} \eta_1, \\[4pt]
\text{(vii)} & \eta_1 \xleftarrow{\gamma_{1,1}} \xi_1 \xleftrightarrow{\phi_{3,1}} \xi_3 \xrightarrow{\gamma_{1,3}} \eta_1,
\end{array}
$$

$$\text{(viii)}\qquad \eta_1 \xleftarrow{\gamma_{1,3}} \xi_3 \xleftrightarrow{\phi_{3,1}} \xi_1 \xrightarrow{\gamma_{1,1}} \eta_1,$$

$$\text{(ix)}\qquad \eta_1 \xleftarrow{\gamma_{1,2}} \xi_2 \xleftrightarrow{\phi_{3,2}} \xi_3 \xrightarrow{\gamma_{1,3}} \eta_1,$$

$$\text{(x)}\qquad \eta_1 \xleftarrow{\gamma_{1,3}} \xi_3 \xleftrightarrow{\phi_{3,2}} \xi_2 \xrightarrow{\gamma_{1,2}} \eta_1,$$

yielding a total expected variance of $(\gamma_{1,1}^2\phi_{1,1} + \gamma_{1,2}^2\phi_{2,2} + \gamma_{1,3}^2\phi_{3,3} + 2\gamma_{1,1}\gamma_{1,2}\phi_{2,1} + 2\gamma_{1,1}\gamma_{1,3}\phi_{3,1} + 2\gamma_{1,2}\gamma_{1,3}\phi_{3,2} + \psi_{1,1})$.

In the case of Figure 5.2c, we may derive the expected covariance of η_1 and η_2 as the sum of

$$\text{(i)}\qquad \eta_1 \xleftarrow{\gamma_{1,1}} \xi_1 \xleftrightarrow{\phi_{2,1}} \xi_2 \xrightarrow{\gamma_{2,2}} \eta_2,$$

$$\text{(ii)}\qquad \eta_1 \xleftarrow{\gamma_{1,1}} \xi_1 \xleftrightarrow{\phi_{3,1}} \xi_3 \xrightarrow{\gamma_{2,3}} \eta_2,$$

$$\text{(iii)}\qquad \eta_1 \xleftarrow{\gamma_{1,2}} \xi_2 \xleftrightarrow{\phi_{2,2}} \xi_2 \xrightarrow{\gamma_{2,2}} \eta_2,$$

$$\text{(iv)}\qquad \eta_1 \xleftarrow{\gamma_{1,2}} \xi_2 \xleftrightarrow{\phi_{3,2}} \xi_3 \xrightarrow{\gamma_{2,3}} \eta_2,$$

giving $[\gamma_{1,1}(\phi_{2,1}\gamma_{2,2}+\phi_{3,1}\gamma_{2,3})+\gamma_{1,2}(\phi_{2,2}\gamma_{2,2}+\phi_{3,2}\gamma_{2,3})]$ for the expected covariance. This expectation, and the preceding ones, can be derived equally (and arguably more easily) by simple matrix algebra. For example, the expected covariance matrix ($\boldsymbol{\Sigma}$) for η_1 and η_2 under the model of Figure 5.2c is given as

$$\boldsymbol{\Sigma} = \boldsymbol{\Gamma\Phi\Gamma'} + \boldsymbol{\Psi},$$

$$= \begin{pmatrix} \gamma_{1,1} & \gamma_{1,2} & 0 \\ 0 & \gamma_{2,2} & \gamma_{3,3} \end{pmatrix} \begin{pmatrix} \phi_{1,1} & \phi_{1,2} & \phi_{1,3} \\ \phi_{2,1} & \phi_{2,2} & \phi_{2,3} \\ \phi_{3,1} & \phi_{3,2} & \phi_{3,3} \end{pmatrix} \begin{pmatrix} \gamma_{1,1} & 0 \\ \gamma_{1,2} & \gamma_{2,2} \\ 0 & \gamma_{2,3} \end{pmatrix}$$
$$+ \begin{pmatrix} \psi_{1,1} & 0 \\ 0 & \psi_{2,2} \end{pmatrix}$$

in which the elements of $\boldsymbol{\Gamma}$ are the paths from the ξ variables (columns) to the η variables (rows); the elements of $\boldsymbol{\Phi}$ are the covariances between the independent variables; and the elements of $\boldsymbol{\Psi}$ are the residual error variances.

5.6   Path Models for the Classical Twin Study

To introduce genetic models and to further illustrate the tracing rules both for standardized variables and unstandardized variables, we examine some simple genetic models of resemblance. The classical twin study, in which MZ twins and DZ twins are reared together in the same home is one of the most powerful designs for detecting genetic and shared environmental effects. Once we have collected such data, they may be summarized as observed covariance matrices (Chapter 2), but in order to test hypotheses we need to derive expected covariance matrices from the model. We first digress briefly to review the biometrical principles outlined in Chapter 3, in order to express the ideas in a path–analytic context.

In contrast to the regression models considered in previous sections, many genetic analyses of family data postulate independent variables (genotypes and environments) as *latent* rather than manifest variables. In other words, the genotypes and environments are not measured directly but their influence is inferred through their effects on the covariances of relatives. However, we can represent these models as path diagrams in just the same way as the regression models. The brief introduction to path-analytic genetic models we give here will be treated in greater detail in Chapter 8, and thereafter.

From quantitative genetic theory (see Chapter 3), we can write equations relating the phenotypes P_i and P_j of relatives i and j (e.g., systolic blood pressures of first and second members of a twin pair), to their underlying genotypes and environments. We may decompose the total genetic effect on a phenotype into that due to the additive effects of alleles at multiple loci, that due to the dominance effects at multiple loci, and that due to the epistatic interactions between loci (Mather and Jinks, 1982). Similarly, we may decompose the total environmental effect into that due to environmental influences shared by twins or sibling pairs reared in the same family ('shared', 'common', or 'between-family' environmental effects), and that due to environmental effects which make family members differ from one another ('random', 'specific', or 'within-family' environmental effects). Thus, the observed phenotypes, P_i and P_j, are assumed to be linear functions of the underlying additive genetic variance (A_i and A_j), dominance variance (D_i and D_j), shared environmental variance (C_i and C_j) and random environmental variance (E_i and E_j). In quantitative genetic studies of human populations, epistatic genetic effects are usually confounded with dominance genetic effects, and so will not be considered further here. Assuming all variables are scaled as deviations from zero, we have

$$P_1 = e_1 E_1 + c_1 C_1 + a_1 A_1 + d_1 D_1$$

and

$$P_2 = e_2 E_2 + c_2 C_2 + a_2 A_2 + d_2 D_2$$

Particularly for pairs of twins, we do not expect the magnitude of genetic or environmental effects to vary as a function of relationship[3] so we set $e_1 = e_2 = e$,

---

[3]i.e. we do not expect different heritabilities for twin 1 and twin 2; however for other relationships such as parents and children, the assumption may not be valid, as could be established empirically if we had genetically informative data in both generations.

$c_1 = c_2 = c$, $a_1 = a_2 = a$, and $d_1 = d_2 = d$. In matrix form, we write

$$
\begin{pmatrix} P_1 \\ P_2 \end{pmatrix} = \begin{pmatrix} e & c & a & d & 0 & 0 & 0 & 0 \\ 0 & 0 & 0 & 0 & e & c & a & d \end{pmatrix} \begin{pmatrix} E_1 \\ C_1 \\ A_1 \\ D_1 \\ E_2 \\ C_2 \\ A_2 \\ D_2 \end{pmatrix}.
$$

Unless two or more waves of measurement are used, or several observed variables index the phenotype under study, residual effects are included in the random environmental component, and are not separately specified in the model.

Figures 5.4a and 5.4b represent two alternative parameterizations of the basic genetic model, illustrated for the case of pairs of monozygotic twins (MZ) or dizygotic twins (DZ), who may be reared together (MZT, DZT) or reared apart (MZA, DZA). In Figure 5.4a, the traditional *path coefficients model*, the variances of the latent variables A_1, C_1, E_1, D_1 and A_2, C_2, E_2, D_2 are standardized ($V_E = V_C = V_A = V_D = 1$, and the path coefficients e, c, a, or d — quantifying the paths from the latent variables to the observed variable, measured on both twins, P_1 and P_2 — are free parameters to be estimated. Figure 5.4b is called a *variance components model* because it fixes $e = c = a = d = 1$, and estimates separate random environmental, shared environmental, additive genetic and dominance genetic variances instead.

The traditional path model illustrates tracing rules for standardized variables, and is straightforward to generalize to multivariate problems; the variance components model illustrates an unstandardized path model. Provided all parameter estimates are non-negative, tracing the paths in either parameterization will give the same solution, with $V_A = a^2$, $V_D = d^2$, $V_C = c^2$ and $V_E = e^2$.

5.6.1   Path Coefficients Model: Example of Standardized Tracing Rules

When applying the tracing rules, it helps to draw out each tracing route to ensure that they are neither forgotten nor traced twice. In the traditional path model of Figure 5.4a, to derive the expected twin covariance for the case of monozygotic twin pairs reared together, we can trace the following routes:

$$
\begin{aligned}
&\text{(i)} && P1 \xleftarrow{\ c\ } C1 \xleftrightarrow{\ 1\ } C2 \xrightarrow{\ c\ } P2 \\
&\text{(ii)} && P1 \xleftarrow{\ a\ } A1 \xleftrightarrow{\ 1\ } A2 \xrightarrow{\ a\ } P2 \\
&\text{(iii)} && P1 \xleftarrow{\ d\ } D1 \xleftrightarrow{\ 1\ } D2 \xrightarrow{\ d\ } P2
\end{aligned}
$$

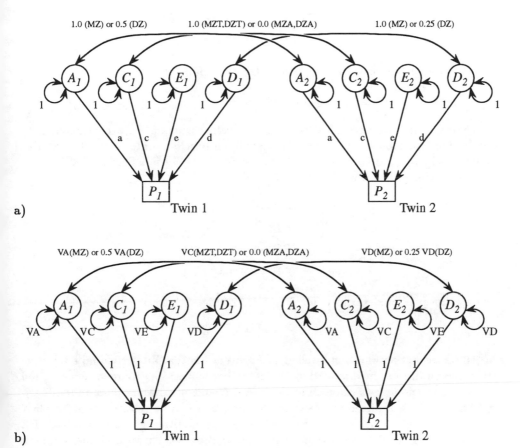

Figure 5.4: Alternative representations of the basic genetic model: a) variance components model, and b) traditional path coefficients model.

so that the expected covariance between MZ twin pairs reared together will be

$$r_{MZ} = c^2 + a^2 + d^2. \tag{5.5}$$

In the case of dizygotic twin pairs reared together, we can trace the following routes:

(i) $P1 \xleftarrow{c} C1 \xleftrightarrow{1} C2 \xrightarrow{c} P2$

(ii) $P1 \xleftarrow{a} A1 \xleftrightarrow{0.5} A2 \xrightarrow{a} P2$

(iii) $P1 \xleftarrow{d} D1 \xleftrightarrow{0.25} D2 \xrightarrow{d} P2$

yielding an expected covariance between DZ twin pairs of

$$r_{DZ} = c^2 + 0.5a^2 + 0.25d^2. \tag{5.6}$$

The expected variance of a variable — again assuming we are working with standardized variables — is derived by tracing all possible routes from the variable back to itself, without violating any of the tracing rules given in Section 5.4.1 above. Thus, following paths from P1 to itself we have

(i) $P1 \xleftarrow{e} E1 \xrightarrow{e} P1$

(ii) $P1 \xleftarrow{c} C1 \xrightarrow{c} P1$

(iii) $P1 \xleftarrow{a} A1 \xrightarrow{a} P1$

(iv) $P1 \xleftarrow{d} D1 \xrightarrow{d} P1$

yielding the predicted variance for $P1$ or $P2$ in Figure 5.4a of

$$V_P = e^2 + c^2 + a^2 + d^2. \tag{5.7}$$

An important assumption implicit in Figure 5.4 is that an individual's additive genetic deviation is uncorrelated with his or her shared environmental deviation (i.e., there are no arrows connecting the latent C and A variables of an individual). In Chapter 17 we shall discuss how this assumption can be relaxed. Also implicit in the coefficient of 0.5 for the covariance of the additive genetic values of DZ twins or siblings is the assumption of random mating, which we shall also relax in Chapter 17.

5.6.2   Variance components model: Example of Unstandardized Tracing Rules

Following the unstandardized tracing rules, the expected covariances of twin pairs in the variance components model of Figure 5.4b, are also easily derived. For the case of monozygotic twin pairs reared together (MZT), we can trace the following routes:

$$\text{(i)} \qquad P1 \xleftarrow{1} C1 \xleftrightarrow{V_C} C2 \xrightarrow{1} P2$$

$$\text{(ii)} \qquad P1 \xleftarrow{1} A1 \xleftrightarrow{V_A} A2 \xrightarrow{1} P2$$

$$\text{(iii)} \qquad P1 \xleftarrow{1} D1 \xleftrightarrow{V_D} D2 \xrightarrow{1} P2$$

so that the expected covariance between MZ twin pairs reared together will be

$$\text{Cov}(MZT) = V_C + V_A + V_D.$$

Only the latter two chains contribute to the expected covariance of MZ twin pairs reared apart, as they do not share their environment. The expected covariance of MZ twin pairs reared apart (MZA)is thus

$$\text{Cov}(MZA) = V_A + V_D.$$

In the case of dizygotic twin pairs reared together (DZT), we can trace the following routes:

$$\text{(i)} \qquad P1 \xleftarrow{1} C1 \xleftrightarrow{V_C} C2 \xrightarrow{1} P2$$

$$\text{(ii)} \qquad P1 \xleftarrow{1} A1 \xleftrightarrow{0.5V_A} A2 \xrightarrow{1} P2$$

$$\text{(iii)} \qquad P1 \xleftarrow{1} D1 \xleftrightarrow{0.25V_D} D2 \xrightarrow{1} P2$$

yielding an expected covariance between DZ twin reared together of

$$\text{Cov}(DZT) = V_C + 0.5V_A + 0.25V_D.$$

Similarly, the expected covariance of DZ twin pairs reared apart (DZA)is

$$\text{Cov}(DZA) = 0.5V_A + 0.25V_D.$$

In deriving expected variances of unstandardized variables, any chain from a dependent variable to an independent variable will include the double-headed arrow from the independent variable to itself (unless it also includes a double-headed arrow connecting that variable to another independent variable) and each path from an dependent variable to an independent variable and back to itself is only counted once. In this example the expected phenotypic variance, for all groups of relatives, is easily derived by tracing all the paths from $P1$ to itself:

$$\text{(i)} \qquad P1 \xleftarrow{1} E1 \xleftrightarrow{V_E} E1 \xrightarrow{1} P1$$

$$\text{(ii)} \qquad P1 \xleftarrow{1} C1 \xleftrightarrow{V_C} C1 \xrightarrow{1} P1$$

$$\text{(iii)} \qquad P1 \xleftarrow{1} A1 \xleftrightarrow{V_A} A1 \xrightarrow{1} P1$$

$$\text{(iv)} \qquad P1 \xleftarrow{1} D1 \xleftrightarrow{V_D} D1 \xrightarrow{1} P1$$

yielding the predicted variance for P1 or P2 in Figure 5.4b of

$$V_P = V_E + V_C + V_A + V_D.$$

The equivalence between Figures 5.4a and 5.4b comes from the biometrical principles outlined in Chapter 3: a^2, c^2, e^2, and d^2 are defined as $\frac{V_A}{V_P}$, $\frac{V_C}{V_P}$, $\frac{V_E}{V_P}$, and $\frac{V_D}{V_P}$, respectively. Since correlations are calculated as covariances divided by the product of the square roots of the variances (see Chapter 2), the twin correlations in Figure 5.4a may be derived using the covariances and variances in Figure 5.4b. Thus, in Figure 5.4b, the correlation for MZ pairs reared together is

$$
\begin{aligned}
r_{\text{MZT}} &= \frac{V_C + V_A + V_D}{\sqrt{(V_C + V_A + V_D + V_E)}\sqrt{(V_C + V_A + V_D + V_E)}} \\
&= \frac{V_C + V_A + V_D}{V_P} \\
&= \frac{V_C}{V_P} + \frac{V_A}{V_P} + \frac{V_D}{V_P} \\
&= c^2 + a^2 + d^2
\end{aligned}
$$

Similarly, the correlations for MZ twins reared apart, and for DZ twins together and apart are

$$
\begin{aligned}
r_{\text{MZA}} &= a^2 + d^2 \\
r_{\text{DZT}} &= c^2 + 0.5a^2 + 0.25d^2 \\
r_{\text{DZA}} &= 0.5a^2 + 0.25d^2,
\end{aligned}
$$

as in the case of Figure 5.4a.

5.7   Identification of models and parameters

One key issue with structural equation modeling is whether a model, or a parameter within a model is *identified*. We say that the free parameters of a model are either (i) overidentified; (ii) just identified; or (iii) underidentified. If all of the parameters fall into the first two classes, we say that the model as a whole is identified, but if one or more parameters are in class (iii), we say that the model is not identified. In this Section, we briefly address the identification of parameters in structural equation models, and illustrate how data from additional types of relative may or may not identify the parameters of a model.

When we applied the rules of standardized path analysis to the simple path coefficient model for twins (Figure 5.4b), we obtained expressions for MZ and DZ covariances and the phenotypic variance:

$$
\begin{aligned}
\text{Cov}(MZ) &= c^2 + a^2 + d^2 & (5.8) \\
\text{Cov}(DZ) &= c^2 + .5a^2 + .25d^2 & (5.9) \\
V_P &= c^2 + a^2 + d^2 + e^2 & (5.10)
\end{aligned}
$$

These three equations have four unknown parameters c, a, d and e, and illustrate the first point about identification. *A model is underidentified if the number of free parameters is greater than the number of distinct statistics that it predicts.* Here there are four unknown parameters but only three distinct statistics, so the model is underidentified.

One way of checking the identification of simple models is to represent the expected variances and covariances as a system of equations in matrix algebra:

$$\mathbf{Ax} = \mathbf{b}$$

where $\mathbf{x}$ is the vector of parameters, $\mathbf{b}$ is the vector of observed statistics, and $\mathbf{A}$ is the matrix of weights such that element A_{ij} gives the coefficient of parameter j in equation i. Then, if the inverse of $\mathbf{A}$ exists, the model is identified. Thus in our example we have:

$$\begin{pmatrix} 1 & 1 & 1 & 0 \\ 1 & .5 & .25 & 0 \\ 1 & 1 & 1 & 1 \end{pmatrix} \begin{pmatrix} c^2 \\ a^2 \\ d^2 \\ e^2 \end{pmatrix} = \begin{pmatrix} b_1 \\ b_2 \\ b_3 \end{pmatrix}. \tag{5.11}$$

Now, what we would really like to find here is the left inverse, $\mathbf{L}$, of $\mathbf{A}$ such that $\mathbf{LA} = \mathbf{I}$. However, it is easy to show that left inverses may exist only when $\mathbf{A}$ has at least as many rows as it does columns (for proof see, e.g., Searle, 1982, p. 147). Therefore, if we are limited to data from a classical twin study, i.e. MZ and DZ twins reared together, it is necessary to assume that one of the parameters a, c or d is zero to identify the model. Let us suppose that we have reason to believe that c can be ignored, so that the equations may be rewritten as:

$$\begin{pmatrix} 1 & 1 & 0 \\ .5 & .25 & 0 \\ 1 & 1 & 1 \end{pmatrix} \begin{pmatrix} c^2 \\ a^2 \\ d^2 \end{pmatrix} = \begin{pmatrix} b_1 \\ b_2 \\ b_3 \end{pmatrix}$$

and in this case, the inverse of $\mathbf{A}$ exists[4]. Another, generally superior, approach to resolving the parameters of the model is to collect new data. For example, if we collected data from separated MZ or DZ twins, then we could add a fourth row to $\mathbf{A}$ in equation 5.11 to get (for MZ twins apart)

$$\begin{pmatrix} 1 & 1 & 1 & 0 \\ 1 & .5 & .25 & 0 \\ 1 & 1 & 1 & 1 \\ 0 & 1 & 1 & 1 \end{pmatrix} \begin{pmatrix} c^2 \\ a^2 \\ d^2 \\ e^2 \end{pmatrix} = \begin{pmatrix} b_1 \\ b_2 \\ b_3 \\ b_4 \end{pmatrix} \tag{5.12}$$

and again the inverse of $\mathbf{A}$ exists. Now it is not necessarily the case that adding another type of relative (or type of rearing environment) will turn an underidentified model into one that is identified! Far from it, in fact, as we show with reference

---

[4]The reader may like to verify this by calculating the determinant according to the method laid out in Section 4.2.2 or with the aid of a computer.

to siblings reared together, and half-siblings and cousins reared apart. Under our simple genetic model, the expected covariances of the siblings and half-siblings are

$$\text{Cov}(Sibs) \quad = \quad c^2 + .5a^2 + .25d^2 \tag{5.13}$$
$$\text{Cov}(Half - sibs) \quad = \quad .25a^2 \tag{5.14}$$
$$\text{Cov}(Cousins) \quad = \quad .125a^2 \tag{5.15}$$
$$V_P \quad = \quad c^2 + a^2 + d^2 + e^2 \tag{5.16}$$

as could be shown by extending the methods outlined in Chapter 3. In matrix form the equations are:

$$\begin{pmatrix} 1 & .5 & .25 & 0 \\ 0 & .25 & 0 & 0 \\ 0 & .125 & 0 & 0 \\ 1 & 1 & 1 & 1 \end{pmatrix} \begin{pmatrix} c^2 \\ a^2 \\ d^2 \\ e^2 \end{pmatrix} = \begin{pmatrix} b_1 \\ b_2 \\ b_3 \\ b_4 \end{pmatrix}. \tag{5.17}$$

Now in this case, although we have as many types of relationship with different expected covariance as there are unknown parameters in the model, we still cannot identify all the parameters, because the matrix **A** is singular. The presence of data collected from cousins does not add any information to the system, because their expected covariance is exactly half that of the half-siblings. In general, if any row (column) of a matrix can be expressed as a linear combination of the other rows (columns) of a matrix, then the matrix is singular and cannot be inverted. Note, however, that just because we cannot identify the model as a whole, it does not mean that none of the parameters can be estimated. In this example, we can obtain a valid estimate of additive genetic variance a^2 simply from, say, eight times the difference of the half-sib and cousin covariances. With this knowledge and the observed full sibling covariance, we could estimate the *combined* effect of dominance and the shared environment, but it is impossible to separate these two sources.

Throughout the above examples, we have taken advantage of their inherent simplicity. The first useful feature is that the parameters of the model only occur in linear combinations, so that, e.g., terms of the form c^2a are not present. While true of a number of simple genetic models that we shall use in this book, it is not the case for them all (see Table 17.2 for example). Nevertheless, some insight may be gained by examining the model in this way, since if we are able to identify both c and c^2a then both parameters may be estimated. Yet for complex systems this can prove a a difficult task, so we suggest an alternative, numerical approach. The idea is to simulate expected covariances for certain values of the parameters, and then see whether a program such as LISREL can recover these values from a number of different starting points. If we find another set of parameter values that generates the same expected variance and covariances, the model is not identified. We shall not go into this procedure in detail here, but simply note that it is very similar to that described for power calculations in Chapter 9.

5.8 Summary

In this chapter we have reviewed briefly the use of path analysis to represent certain linear and genetic models. We have discussed the conventions of path analysis, and shown how it may be used to derive the covariance matrices predicted under a particular model. We emphasize that the systems described here have been chosen as simple examples to illustrate elementary principles of path analysis. Although these examples are somewhat simplistic in the sense that they do not elucidate many of the characteristics of which structural equation models are capable, familiarity with them should provide sufficient skills for comprehension of other, more advanced, genetic models described in this text and for development of one's own path models.

However, one aspect of structural models which has not been discussed in this chapter is that of *multiple indicators*. While not strictly a feature of path analysis, multiple indicator models, — those with more than one measure for each dependent or independent variable — warrant some attention because they are used often in genetic analyses of twin data, and in analyses of behavioral data in general. Our initial regression examples from Figures 5.2 and 5.3 assumed that we had only a single measure for each variable (systolic blood pressure, sodium intake, etc), and could ignore measurement error in these observed variables. Inclusion of multiple indicators allows for explicit representation of assumptions about measurement error in a model. In our regression example of Figures 5.2d and 5.3, for example, we might have several measures of our independent (ξ) variables, a number of measures of sodium intake (e.g., diet diary and urinary sodium), multiple measures of exercise (e.g., exercise diary and frequency checklist), and numerous measures of obesity (e.g., self-report body mass index, measures of skin-fold thickness). Likewise, we might have many estimates of our dependent η variables, such as repeated measures of blood pressure, and several tests for coronary artery disease. Figure 5.5 expands Figure 5.2a by illustrating the cases of (i) one variable per construct, (ii) two variables per construct, and (iii) three or more observed variables per construct.

Covariance and variance expectations for multiple indicator models such as those shown in Figure 5.5 follow without exception from the path tracing rules outlined earlier in this chapter. However, the increase in number of variables in these models often results in substantial increases in model complexity. One of the important attractions of the LISREL model to behavior geneticists has been that it allows for multiple indicators with relative ease in model specification, as such effects are built-in to the "LISREL Measurement Model." It is to these models, and to the LISREL model in general, that we now turn.

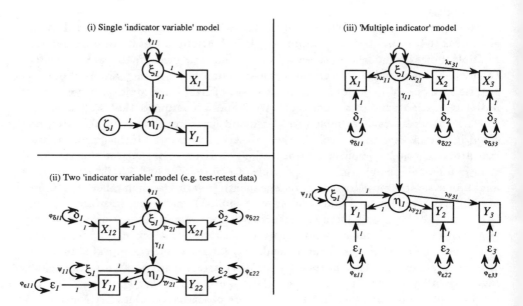

Figure 5.5: Multiple indicators in regression path models.

Chapter 6

LISREL Models and Methods

6.1 Introduction

In this Chapter we develop the LISREL model formally, and assume some knowledge of elementary statistics. While understanding the model will prove useful in the long run, it is not strictly prerequisite for the LISREL applications in this book. It provides a valuable reference section and guide to the statistical theory behind applied model-fitting, especially in conjunction with our first application of the package in Section 8.4. The less mathematically-minded reader may wish to skim this Chapter for now, and return to it when they feel more comfortable with the practical use of LISREL for simple models.

The LISREL model is a formal mathematical model which has to be given substantive content in each application. The meaning of the terms involved in the model varies from one application to another. The formal LISREL model defines a large class of models within which one can work and this class contains several useful subclasses as special cases.

In its most general form, the LISREL model consists of a set of linear structural equations. Variables in the equation system may be either directly observed variables or unmeasured latent (theoretical) variables that are not observed but relate to observed variables. The model assumes that there is a "causal" structure among a set of latent variables, and that the observed variables are indicators or symptoms of the latent variables. Sometimes the latent variables appear as linear composites of observed variables, at others they are intervening variables in a "causal chain." The LISREL methodology is particularly designed to accommodate models that include latent variables, measurement errors, and reciprocal causation.

In addition, LISREL covers a wide range of models useful in the social and behavioral sciences, including confirmatory factor analysis, path analysis, econometric models for time series data, recursive and non-recursive models for cross-sectional and longitudinal data, and covariance structure models.

The basic LISREL model was introduced by Jöreskog (1973). Other descriptions of it are given by Jöreskog (1977, 1978, 1981). A more recent and complete description of it is found in Jöreskog and Sörbom (1989), which also contains a large bibliography of LISREL-related literature. The LISREL model defined in this chapter is the one introduced in LISREL 8 (Jöreskog and Sörbom, 1992), which includes a small extension of the LISREL 7 model defined in Jöreskog and Sörbom (1989).

6.2   The LISREL Model

In most applications of LISREL, including those of this book, there is no interest in mean values of latent variables and intercept terms in the equations. We shall therefore assume that all variables, observed as well as latent, are measured in deviations from their means. The LISREL model may then be defined as follows.

Consider random vectors $\eta' = (\eta_1, \eta_2, \ldots, \eta_m)$ and $\xi' = (\xi_1, \xi_2, \ldots, \xi_n)$ of latent dependent and independent variables, respectively, and the following system of linear structural relations

$$\eta = \mathbf{B}\eta + \mathbf{\Gamma}\xi + \zeta, \tag{6.1}$$

where $\mathbf{B}(m \times m)$ and $\mathbf{\Gamma}(m \times n)$ are coefficient matrices and $\zeta' = (\zeta_1, \zeta_2, \ldots, \zeta_m)$ is a random vector of residuals (errors in equations, random disturbance terms). The elements of $\mathbf{B}$ represent direct effects of η-variables on other η-variables and the elements of $\mathbf{\Gamma}$ represent direct effects of ξ-variables on η-variables. It is assumed that ζ is uncorrelated with ξ and that $\mathbf{I}$ - $\mathbf{B}$ is non-singular.

Vectors η and ξ are not observed, but instead vectors $\mathbf{y}' = (y_1, y_2, \ldots, y_p)$ and $\mathbf{x}' = (x_1, x_2, \ldots, x_q)$ are observed, such that

$$\mathbf{y} = \mathbf{\Lambda}_y\eta + \epsilon, \tag{6.2}$$

and

$$\mathbf{x} = \mathbf{\Lambda}_x\xi + \delta, \tag{6.3}$$

where ϵ and δ are vectors of error terms (errors of measurement or measure-specific components). These equations represent the multivariate regressions of $\mathbf{y}$ on η and of $\mathbf{x}$ on ξ, respectively. It is convenient to refer to $\mathbf{y}$ and $\mathbf{x}$ as the observed variables and η and ξ as the latent variables.

In summary, the full LISREL model is defined by the three equations,

Structural Equation Model: $\eta = \mathbf{B}\eta + \mathbf{\Gamma}\xi + \zeta$
Measurement Model for y : $\mathbf{y} = \mathbf{\Lambda}_y\eta + \epsilon$
Measurement Model for x : $\mathbf{x} = \mathbf{\Lambda}_x\xi + \delta$

with the assumptions,

1. ζ is uncorrelated with ξ

2. ϵ is uncorrelated with η

3. δ is uncorrelated with ξ

4. ζ is uncorrelated with ϵ and δ

5. $\mathbf{I} - \mathbf{B}$ is non-singular.

Let $\mathbf{\Phi}(n \times n)$ and $\mathbf{\Psi}(m \times m)$ be the covariance matrices of ξ and ζ, respectively, let $\mathbf{\Theta}_\epsilon(p \times p)$ and $\mathbf{\Theta}_\delta(q \times q)$ be the covariance matrices of ϵ and δ, respectively, and let $\mathbf{\Theta}_{\delta\epsilon}(q \times p)$ be the covariance matrix between δ and ϵ. Then, using the assumptions listed above, the expected covariance matrix $\mathbf{\Sigma}[(p + q) \times (p + q)]$ of $(\mathbf{y}', \mathbf{x}')'$ may be obtained in the following manner.

The system of linear equations shown in Eq. 6.1 may be rearranged to get η on the lefthand side of the equation

$$\eta - \mathbf{B}\eta = \mathbf{\Gamma}\xi + \zeta,$$

which can be written as

$$(\mathbf{I} - \mathbf{B})\eta = \mathbf{\Gamma}\xi + \zeta.$$

Premultiplying both sides by $(\mathbf{I} - \mathbf{B})^{-1}$ gives

$$(\mathbf{I} - \mathbf{B})^{-1}(\mathbf{I} - \mathbf{B})\eta = (\mathbf{I} - \mathbf{B})^{-1}(\mathbf{\Gamma}\xi + \zeta),$$

which, since $\mathbf{X}^{-1}\mathbf{X} = \mathbf{I}$ by definition of an inverse matrix, simplifies to

$$\eta = (\mathbf{I} - \mathbf{B})^{-1}(\mathbf{\Gamma}\xi + \zeta).$$

The expected covariance matrix of the ξ variables is given by $\mathbf{\Phi}$, since $\mathcal{E}(\xi\xi') = \mathbf{\Phi}$, by definition. To derive the expected covariance matrix of the η variables, recall that this is given by $\mathcal{E}(\eta\eta')$ and, by substitution

$$\mathcal{E}(\eta\eta') = \mathcal{E}[(\mathbf{I} - \mathbf{B})^{-1}(\mathbf{\Gamma}\xi + \zeta)((\mathbf{I} - \mathbf{B})^{-1}(\mathbf{\Gamma}\xi + \zeta))'].$$

Using two properties of the transpose operation, namely $(\mathbf{A} + \mathbf{B})' = \mathbf{A}' + \mathbf{B}'$, and $(\mathbf{CD})' = \mathbf{D}'\mathbf{C}'$, this simplifies to

$$\mathcal{E}(\eta\eta') = \mathcal{E}[(\mathbf{I} - \mathbf{B})^{-1}(\mathbf{\Gamma}\xi + \zeta)(\xi'\mathbf{\Gamma}' + \zeta')(\mathbf{I} - \mathbf{B})^{-1'}].$$

Remembering from elementary statistics that $\mathcal{E}(k \cdot g(x)) = k \cdot \mathcal{E}(g(x))$, and $\mathcal{E}(g(x) + h(y)) = \mathcal{E}(g(x)) + \mathcal{E}(h(y))$, this further reduces to

$$\mathcal{E}(\eta\eta') = (\mathbf{I} - \mathbf{B})^{-1}[\mathcal{E}(\mathbf{\Gamma}\xi\xi'\mathbf{\Gamma}') + \mathcal{E}(\mathbf{\Gamma}\xi\zeta') + \mathcal{E}(\zeta\xi'\mathbf{\Gamma}') + \mathcal{E}(\zeta\zeta')](\mathbf{I} - \mathbf{B})^{-1'}$$

which, since $\mathcal{E}(\boldsymbol{\xi}\boldsymbol{\xi}') = \boldsymbol{\Phi}$, $\mathcal{E}(\boldsymbol{\zeta}\boldsymbol{\zeta}') = \boldsymbol{\Psi}$, and $\mathcal{E}(\boldsymbol{\xi}\boldsymbol{\zeta}') = \mathcal{E}(\boldsymbol{\zeta}'\,\boldsymbol{\xi}) = \mathbf{0}$, by definition, simplifies to

$$\mathcal{E}(\boldsymbol{\eta}\boldsymbol{\eta}') = (\mathbf{I} - \mathbf{B})^{-1}(\boldsymbol{\Gamma}\boldsymbol{\Phi}\boldsymbol{\Gamma}' + \boldsymbol{\Psi})(\mathbf{I} - \mathbf{B})^{-1'}.$$

This expression gives us the expected covariance matrix for the dependent variables.

In similar fashion, we can derive the expected covariances of the independent $\boldsymbol{\xi}$ variables with the dependent $\boldsymbol{\eta}$ variables,

$$
\begin{aligned}
\mathcal{E}(\boldsymbol{\xi}\boldsymbol{\eta}') &= \mathcal{E}[\boldsymbol{\xi}((\mathbf{I} - \mathbf{B})^{-1}(\boldsymbol{\Gamma}\boldsymbol{\xi} + \boldsymbol{\zeta}))'] \\
&= \boldsymbol{\Phi}\boldsymbol{\Gamma}'(\mathbf{I} - \mathbf{B})^{-1'}.
\end{aligned}
$$

Incorporating the measurement models for the x- and y-variables from equations 6.2 and 6.3 yields the expected covariance matrix

$$\boldsymbol{\Sigma} = \begin{pmatrix} \boldsymbol{\Lambda}_y \mathbf{A}(\boldsymbol{\Gamma}\boldsymbol{\Phi}\boldsymbol{\Gamma}' + \boldsymbol{\Psi})\mathbf{A}'\boldsymbol{\Lambda}_y' + \boldsymbol{\Theta}_\epsilon & \boldsymbol{\Lambda}_y \mathbf{A}\boldsymbol{\Gamma}\boldsymbol{\Phi}\boldsymbol{\Lambda}_x' + \boldsymbol{\Theta}_{\delta\epsilon}' \\ \boldsymbol{\Lambda}_x \boldsymbol{\Phi}\boldsymbol{\Gamma}'\mathbf{A}'\boldsymbol{\Lambda}_y' + \boldsymbol{\Theta}_{\delta\epsilon} & \boldsymbol{\Lambda}_x \boldsymbol{\Phi}\boldsymbol{\Lambda}_x' + \boldsymbol{\Theta}_\delta \end{pmatrix}, \qquad (6.4)$$

where $\mathbf{A} = (\mathbf{I} - \mathbf{B})^{-1}$.

The elements of $\boldsymbol{\Sigma}$ are functions of the elements of $\boldsymbol{\Lambda}_y$, $\boldsymbol{\Lambda}_x$, $\mathbf{B}$, $\boldsymbol{\Gamma}$, $\boldsymbol{\Phi}$, $\boldsymbol{\Psi}$, $\boldsymbol{\Theta}_\epsilon$, $\boldsymbol{\Theta}_\delta$, and $\boldsymbol{\Theta}_{\delta\epsilon}$. In applications, some of these elements are fixed and equal to assigned values. In particular, this is so for elements of $\boldsymbol{\Lambda}_y$, $\boldsymbol{\Lambda}_x$, $\mathbf{B}$, and $\boldsymbol{\Gamma}$, but it is possible to have fixed values in the other matrices also. For the remaining non-fixed elements, one or more subsets may have identical but unknown values. Thus, the elements in $\boldsymbol{\Lambda}_y$, $\boldsymbol{\Lambda}_x$, $\mathbf{B}$, $\boldsymbol{\Gamma}$, $\boldsymbol{\Phi}$, $\boldsymbol{\Psi}$, $\boldsymbol{\Theta}_\epsilon$, $\boldsymbol{\Theta}_\delta$, and $\boldsymbol{\Theta}_{\delta\epsilon}$ are of three kinds:

- *fixed parameters* that have been assigned specified values,

- *constrained parameters* that are unknown but equal to one or more other parameters, and

- *free parameters* that are unknown and not constrained to be equal to any other parameter.

With LISREL 8 it is also possible to specify that any element in the parameter matrices be a linear or nonlinear function of free parameters, see Jöreskog and Sörbom (1992) for a complete description, and Chapter 16 of this text for a genetic example.

6.3   Path Diagrams

In presenting and discussing a LISREL model it is often useful to draw a path diagram. The path diagram effectively communicates the basic conceptual ideas of the model. However, the path diagram can do more than that, as shown in the preceding chapter. If the path diagram is drawn correctly and includes sufficient

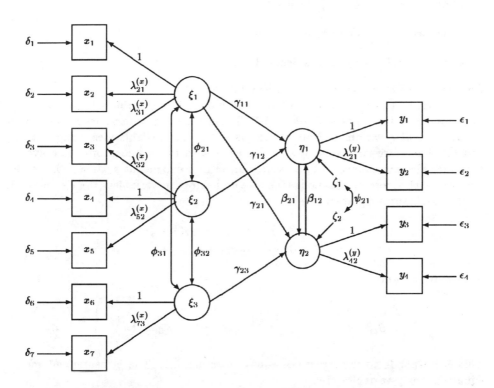

Figure 6.1: Path diagram for hypothetical model.

detail, it can represent exactly the corresponding algebraic equations of the model and the assumptions about the error terms in these equations.

We use an hypothetical model to illustrate the general LISREL model and its basic ingredients. The path diagram for this hypothetical model is given in Figure 6.1. If tracing rules are followed in the path diagram, it is possible to derive the model equations from the path diagram and to derive the LISREL parameter matrices.

In LISREL, coefficients are associated to each arrow as follows:

- An arrow from ξ_i to x_b is denoted $\lambda_{bi}^{(x)}$

- An arrow from η_g to y_a is denoted $\lambda_{ag}^{(y)}$

- An arrow from η_h to η_g is denoted β_{gh}

- An arrow from ξ_i to η_g is denoted γ_{gi}

- An arrow from ξ_j to ξ_i is denoted ϕ_{ij}

- An arrow from ζ_h to ζ_g is denoted ψ_{gh}

- An arrow from δ_b to δ_a is denoted $\theta_{ab}^{(\delta)}$

- An arrow from ϵ_d to ϵ_c is denoted $\theta_{cd}^{(\epsilon)}$

The last four arrows are always two-way arrows.

Following the tracing rules outlined in Chapter 5, we can now write the equations for the path diagram in Figure 6.1. There are seven x-variables as indicators of three latent ξ-variables. Note that x_3 is a complex variable measuring both ξ_1 and ξ_2. There are two latent η-variables each with two y-indicators. The five latent variables are connected in a two-equation interdependent system. The model involves both errors in equations (the ζ's) and errors in variables (the ϵ's and δ's).

The structural equations are

$$\eta_1 = \beta_{12}\eta_2 + \gamma_{11}\xi_1 + \gamma_{12}\xi_2 + \zeta_1$$
$$\eta_2 = \beta_{21}\eta_1 + \gamma_{21}\xi_1 + \gamma_{23}\xi_3 + \zeta_2$$

or in matrix form

$$\begin{pmatrix} \eta_1 \\ \eta_2 \end{pmatrix} = \begin{pmatrix} 0 & \beta_{12} \\ \beta_{21} & 0 \end{pmatrix} \begin{pmatrix} \eta_1 \\ \eta_2 \end{pmatrix} + \begin{pmatrix} \gamma_{11} & \gamma_{12} & 0 \\ \gamma_{21} & 0 & \gamma_{23} \end{pmatrix} \begin{pmatrix} \xi_1 \\ \xi_2 \\ \xi_3 \end{pmatrix} + \begin{pmatrix} \zeta_1 \\ \zeta_2 \end{pmatrix}.$$

This corresponds to the structural equation model 6.1. The measurement model equations for y-variables are

$$y_1 = \eta_1 + \epsilon_1$$
$$y_2 = \lambda_{21}^{(y)}\eta_1 + \epsilon_2$$
$$y_3 = \eta_2 + \epsilon_3$$
$$y_4 = \lambda_{42}^{(y)}\eta_2 + \epsilon_4$$

or in matrix form

$$\begin{pmatrix} y_1 \\ y_2 \\ y_3 \\ y_4 \end{pmatrix} = \begin{pmatrix} 1 & 0 \\ \lambda_{21}^{(y)} & 0 \\ 0 & 1 \\ 0 & \lambda_{42}^{(y)} \end{pmatrix} \begin{pmatrix} \eta_1 \\ \eta_2 \end{pmatrix} + \begin{pmatrix} \epsilon_1 \\ \epsilon_2 \\ \epsilon_3 \\ \epsilon_4 \end{pmatrix}$$

and the measurement model equations for x-variables are

$$\begin{aligned}
x_1 &= \xi_1 + \delta_1 \\
x_2 &= \lambda_{21}^{(x)}\xi_1 + \delta_2 \\
x_3 &= \lambda_{31}^{(x)}\xi_1 + \lambda_{32}^{(x)}\xi_2 + \delta_3 \\
x_4 &= \xi_2 + \delta_4 \\
x_5 &= \lambda_{52}^{(x)}\xi_2 + \delta_5 \\
x_6 &= \xi_3 + \delta_6 \\
x_7 &= \lambda_{73}^{(x)}\xi_3 + \delta_7
\end{aligned}$$

or in matrix form

$$\begin{pmatrix} x_1 \\ x_2 \\ x_3 \\ x_4 \\ x_5 \\ x_6 \\ x_7 \end{pmatrix} = \begin{pmatrix} 1 & 0 & 0 \\ \lambda_{21}^{(x)} & 0 & 0 \\ \lambda_{31}^{(x)} & \lambda_{32}^{(x)} & 0 \\ 0 & 1 & 0 \\ 0 & \lambda_{52}^{(x)} & 0 \\ 0 & 0 & 1 \\ 0 & 0 & \lambda_{73}^{(x)} \end{pmatrix} \begin{pmatrix} \xi_1 \\ \xi_2 \\ \xi_3 \end{pmatrix} + \begin{pmatrix} \delta_1 \\ \delta_2 \\ \delta_3 \\ \delta_4 \\ \delta_5 \\ \delta_6 \\ \delta_7 \end{pmatrix}$$

These equations correspond to 6.2 and 6.3, respectively.

One λ in each column of Λ_y and Λ_x has been set equal to 1 to fix the scales of measurement in the latent variables.

In these equations, note that the second subscript on each coefficient is always equal to the subscript of the variable that follows the coefficient. This can serve as a check that everything is correct. Furthermore, in the matrices B, Γ, Λ_y, and Λ_x, subscripts on each coefficient, which were originally defined in the path diagram, now correspond to the row and column of the matrix in which they appear. Also note that arrows which are not included in the path diagram correspond to zeros in these matrices.

Each of the parameter matrices contains fixed elements (the zeros and ones) and free parameters (the coefficients with two subscripts).

The four remaining parameter matrices are the symmetric matrices

$$\Phi = \begin{pmatrix} \phi_{11} & & \\ \phi_{21} & \phi_{22} & \\ \phi_{31} & \phi_{32} & \phi_{33} \end{pmatrix},$$

the covariance matrix of ξ,

$$\Psi = \begin{pmatrix} \psi_{11} & \\ \psi_{21} & \psi_{22} \end{pmatrix},$$

Table 6.1: Parameter Matrices in LISREL: Their Possible Forms and Default Values

Name	Math Symbol	LISREL Name	Order	Possible Forms	Def. Form	Def. Mode
LAMBDA-Y	Λ_y	LY	NY×NE	ID,IZ,ZI,DI,FU	FU	FI
LAMBDA-X	Λ_x	LX	NX×NK	ID,IZ,ZI,DI,FU	FU	FI
BETA	$\mathbf{B}$	BE	NE×NE	ZE,SD,FU	ZE	FI
GAMMA	Γ	GA	NE×NK	ID,IZ,ZI,DI,FU	FU	FR
PHI	Φ	PH	NK×NK	ID,DI,SY,ST	SY	FR
PSI	Ψ	PS	NE×NE	ZE,DI,SY	SY	FR
THETA-EPSILON	Θ_ϵ	TE	NY×NY	ZE,DI,SY	DI	FR
THETA-DELTA	Θ_δ	TD	NX×NX	ZE,DI,SY	DI	FR
THETA-DELTA-EPSILON	$\Theta_{\delta\epsilon}$	TH	NX×NY	ZE[1]	ZE	FI

[1] Any element of $\Theta_{\delta\epsilon}$ may be declared free

the covariance matrix of ζ, and the diagonal matrices

$$\Theta_\epsilon = \text{diag}(\theta_{11}^{(\epsilon)}, \theta_{22}^{(\epsilon)}, \ldots, \theta_{44}^{(\epsilon)}) ,$$

the covariance matrix of ϵ and

$$\Theta_\delta = \text{diag}(\theta_{11}^{(\delta)}, \theta_{22}^{(\delta)}, \ldots, \theta_{77}^{(\delta)}) ,$$

the covariance matrix of δ.

6.3.1 Default Values for Parameter Matrices

There are nine parameter matrices in LISREL: $\Lambda_y, \Lambda_x, \mathbf{B}, \Gamma, \Phi, \Psi, \Theta_\epsilon, \Theta_{\delta\epsilon}$ and Θ_δ. The LISREL names for these parameter matrices, their possible forms and default values are given in Table 6.1.

One can make any number of specifications of the form

    MN = AA,BB

where MN is a matrix name (column 3), AA is a matrix form (column 5) and BB is FR (free) or FI (fixed) (column 7). Either AA or BB may be omitted in which case the defaults of Table 6.1 are used. The order of AA and BB is immaterial so that the above specification can also be written MN=BB,AA.

The meanings of the possible form values are as follows:

- ZE = **0** (zero matrix)

- ID = **I** (identity matrix)

- IZ =(**I** **0**) or $\begin{pmatrix} \mathbf{I} \\ \mathbf{0} \end{pmatrix}$ (partitioned identity and zero)

- ZI = (**0** **I**) or $\begin{pmatrix} \mathbf{0} \\ \mathbf{I} \end{pmatrix}$ (partitioned zero and identity)

- DI = a diagonal matrix

- SD = a full square matrix with fixed zeros in and above the diagonal and all elements under the diagonal free (refers to **B** only)

- SY = a symmetric matrix which is not diagonal

- ST = a symmetric matrix with fixed ones in the diagonal (a correlation matrix)

- FU = a rectangular or square non-symmetric matrix.

The eight parameter matrices are stored in the order Λ_y, Λ_x, **B**, Γ, Φ, Ψ, Θ_ϵ, $\Theta_{\delta\epsilon}$, Θ_δ, and within each matrix, elements are ordered row-wise. Only the lower triangular parts of the symmetric matrices Φ, Ψ, Θ_ϵ, and Θ_δ are stored in memory. Matrices which are specified to be **I** (ID) or **0** (ZE) are not stored in memory.

6.4 Submodels

The general LISREL model involves four kinds of variables in addition to the error variables ζ, ϵ, and δ; namely y-variables, x-variables, η-variables and ξ-variables. The notation for the number of each of these is given in Table 6.2.

Table 6.2: Notation for Number of Variables

	Mathematical Notation	LISREL Notation
Number of y-variables	p	NY
Number of x-variables	q	NX
Number of η-variables	m	NE
Number of ξ-variables	n	NK

The general model subsumes many models as special cases. A submodel will be obtained when one or more of NY, NX, NE and NK are zero or are not specified.

This means that one or more of the four types of variables are not included in the model. Thus each submodel involves only some of the eight parameter matrices. The default values for NY, NX, NE, and NK have been chosen so as to be able to specify the most common submodels with a minimum of input. A researcher who is only interested in a particular submodel needs only be concerned with a subset of the eight parameter matrices and does not have to understand the full model.

A summary of the different submodels is given in Table 6.3.

Table 6.3: Submodels in LISREL

Type	Specified	Default	Model	Parameters
1	NX,NK	NY,NE	$x = \Lambda_x \xi + \delta$	$\Lambda_x, \Phi, \Theta_\delta$
2	NY,NX	NE,NK	$y = By + \Gamma x + \zeta$	B, Γ, Ψ
3A	NY,NE,NK	NX	$y = \Lambda_y A(\Gamma \xi + \zeta) + \epsilon$	$\Lambda_y, B, \Gamma, \Phi, \Psi, \Theta_\epsilon$
3B	NY,NE	NX,NK	$y = \Lambda_y A\zeta + \epsilon$	$\Lambda_y, B, \Psi, \Theta_\epsilon$

Note: $A = (I - B)^{-1}$.

The common types of submodels are as follows.

6.4.1   Submodel 1: only x- and ξ-variables

When only NX and NK are specified, the program assumes the model

$$x = \Lambda_x \xi + \delta \qquad (6.5)$$

i.e., a measurement model or a factor analysis model for x-variables. In this case there is no structural equation model of the form 6.1 and there are no y-variables or η-variables and consequently no measurement model of the form 6.2. Only one of the three equations 6.1, 6.2, and 6.3, namely 6.3, is in operation. The only parameter matrices included in this submodel are Λ_x, Φ, and Θ_δ. The implied covariance matrix under this model is

$$\Sigma = \Lambda_x \Phi \Lambda_x' + \Theta_\delta .$$

6.4.2   Submodel 2: only y- and x-variables

When only NY and NX are specified, the program assumes the model

$$y = By + \Gamma x + \zeta \qquad (6.6)$$

i.e., a structural equation model or a path analysis model for directly observed variables. If, in addition, $B = 0$, one can have multivariate or univariate regression models and other forms of the multivariate general linear model. Technically, when NE and NK are not specified, the program sets $NE = NY$, $NK = NX$, $\Lambda_y = I$, $\Lambda_x = I$, $\Theta_\epsilon = 0$, $\Theta_\delta = 0$ and $\Phi = S_{xx}$. The only matrices involved in this submodel are B, Γ, Φ, and Ψ. The implied covariance matrix is

$$\Sigma = (I - B)^{-1}(\Gamma \Phi \Gamma' + \Psi)(I - B')^{-1} .$$

6.4.3   Submodel 3A: only y-, η-, and ξ-variables

When only NY, NE, and NK are specified, the program assumes the model

$$\eta = B\eta + \Gamma\xi + \zeta \tag{6.7}$$

$$y = \Lambda_y \eta + \epsilon \tag{6.8}$$

or equivalently,

$$y = \Lambda_y(I - B)^{-1}(\Gamma\xi + \zeta) + \epsilon . \tag{6.9}$$

Note that the model can have ξ-variables even when there are no x-variables.

   This submodel involves the parameter matrices Λ_y, B, Γ, Φ, Ψ, and Θ_ϵ and the implied covariance matrix is

$$\Sigma = \Lambda_y(I - B)^{-1}(\Gamma \Phi \Gamma' + \Psi)(I - B')^{-1}\Lambda_y' + \Theta_\epsilon.$$

When $B = 0$, Eq. 6.9 becomes

$$y = \Lambda_y(\Gamma\xi + \zeta) + \epsilon , \tag{6.10}$$

with parameter matrices: Λ_y, Γ, Φ, Ψ, and Θ_ϵ and covariance matrix

$$\Sigma = \Lambda_y(\Gamma \Phi \Gamma' + \Psi)\Lambda_y' + \Theta_\epsilon .$$

This is a second-order factor analysis model for y-variables with first-order factor loadings given by Λ_y and second-order factor loadings given by Γ.

6.4.4   Submodel 3B: only y- and η-variables

When only NY and NE are specified, the program assumes the model

$$y = \Lambda_y \eta + \epsilon \tag{6.11}$$

$$\eta = B\eta + \zeta \tag{6.12}$$

or equivalently

$$y = \Lambda_y(I - B)^{-1}\zeta + \epsilon , \tag{6.13}$$

with implied covariance matrix

$$\Sigma = \Lambda_y(I - B)^{-1}\Psi(I - B')^{-1}\Lambda_y' + \Theta_\epsilon .$$

This is just the special case of submodel 3A without ξ-variables. In this case the parameter matrices are Λ_y, B, Ψ, and Θ_ϵ. When $B = 0$, this model reduces to

$$y = \Lambda_y \zeta + \epsilon \qquad (6.14)$$

with parameter matrices Λ_y, Ψ, and Θ_ϵ, and covariance matrix

$$\Sigma = \Lambda_y \Psi \Lambda_y' + \Theta_\epsilon \, .$$

This, of course, is a factor analysis model for a set of y-variables, in which the matrix Ψ plays the role of a factor covariance or correlation matrix. To analyze a factor analysis model, one can use either model 6.5 or model 6.14 but because Φ may be specified to be a correlation matrix, it is slightly more convenient to use model 6.5.

6.5   Twin Model Example

In the simplest type of twin design, the observed phenotypes P_1 and P_2 of twin 1 and twin 2 in a twin pair are postulated to depend on additive genes A_1 and A_2, common environments C_1 and C_2, and unique environments E_1 and E_2. A path diagram is shown in Figure 6.2; this is an equivalent representation to that shown in the previous chapter, Figure 5.4b, in the absence of dominance effects.

This model may be represented in various ways in LISREL. For example we may use submodel 1 and treat A_1, C_1, C_2, and A_2 as ξ-variables and E_1 and E_2 as δ-variables. Assuming that all these variables are standardized, the three parameter matrices Λ_x, Φ, and Θ_δ are specified as

$$\Lambda_x = \begin{pmatrix} a & c & 0 & 0 \\ 0 & 0 & c & a \end{pmatrix}$$

$$\Phi = \begin{pmatrix} 1 & & & \\ 0 & 1 & & \\ 0 & 1 & 1 & \\ x & 0 & 0 & 1 \end{pmatrix}$$

$$\Theta_\delta = \mathrm{diag}(e^2, e^2) \, ,$$

where $x = 1$ for monozygotic twins and $x = \frac{1}{2}$ for dizygotic twins, corresponding to the degree of genetic relatedness.

Alternatively, we may include E_1 and E_2 among the ξ-variables and let δ be zero. Let $\xi' = (A_1, C_1, C_2, A_2, E_1, E_2)$. Then we need only be concerned with two parameter matrices, namely

$$\Lambda_x = \begin{pmatrix} a & c & 0 & 0 & e & 0 \\ 0 & 0 & c & a & 0 & e \end{pmatrix} \, ,$$

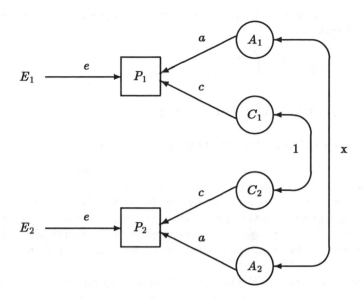

Figure 6.2: Simple twin model with additive genes, common and unique environments.

$$\Phi = \begin{pmatrix} 1 & & & & & \\ 0 & 1 & & & & \\ 0 & 1 & 1 & & & \\ x & 0 & 0 & 1 & & \\ 0 & 0 & 0 & 0 & 1 & \\ 0 & 0 & 0 & 0 & 0 & 1 \end{pmatrix}.$$

Similarly, we may treat the model as a submodel 3a with $\Lambda_y = I$, $B = 0$, $\Psi = 0$, $\Theta_\epsilon = 0$,

$$\Gamma = \begin{pmatrix} a & c & 0 & 0 & e & 0 \\ 0 & 0 & c & a & 0 & e \end{pmatrix},$$

$$\Phi = \begin{pmatrix} 1 & & & & & \\ 0 & 1 & & & & \\ 0 & 1 & 1 & & & \\ x & 0 & 0 & 1 & & \\ 0 & 0 & 0 & 0 & 1 & \\ 0 & 0 & 0 & 0 & 0 & 1 \end{pmatrix}.$$

Still another way to represent the model as a submodel 3a is to let $\Lambda_y = I$, $B = 0$, $\Gamma = I$,

$$\Phi = \begin{pmatrix} a^2 & \\ xa^2 & a^2 \end{pmatrix}, \Psi = \begin{pmatrix} c^2 & \\ c^2 & c^2 \end{pmatrix}, \Theta_\epsilon = \begin{pmatrix} e^2 & \\ e^2 & e^2 \end{pmatrix}.$$

In all these specifications of the same model, the implied covariance matrix of the observed phenotypes is

$$\Sigma = \left(\begin{array}{cc} a^2 + c^2 + e^2 & \\ xa^2 + c^2 + e^2 & a^2 + c^2 + e^2 \end{array} \right) .$$

6.6   Practical Model Fitting

6.6.1   Estimating Parameters of the Model

The term covariance matrix is used here in the general sense of a moment matrix, which may be a matrix of moments about zero, a matrix of variances and covariances, or a matrix of correlations. In the following, the matrix to be analyzed is denoted **S** regardless of the type of moment matrix. Here we assume that the mean vector is unconstrained, so the estimation is essentially that of fitting the covariance matrix Σ in equation 6.4 implied by the model to the sample covariance matrix **S**.

LISREL can obtain seven kinds of estimates of parameters:

- Instrumental Variables (IV)

- Two-Stage Least Squares (TSLS)

- Unweighted Least Squares (ULS)

- Generalized Least Squares (GLS)

- Maximum Likelihood (ML)

- Generally Weighted Least Squares (WLS)

- Diagonally Weighted Least Squares (DWLS)

Under general assumptions, all seven methods give consistent estimates of parameters. This means that they will be close to the true parameter values in large samples (assuming, of course, that the model is correct). The seven types of estimates differ in several respects. The TSLS and IV methods are procedures which are non-iterative and very fast. The ULS, GLS, ML, WLS, and DWLS estimates are obtained by means of an iterative procedure which minimizes a particular fit function by successively improving the parameter estimates. Initial values for the iterative procedures are provided by IV or TSLS. Because NK > NX and/or NE > NY in the type of applications considered in this book, IV and TSLS does not work (see Jöreskog and Sörbom, 1989, pp. 25 - 27). In these applications, initial values are either obtained by ULS or provided by the user. Here we describe briefly the fit functions available in LISREL; we give a more complete description of these functions in the next chapter.

Specific Fit Functions

The "classical" methods are ULS, GLS and ML. The fit function for ULS is

$$F = \frac{1}{2}tr[(\mathbf{S} - \mathbf{\Sigma})^2] \,, \tag{6.15}$$

i.e., half the sum of squares of all the elements of the matrix $\mathbf{S} - \mathbf{\Sigma}$.

The fit function for GLS,

$$F = \frac{1}{2}tr[(\mathbf{I} - \mathbf{S}^{-1}\mathbf{\Sigma})^2] \,, \tag{6.16}$$

uses sums of squares weighted by the inverse of the sample covariance matrix $\mathbf{S}$.

Finally, ML minimizes the function

$$F = \log|\mathbf{\Sigma}| + tr(\mathbf{S}\mathbf{\Sigma}^{-1}) - \log|\mathbf{S}| - (p + q) \,, \tag{6.17}$$

where, for a square matrix $\mathbf{A}$, $|\mathbf{A}|$ denotes the determinant of $\mathbf{A}$ and $tr(\mathbf{A})$ denotes the sum of the diagonal elements of $\mathbf{A}$. Each of the three equations represents a function of the independent parameters θ, i.e., the free and constrained elements in $\mathbf{\Lambda}_y$, $\mathbf{\Lambda}_x$, $\mathbf{B}$, $\mathbf{\Gamma}$, $\mathbf{\Phi}$, $\mathbf{\Psi}$, $\mathbf{\Theta}_\epsilon$, $\mathbf{\Theta}_{\delta\epsilon}$, and $\mathbf{\Theta}_\delta$, and is minimized with respect to these. The fit functions are always non-negative; they are equal to zero only when there is a perfect fit, in which case the fitted $\mathbf{\Sigma}$ equals $\mathbf{S}$.

The fit function for ULS is justified when all variables are measured in the same units. The fit function for ML is derived from the maximum likelihood principle based on the assumption that the observed variables have a multinormal distribution (see, e.g., Jöreskog, 1967). The GLS estimator is a straightforward application of Aitken's (1934) generalized least-squares principle (cf. Jöreskog and Goldberger, 1972, and Browne, 1974). GLS and ML estimates have similar asymptotic properties. Under the assumption of multivariate normality, both estimators are optimal in the sense of being most precise in large samples. LISREL provides large sample standard errors for ULS, GLS, and ML parameter estimates under normal theory. A standard error is a measure of the precision of a parameter estimate.

The fit function for ML or GLS also may be used to compute parameter estimates even if the distribution of the observed variables deviates from normality. Even standard errors and chi-squared goodness-of-fit measures may be used if interpreted with caution. ML and GLS estimates have been found to be robust against non-normality, see e.g., Monte Carlo studies by Boomsma (1983) and Harlow (1985) and theoretical studies by Browne (1987) and Anderson and Amemiya (1985). However, if the distributions deviate from normality it *may* be best to use the general WLS method with an asymptotic covariance matrix $\mathbf{W}$ produced by PRELIS (Jöreskog and Sörbom, 1988). This is particularly important if one wants asymptotically correct standard errors of parameter estimates and chi-squared goodness-of-fit measures. The WLS method should also be used when polychoric (tetrachoric) and polyserial correlations are analyzed and when product moment correlations based on normal scores are analyzed. The general family of WLS fit functions are described in greater detail in the next chapter.

Minimization and the Information Matrix

The fit function $F(\theta)$ is minimized by an iterative procedure which, starting at the initial estimates $\theta^{(1)}$, generates successively new points $\theta^{(2)}$, $\theta^{(3)}$... in the parameter space such that $F(\theta^{(s+1)}) < F(\theta^{(s)})$, until convergence is obtained. The minimization method makes use of the first-order derivatives and approximations (probability limits) to the second-order derivatives of F. For the ML and GLS methods, the approximation to the second-order derivatives is the information matrix which is nearly always positive definite if the model is identified. The information matrix is used to compute standard errors for all the parameters. The whole estimated covariance or correlation matrix of all the estimated parameters may also be obtained.

It can happen that there are several local minima of the fit function. The only way to avoid this is to have a model which is appropriate for the data and a large random sample. Experience indicates, however, that multiple solutions very seldom occur, and when they do, it is usually with solutions on the boundary of or outside the admissible parameter space.

Admissibility Test

The computer program does not in general constrain the solution to be admissible. There is, however, a built-in admissibility check which will stop the iterations after a specified number of iterations (default = 10) if the solution becomes non-admissible. The *admissibility* check is that

1. Λ_y and Λ_x have full column ranks and no rows of only zeros.
2. Φ, Ψ, Θ_ϵ, and Θ_δ are positive definite.

There are situations where one wants to have a non-admissible solution intentionally, so there are provisions to set the admissibility check off (i.e., setting AD=OFF on the OU line)[1].

6.6.2   Assessment of Fit

After the fit function has been minimized, the fit of the model to data may be assessed by means of a χ^2 measure of fit. For ML, GLS, and WLS, the χ^2-measure is $(N-1)$ times the minimum value of the fit function for the specified model. The χ^2-measure is distributed asymptotically as a chi-square distribution under certain conditions.

If the model is correct and the sample size is sufficiently large, the χ^2-measure may be derived as a likelihood ratio test statistic for testing the model against the alternative that Σ is unconstrained. The degrees of freedom for χ^2 are

$$df = \frac{1}{2}(p+q)(p+q+1) - t \,, \qquad (6.18)$$

---

[1] This is often the case in twin models. Because LISREL 7 will halt execution if the admissibility test fails, it is important to set AD=OFF on the OU card.

where $p + q$ is the number of observed variables analyzed and t is the total number of independent parameters estimated. The P-value reported by the program is the probability level of χ^2; that is, the probability of obtaining a χ^2-value larger than the value actually obtained, given that the model is correct.

Although the χ^2-measure may be viewed theoretically as a test statistic for testing the hypothesis that Σ is of the form implied by the model against the alternative that Σ is unconstrained (see Jöreskog, 1977), it should be emphasized that such a use of χ^2 is not valid in most applications. In most empirical work, the model is only tentative and is only regarded as an approximation to reality. From this point of view the statistical problem is not one of testing a given hypothesis (which a priori may be considered false), but rather one of fitting the model to the data and to decide whether the fit is adequate or not.

Instead of regarding χ^2 as a test statistic, one should regard it as a goodness (or badness)-of-fit measure in the sense that large χ^2-values correspond to bad fit and small χ^2-values to good fit. The degrees of freedom serve as a standard by which to judge whether χ^2 is large or small. The χ^2-measure is sensitive to sample size and very sensitive to departures from multivariate normality of the observed variables. Large sample sizes and departures from normality tend to increase χ^2 over and above what can be expected due to specification error in the model. One reasonable way to use χ^2-measures in comparative model fitting is to use χ^2-differences in the following way. If a value of χ^2 is obtained, which is large compared to the number of degrees of freedom, the fit may be examined and assessed by an inspection of the fitted residuals, the standardized residuals, and the modification indices. Often these quantities will suggest ways to relax the model somewhat by introducing more parameters. The new model usually yields a smaller χ^2. A large drop in χ^2, compared to the difference in degrees of freedom, indicates that the changes made in the model represent a real improvement. On the other hand, a drop in χ^2 close to the difference in number of degrees of freedom indicates that the improvement in fit is obtained by "capitalizing on chance," and the added parameters may not have real significance and meaning.

6.6.3 Tests of Hypotheses

Once the validity of a model has been reasonably well established, various structural hypotheses about the parameters $\theta(t \times 1)$ in this model may be tested. One can test hypotheses of the forms

- that certain θ's have particular values

- that certain θ's are equal

- that certain θ's are specified linear or nonlinear functions of of other parameters

Each of these two types of hypotheses leads to a model with fewer parameters ν, where ν $(u \times 1)$ is a subset of the parameters in θ, $u < t$. In conventional statistical terminology, the model with parameters ν is called the *null hypothesis* H_0 and the model with parameters θ is called the *alternative hypothesis* H_1. Let χ_0^2 and χ_1^2 be the χ^2 goodness-of-fit measures for models H_0 and H_1, respectively. The test statistic for testing H_0 against H_1 is then

$$D^2 = \chi_0^2 - \chi_1^2 \qquad (6.19)$$

which is used as χ^2 with $d = t - u$ degrees of freedom. The degrees of freedom can also be computed as the difference between the degrees of freedom associated with χ_0^2 and χ_1^2. To use the test statistic formally, one chooses a significance level α (probability of type I error) and rejects H_0 if D^2 exceeds the $(1-\alpha)$-percentile of the χ^2 distribution with d degrees of freedom.

The test statistic D^2 can only be used with GLS, ML and WLS and is valid under the following assumptions:

- with GLS and ML if the observed variables have a multivariate normal distribution and the sample covariance matrix is analyzed; with WLS if the correct weight matrix is used

- if the model H_0 is true

- if the sample size is large

The most common type of hypothesis H_0 postulates that a single parameter θ be restricted to a specified value θ_0, usually zero. The corresponding alternative hypothesis H_1 specifies θ as a free parameter in the same model. D^2 is then distributed as χ^2 with 1 degree of freedom.

6.7 Problems with Analysis of Correlation Matrices

The general rule is that the covariance matrix should be analyzed. However, in many applications, units of measurements in the observed variables have no definite meaning and are often arbitrary or irrelevant. For these reasons, for convenience, and for interpretational purposes, the correlation matrix is often analyzed as if it is a covariance matrix. This is a common practice.

The analysis of correlation matrices is problematic in several ways. As pointed out by Cudeck (1989), such an analysis may

(a) modify the model being analyzed,

(b) produce incorrect χ^2 and other goodness-of-fit measures, and

(c) give incorrect standard errors.

Problem (a) can occur when the model includes constrained parameters. For example, if $\lambda_{11}^{(x)}$ and $\lambda_{21}^{(x)}$ are constrained to be equal but the variances $\sigma_{11}^{(xx)}$ and $\sigma_{22}^{(xx)}$ are not equal, then analysis of the correlation matrix will give estimates of

$$\lambda_{11}^{(x)}/\sqrt{\sigma_{11}^{(xx)}} \text{ and } \lambda_{21}^{(x)}/\sqrt{\sigma_{22}^{(xx)}}$$

which are not equal. Correlation matrices should not be analyzed if the model contains equality constraints of this kind.

The main question is whether the standard errors and χ^2 goodness-of-fit measures produced when correlation matrices are analyzed are asymptotically correct. The exact conditions under which this is the case are extremely complicated and give little practical guidance. However, two crucial conditions are

- that the model is scale invariant (see Chapter 7 for discussion)

- that the condition

$$diag(\hat{\Sigma}) = diag(\mathbf{S}) \tag{6.20}$$

holds.

Condition 6.20 can be checked by examining the fitted residuals. For the ML method, this condition is expected to hold if the diagonal elements of Θ_ϵ and Θ_δ are free parameters and the joint covariance matrix of η and ξ is unconstrained.

To clarify the issue further, we distinguish between covariance and correlation structures. In principle, all LISREL models are covariance structures, where the variances of Σ as well as the covariances are functions of correlation structure, and the diagonal elements of Σ are constants independent of parameters. We now distinguish between four possible cases.

A A sample covariance matrix is used to estimate a covariance structure.

B A sample correlation matrix is used to estimate a covariance structure.

C A sample covariance matrix is used to estimate a correlation structure.

D A sample correlation matrix is used to estimate a correlation structure.

Case A is the standard case in LISREL. Because asymptotic variances and covariances of sample variances and covariances often tend to be of the form (6.21 below) chi-squares and standard errors can be used in most cases to evaluate the fit of the model.

Case B is a very common situation. If asymptotic variances and covariances of sample correlations are not of the form

$$\text{ACov}(s_{gh}, s_{ij}) = (1/N)(\sigma_{gi}\sigma_{hj} + \sigma_{gj}\sigma_{hi}), \tag{6.21}$$

where s_{gh} and s_{ij} are typical elements of $\mathbf{S}$, then standard normal asymptotic theory is not valid (see Chapter 7 for a detailed description of asymptotic variances/covariances). However, if the model is scale invariant and if the ML method produces estimates such that

$$diag(\hat{\mathbf{\Sigma}}) = \mathbf{I},$$

then standard errors and χ^2 goodness-of-fit measures *still may be asymptotically correct*. However, this property does not hold when such models are estimated with GLS.

In Case C, if the model is defined as a *correlation structure* $\mathbf{P}(\boldsymbol{\theta})$, with diagonal elements equal to 1 (i.e., *the diagonal elements are not functions of parameters*), it may be formulated as a covariance structure

$$\mathbf{\Sigma} = \mathbf{D}_\sigma \mathbf{P}(\boldsymbol{\theta}) \mathbf{D}_\sigma, \tag{6.22}$$

where $\mathbf{D}_\sigma$ is a diagonal matrix of population standard deviations σ_1, σ_2,..., σ_k of the observed variables, which are regarded as free parameters. The covariance structure 6.22 has parameters σ_1, σ_2,..., σ_k, θ_1, θ_2,..., θ_t. Such a model may be estimated correctly using the sample covariance matrix $\mathbf{S}$. However, the standard deviations σ_1, σ_2,..., σ_k as well as $\boldsymbol{\theta}$ must be estimated from data and the estimate of σ_i does not necessarily equal the corresponding standard deviation s_{ii} in the sample. When $\mathbf{P}(\boldsymbol{\theta})$ is estimated directly from the sample correlation matrix $\mathbf{R}$, standard errors and χ^2 goodness-of-fit values will not in general be correct.

Consider Case D. To obtain correct asymptotic standard errors in LISREL for a *correlation structure* when the matrix is analyzed, the WLS method must be used with a weight matrix $\mathbf{W}^{-1}$, where $\mathbf{W}$ is a consistent estimate of the asymptotic covariance matrix of *the correlations being analyzed*. Such a $\mathbf{W}$ may be obtained with PRELIS under non-normal theory. PRELIS can estimate such a $\mathbf{W}$ also for a correlation matrix containing polychoric and/or polyserial correlations.

The asymptotic covariance matrix $\mathbf{W}$ produced by PRELIS is a consistent estimate of the covariance matrix of

$$\mathbf{r} = (r_{21}, r_{31}, r_{32}, r_{41}, r_{42}, r_{43}, \ldots)$$

The diagonal elements of the correlation matrix *are not included* in this vector. The number of distinct elements in $\mathbf{W}$ is

$$\frac{1}{2}k(k-1)[\frac{1}{2}k(k-1)+1],$$

where $k = p + q$ is the number of observed variables in the model. In fitting a correlation structure $\mathbf{P}(\boldsymbol{\theta})$ to a correlation matrix using WLS, LISREL minimizes the fit function [cf. Chapter 7, Eq. 7.1]

$$
\begin{aligned}
F(\boldsymbol{\theta}) &= (\mathbf{r} - \boldsymbol{\rho})' \mathbf{W}^{-1} (\mathbf{r} - \boldsymbol{\rho}) \\
&= \sum_{g=2}^{k} \sum_{h=1}^{g-1} \sum_{i=2}^{k} \sum_{j=1}^{i-1} w^{gh,ij} (r_{gh} - \rho_{gh})(r_{ij} - \rho_{ij})
\end{aligned}
\tag{6.23}
$$

where
$$\rho' = (\rho_{21}(\theta), \rho_{31}(\theta), \rho_{32}(\theta), \rho_{41}(\theta), \ldots, \rho_{k,k-1}(\theta)) .$$

This approach assumes that the diagonal elements of $\mathbf{P}(\theta)$ are fixed ones and not functions of parameters.

WLS may also be used to fit ordinary LISREL models (i.e., *covariance structures*) to sample correlation matrices (Case B). This is especially useful when polychoric and polyserial correlations are analyzed. A small problem arises here because the fit function 6.23 is not a function of the diagonal elements of $\mathbf{P}(\theta)$, and, as a consequence, parameters such as the diagonal elements of Θ_ϵ and Θ_δ cannot be estimated directly. However, they can of course be estimated afterwards. For example, in Submodel 1, one can estimate Θ_δ as

$$\hat{\Theta}_\delta = \mathbf{I} - diag(\hat{\Lambda}_x \hat{\Phi} \hat{\Lambda}_x')$$

A better and more general approach is to add the term

$$\sum_{i=1}^{k} [1 - \sigma_{ii}(\theta)]^2 \tag{6.24}$$

to the fit function 6.23. The program does this automatically when the diagonal elements of Σ are functions of parameters. The advantages of this approach are:

- Estimates of all parameters can be obtained directly even when constraints are imposed

- When the diagonal elements of Θ_ϵ and Θ_δ are free parameters, the WLS solution will satisfy
$$diag(\hat{\Sigma}) = \mathbf{I} .$$

This approach can be generalized further by replacing the 1 in 6.24 by a variance s_{ii} which has been estimated or obtained separately from the correlations. Such variances can be obtained with PRELIS for ordinal variables for which the thresholds are assumed to be equal.

6.8 Multi-Sample Analysis

In this chapter the LISREL model has been described as it applies to analyze data from a single sample. However, LISREL also can be used to analyze data from several samples simultaneously according to LISREL models for each group with some or all parameters constrained to be equal over groups. In fact, all examples and analyses reported in this book are multi-sample analyses, where the samples represent different kinds of twin groups (MZ twins reared together or apart, DZ twins reared together or apart, same- or opposite-sex DZ twins, etc.).

Consider a set of G populations. It is assumed that a number of variables have been measured on a number of individuals from each population and that a LISREL model of the form 6.1, 6.2, and 6.3 holds in each group. The model for group g is defined by the parameter matrices

$$\Lambda_y^{(g)}, \ \Lambda_x^{(g)}, \ \mathbf{B}^{(g)}, \ \Gamma^{(g)}, \ \Phi^{(g)}, \ \Psi^{(g)}, \ \Theta_\epsilon^{(g)}, \ \Theta_{\delta\epsilon}^{(g)}, \ \Theta_\delta^{(g)} \ ,$$

where the superscript (g) refers to the gth group, $g = 1, 2, ..., G$. Each of these matrices may contain fixed, free, and constrained parameters as before. If there are no constraints across groups, each group can be analyzed separately. However, if there are constraints across groups, as in the case of the twin model discussed earlier, the data from all groups must be analyzed simultaneously to get fully efficient estimates of the parameters.

To estimate all the models simultaneously, LISREL minimizes the fit function

$$F = \sum_{g=1}^{G} (N_g/N) F_g(\mathbf{S}^{(g)}, \mathbf{\Sigma}^{(g)}, \mathbf{W}^{(g)}) \ , \tag{6.25}$$

where F_g is any of the fit functions defined in Section 6.6.1, i.e., ULS, GLS, ML, DWLS and WLS. Here N_g is the sample size in group g and $N = N_1 + N_2 + ... + N_G$ is the total sample size; $\mathbf{S}^{(g)}$ and $\mathbf{\Sigma}^{(g)}$ are the sample and population covariance matrices in group g, and $\mathbf{W}^{(g)}$ is the weight matrix for group g.

As before, the χ^2 goodness-of-fit measure is defined as $N-1$ times the minimum of F. This is a measure of the fit of all LISREL models in all groups, including all constraints, to the data from all groups. The degrees of freedom are

$$df = \frac{1}{2} G(p+q)(p+q+1) - t \ , \tag{6.26}$$

where t is the total number of independent parameters estimated in all groups. Thus, in a multi-sample analysis, only one χ^2 goodness-of-fit measure is given.

Chapter 7

Model Fitting Functions and Optimization

In the previous chapter we described the LISREL model and outlined the functions therein that may be used to fit a model to data. We now describe these fitting functions in greater detail, and with special emphasis on the genetic analysis of twin data. We also discuss how the fitting functions are used to generate optimal estimates of genetic parameters in the twin design. Again, understanding of these issues is not essential for the use of LISREL to fit models to data; we provide this Chapter for those readers wishing to further their knowledge of *how* LISREL does what it does, and the statistical theory behind the choice of fit functions for particular types of data.

7.1 Introduction

Testing a theory regarding the causes of human variation requires using the theory to generate a hypothesis, translating the hypothesis into explicit mathematical expressions, and fitting these expressions to observed data. Getting from theory to model is referred to as *model building*; fitting the model to the observed data is referred to as *model fitting*. It is important to realize that theory, hypotheses implied by theory, and the mathematical expressions representing the hypotheses are all prerequisites to actual model fitting. Furthermore, the acceptability of a given model depends on how well it meets four criteria (Eaves *et al.*, 1989a) . A good model should:

- fit the data
- be consistent
- be simple

131

- have parameters that are statistically significant

An ill-fitting model implies that the theory which generated the model is wrong or requires modification. Consistency means that the model does not violate theoretical constraints. For example, a model that predicts genetic dominance variation in the absence of additive genetic variation is extremely unlikely (see Falconer, 1990, Figure 8.1). Simple models are to be preferred to complex models because they are easier to falsify and they are more informative. Finally, the parameters in the model must be statistically significant. A parameter that does not deviate significantly from zero should be removed from the model and this in turn should have consequences for the theory.

Considering these criteria, we note that the results from model fitting should "feedback" to the theory and the activity of model building. We discussed the relationship between model fitting and model building in some detail in Section 1.3 of Chapter 1, particularly Figure 1.6. The interpretation of model failure (or success) is part of the elaboration/decision process that leads to new theories.

7.2 Fitting Models to Data

The minimal requirements for model fitting include a hypothesis upon which to base the model and observed data to test the model. In genetic covariance structure analysis, hypotheses concern the genetic and environmental contributions to phenotypic variance and covariance. For example, one may suppose that individual differences in some continuously varying character, P, are due to additive genetic (G) and unshared environmental influences (E). We translate this hypothesis into the simple model for subject i:

$$P_i = aG_i + eE_i$$

where P_i, G_i, and E_i all represent deviation scores or measurements from the mean values; that is, the means of these variables are zero. The symbols a and e represent the regression coefficients of the phenotype P on the standardized variables G and E. This model implies the following decomposition of the phenotypic variance:

$$
\begin{aligned}
\text{var}(P) &= a^2\text{var}(G) + e^2\text{var}(E) \\
&= a^2 \times 1 + e^2 \times 1 \\
&= a^2 + e^2 ,
\end{aligned}
$$

if $\text{var}(G) = \text{var}(E) = 1$.

To test this model, one collects measurements of the phenotype in a representative sample according to some research design which, under given assumptions, enables one to identify (i.e., uniquely estimate) the regression coefficients a and e. In the twin method, for example, one obtains data from representative samples of

MZ and DZ twins (e.g. Falconer, 1990, Chapter 10). The measurements obtained in these samples are summarized in covariance matrices S_{MZ} and S_{DZ}:

$$S_{\text{MZ}} = \begin{pmatrix} \text{var}(P_{\text{MZ1}}) & \\ \text{cov}(P_{\text{MZ1}}, P_{\text{MZ2}}) & \text{var}(P_{\text{MZ2}}) \end{pmatrix}$$

$$S_{\text{DZ}} = \begin{pmatrix} \text{var}(P_{\text{DZ1}}) & \\ \text{cov}(P_{\text{DZ1}}, P_{\text{DZ2}}) & \text{var}(P_{\text{DZ2}}) \end{pmatrix}$$

For each of the elements in these covariance matrices, we can write a mathematical expression in which the observed statistics, the covariance and variances, are related to a number of known and unknown parameters. The parameters are collected in the vector Θ, which can be partitioned into a vector of known (fixed) parameters, Θ_{fi}, and a vector of unknown (free) parameters, Θ_{fr}. Thus, $\Theta = (\Theta'_{fi}, \Theta'_{fr})$. The expected covariances, Σ_{MZ} and Σ_{DZ}, are functions of these parameters:

$$\Sigma_{\text{MZ}} = \begin{pmatrix} a^2\text{var}(G) + e^2\text{var}(E) & \\ a^2\text{var}(G) & a^2\text{var}(G) + e^2\text{var}(E) \end{pmatrix}$$

$$= \begin{pmatrix} a^2 + e^2 & \\ a^2 & a^2 + e^2 \end{pmatrix}$$

and

$$\Sigma_{\text{DZ}} = \begin{pmatrix} a^2\text{var}(G) + e^2\text{var}(E) & \\ .5a^2\text{var}(G) & a^2\text{var}(G) + e^2\text{var}(E) \end{pmatrix}$$

$$= \begin{pmatrix} a^2 + e^2 & \\ .5a^2 & a^2 + e^2 \end{pmatrix}$$

so we have $\Theta' = (\Theta'_{fi}, \Theta'_{fr})$, where

$$\Theta_{fi} = (r_A(\text{MZ}), r_A(\text{DZ}), \text{var}(G), \text{var}(E))',$$

and

$$\Theta_{fr} = (a, e)',$$

in which $r_A(\text{MZ})$ and $r_A(\text{DZ})$ represent correlations among additive genetic values for MZ and DZ twins. The parameters in Θ_{fi} are known on theoretical or statistical grounds. The variances of the latent additive and environmental variables, G and E, are standardized because it is not possible to identify the variances of what are essentially unobserved variables (e.g., Long, 1983). The additive genetic correlation of the MZ twin is unity because the members of a MZ twin pair are genetically identical. The additive genetic correlation of the DZ twin pairs equals .5 under the assumption of random mating. Thus, we arrive at values for the fixed or known parameters, $\Theta_{fi} = (1.0, 0.5, 1.0, 1.0)'$.

Now, a model fitting function is defined as some function of the differences between the expected statistics and the observed statistics, and optimization is concerned with finding values for the unknown parameters, Θ_{fr}, that minimize these differences. In our example, the expected statistics, which depend on the value the vector Θ, are collected in the expected covariance matrices Σ_{MZ} and Σ_{DZ}. We wish to find estimates for a and e such that the discrepancies $\Sigma_{MZ} - S_{MZ}$ and $\Sigma_{DZ} - S_{DZ}$ are minimal. We can then consider the *size* of these differences; if they are small we can conclude that the data support the hypothesis; if the differences are large, the hypothesis is rejected. Use of an appropriate function enables us to statistically quantify the terms 'large' and 'small' in this context.

7.3   Weighted Least Squares Fitting Functions

We will consider various ways of defining fitting functions to quantify the afore-mentioned discrepancies, which depend on the unknown vector Θ_{fr}. As above, we assume that the observed data are summarized in dispersion matrices (e.g., covariance matrices).

The best known functions are the Unweighted Least Squares (ULS), General-ized Least Squared (GLS), and Maximum Likelihood (ML), all of which are avail-able in LISREL (see Chapter 6). These are all special cases of a more general function called Weighted Least Squares (WLS), which we consider first because of its generality and intuitive appeal. Subsequently we will examine the well-known formulations of the ULS, GLS, and ML functions, before returning to WLS.

Let s and σ contain the non-duplicate elements (i.e., the diagonal and subdi-agonal elements) of the observed covariance matrix S and the model matrix Σ, respectively. The order of S is k, so that S and Σ have $\frac{1}{2}k(k+1)$ non-duplicate elements, and the vector s (and, of course, σ) is $q = (k \times 1)$ dimensional. For example, the vector σ of the matrix Σ_{MZ} is

$$
\sigma = \begin{pmatrix} \Sigma_{MZ_{(1,1)}} \\ \Sigma_{MZ_{(2,1)}} \\ \Sigma_{MZ_{(2,2)}} \end{pmatrix}
$$
$$
= \begin{pmatrix} a^2 + e^2 \\ a^2 \\ a^2 + e^2 \end{pmatrix}
$$

where $\Sigma_{MZ(i,j)}$ is the element in the ith row and j^{th} column of the matrix Σ_{MZ}. Let **W** denote a $(q \times q)$ positive definite symmetric matrix, where $q = \frac{1}{2}k(k+1)$. The most general formulation is given by the WLS function:

$$
F(\theta) = (s - \sigma)' \mathbf{W}^{-1} (s - \sigma) \tag{7.1}
$$
$$
= \sum_{g=1}^{k} \sum_{h=1}^{g} \sum_{i=1}^{k} \sum_{j=1}^{i} w^{gh,ij} (s_{gh} - \sigma_{gh})(s_{ij} - \sigma_{ij}) ,
$$

where

$$
s' = (s_{11}, s_{21}, s_{22}, s_{31}, ..., s_{kk}) ,
$$

is a vector of the elements in the lower half, including the diagonal, of the covariance matrix $\mathbf{S}$ used to fit the model to the data;

$$\sigma' = (\sigma_{11}, \sigma_{21}, \sigma_{22}, \sigma_{31}, ..., \sigma_{kk}) \,,$$

is the vector of corresponding elements of $\Sigma(\theta)$ reproduced from the model parameters θ, and $w^{gh,ij}$ is a typical element of the matrix $\mathbf{W}^{-1}$.

For example, if we let $k = 3$, $\mathbf{d}' = (s_1 - \sigma_1, s_2 - \sigma_2, s_3 - \sigma_3)'$, and we represent a particular element in $\mathbf{W}^{-1}$ by $\mathbf{W}_{i,j}^{-1}$ ($i = 1, 3$ and $j = 1, 3$), we have:

$$
\begin{aligned}
F(\text{WLS}) \quad = \quad & d_1^2 \mathbf{W}_{1,1}^{-1} + 2d_1 d_2 \mathbf{W}_{2,1}^{-1} + d_2^2 \mathbf{W}_{2,2}^{-1} + 2d_1 d_3 \mathbf{W}_{3,1}^{-1} + \qquad (7.2) \\
& 2d_2 d_3 \mathbf{W}_{3,2}^{-1} + d_3^2 \mathbf{W}_{3,3}^{-1}
\end{aligned}
$$

(remember $\mathbf{W}_{2,1}^{-1} = \mathbf{W}_{1,2}^{-1}$ because $\mathbf{W}^{-1}$ is symmetric). The rationale of the function is easy to see: the discrepancies between the observed and the model statistic are squared and weighted by the inverse of some positive definite symmetric matrix $\mathbf{W}$. It is the choice of this matrix that determines the fitting function. The ideal selection of $\mathbf{W}$ is one that takes into account the precision and the variances and covariances of the estimates in $(\mathbf{d} = \mathbf{s} - \sigma)$. It is also easy to see that when the fit is perfect this function is zero, because then the elements of $\mathbf{d}$ are all zero.

To obtain consistent parameter estimates, any positive definite matrix $\mathbf{W}$ may be used. Under very general assumptions, if the model holds in the population and if the sample variances and covariances in $\mathbf{S}$ converge in probability to the corresponding elements in the population covariance matrix Σ as the sample size increases, any fit function with a positive definite $\mathbf{W}$ will give a consistent estimator of θ. In practice, the numerical results obtained with one fit function often are so close to those of another that we get the same substantive interpretations of the results.

Analysis of Multiple Groups

In the preceding chapter we noted that genetic covariance structure analyses are, more often than not, multiple group analyses. In the simple example given here we have two covariance matrices, $\mathbf{S}_{\text{MZ}}$ and $\mathbf{S}_{\text{DZ}}$. Generally, to obtain a multi-group fitting function, that of each group is weighted by its number of cases and summed:

$$F = (1/N) \sum_{g=1}^{G} N_g F_g \,, \qquad (7.3)$$

where G is the number of groups, N_g represents the number of cases in group g, F_g the value of the fitting function calculated in group g, and N is the total number of cases, $N = \sum_{g=1}^{G} N_g$. For example, to obtain a multi-group WLS function we calculate

$$F(\text{WLS}) = (1/N) \sum_{g=1}^{G} N_g [(\mathbf{s}_g - \sigma_g)' \mathbf{W}_g^{-1} (\mathbf{s}_g - \sigma_g)] \,. \qquad (7.4)$$

The generalized formulation in (7.4) of the fitting function (7.1) has the advantage that it is conceptually easy to understand as a least squares function. However, it is computationally inconvenient because the order of $\mathbf{W}$ can become prohibitively large as the size of $\mathbf{W}$ increases rapidly with k, demanding enormous amounts of computer memory when k is at all large. Consequently, the most common fitting functions mentioned above are not written in this format, but in a more efficient one that we turn to now. To facilitate this discussion, we assume temporarily that the data

1. vary continuously (opposed to, e.g., dichotomous data),

2. are summarized in a covariance matrix (as opposed to, say, a correlation matrix),

3. follow a multivariate normal distribution.

The third assumption is very important because several of the alternative formulations of the fitting function are possible only under this assumption. Each method and its characteristics will be discussed individually. Then, these assumptions will be relaxed and we will return to the WLS function.

7.3.1   Unweighted Least Squares Fitting Function (ULS)

The ULS function is defined as

$$
\begin{aligned}
F(\text{ULS}) &= (\mathbf{s} - \boldsymbol{\sigma})'\mathbf{I}^{-1}(\mathbf{s} - \boldsymbol{\sigma}) \\
&= (\mathbf{s} - \boldsymbol{\sigma})'(\mathbf{s} - \boldsymbol{\sigma}),
\end{aligned} \tag{7.5}
$$

or in its more familiar form:

$$
F(\text{ULS}) = \frac{1}{2}tr[(\mathbf{S} - \boldsymbol{\Sigma})^2]. \tag{7.6}
$$

Note that the weight matrix used in ULS is an identity matrix ($\mathbf{W} = \mathbf{I}$). Thus, this function minimizes one-half the sum of squares of each of the elements in the residual matrix $\mathbf{S} - \boldsymbol{\Sigma}$. Finding the values for $\boldsymbol{\Theta}_{fr}$ that minimize this function yields ULS parameter estimates, $\hat{\boldsymbol{\Theta}}(ULS)$. It can be verified easily that $F(\text{ULS})$ has as its theoretical minimum zero. The ULS function has advantages and disadvantages. Its advantages are:

1. It has good convergence properties; that is to say it is not difficult to minimize.

2. It is simple to program and computationally undemanding.

3. It yields consistent parameter estimates, so as the sample size increases (or, more generally, the information that the estimator uses increases), the estimates $\hat{\boldsymbol{\Theta}}(\text{ULS})$ converge to $\boldsymbol{\Theta}_{fr}$ stochastically with probability 1.0. This characteristic is not conditional on distributional assumptions.

4. It will work under a wide variety of conditions, including non-positive definite states of the input or model covariance matrices.

Its disadvantages are:

1. No statistical inference. It does not generally yield a statistic to rigorously test the overall goodness of fit of the specified model. Therefore, once estimates have been obtained, there is no formal criterion to decide whether or not to reject the specified hypothesis.

2. The parameter estimates are *scale dependent* (see Browne, 1982; Krane and McDonald, 1978). Let **D** be a diagonal matrix of positive scale factors. Scale dependence implies that the results obtained by analyzing **S** and those obtained by analyzing **DSD′** are not properly related. Given one solution and knowledge of the matrix **D**, one cannot derive the other solution. This is a serious disadvantage: if two researchers investigate identical phenotypes with different scales, their results and conclusions regarding the quantitative genetic decomposition of the phenotypic variance may differ!

3. Standard errors of the estimates are not generally available.

4. The ULS estimator is not as efficient as others. That is to say, *ceteris paribus*, the precision of the ULS estimates is not as great as that obtained by the other methods.

The problems associated with ULS stem from the fact that all the discrepancies **S** - **Σ** contribute equally to the fitting function (the choice of **W** = **I** leads to this equal weighting). In other words, no consideration is given to the fact that there might be differences in the precision with which an element in **S** is estimated (Jöreskog, 1988). It is desirable to take into account such differences by weighting the discrepancies in a manner that reflects the precision and interdependence of the estimates in **S**. The next fitting function, GLS, carries out just such a weighting.

7.3.2 Generalized Least Squares (GLS)

The GLS function has the following form:

$$F(\text{GLS}) = (s - \sigma)'\mathbf{W}_{(\text{GLS})}^{-1}(s - \sigma), \qquad (7.7)$$

and a more convenient form:

$$F(\text{GLS}) = \frac{1}{2}tr[(\mathbf{I} - \mathbf{S}^{-1}\mathbf{\Sigma})^2]. \qquad (7.8)$$

The matrix **W**(GLS) in (7.7) contains the covariances and variances of the terms in s. Due to the assumption of multivariate normality many of these terms are known (in the same sense that the skewness and kurtosis of a normally distributed variable are known) and the more convenient form in (7.8) results. We now see that the matrix S^{-1} functions as a weight matrix for the residual matrix $S - \Sigma$. The theoretical minimum is zero, as can be readily verified. Under the distributional assumption noted above, this estimator has a number of advantages over the ULS function. The advantages of GLS are

1. Scale invariance (in the sense defined above: $F(\text{GLS})[S; \Sigma] = F(\text{GLS})[DSD; D\Sigma D]$).

2. The asymptotic covariance matrix of the estimates $\hat{\Theta}(\text{GLS})$ is known so that standard errors are available.

3. An overall goodness of fit test statistic is available (chi-squared) so that one may have a formal criterion to determine the tenability of the hypothesis (statistical inference).

4. The GLS estimator is consistent and has greater efficiency than ULS.

A clear disadvantage of GLS is that the violation of the distributional assumptions lead to incorrect overall test statistic and standard errors. Also, S must be positive definite, although this can hardly be called a disadvantage.

7.3.3   Maximum Likelihood (ML)

The ML function (or likelihood ratio function) is perhaps the most frequently used fitting function. It is defined as

$$F(\text{ML}) = (s - \sigma)' W_{(\text{ML})}^{-1} (s - \sigma), \tag{7.9}$$

and in its more convenient form as

$$F(\text{ML}) = \frac{1}{2} tr[((S - \Sigma)\Sigma^{-1})^2]. \tag{7.10}$$

Finally, in a more familiar form:

$$F(\text{ML}) = \log |\Sigma| + tr(S\Sigma^{-1}) - \log |S| - p, \tag{7.11}$$

where p is the order of input covariance matrix S. The latter formulation is less obvious than the two equivalents. Bollen (1989, Appendix 4A & 4B) gives an excellent derivation of this formulation of the ML function. The matrix $W_{(\text{ML})}^{-1}$ now contains the inverse of the variances and covariances among the elements in the matrix Σ.

The advantages of this fitting function are the same as the GLS function and, like GLS, the major disadvantage is the distributional assumption of multivariate normality. Compared to GLS, ML has the computational disadvantage that Σ has to be inverted at each iteration, but aside from this these fitting functions are very similar (Browne, 1974).

7.3.4 Fitting Functions Including Means

The fit functions we have discussed so far are for covariance structures *only*; they are augmented if we fit models to observed means as well as covariances (see Section 8.8 and Chapter 15). When means are involved, the fit functions are augmented by a term of the form:

$$F(\text{mean}) = \frac{1}{2}(z - \mu)'W^{-1}(z - \mu) \qquad (7.12)$$

where z and μ are respectively the vectors of observed and expected means, and W^{-1} is the observed covariance matrix for ULS, GLS, DWLS and WLS, but is the expected covariance matrix for ML. Note that just like the General WLS function for covariances, equation 7.12 evaluates to zero when the observed and expected means are equal. Thus when $z = \mu$ we are left with a function of the covariance structure alone.

7.3.5 Weighted Least Squares (WLS) Revisited

So far we have been concerned with normally distributed continuously varying variables and we have assumed that the data are summarized in a covariance matrix. We now return to the general and useful fitting function called the weighted least squares function, WLS. The WLS function can be used in many situations; for example, when the data are summarized in a correlation matrix, when the data follow an arbitrary distribution, or when the data are discrete (dichotomous or polychotomous). In (7.1) we presented the WLS function

$$F(\text{WLS}) = (s - \sigma)'W^{-1}(s - \sigma) \qquad (7.13)$$

This function is quite general because it can accommodate, by suitable choice of a W matrix, many types of data summary (correlation, covariance), and data following almost any distribution. The issue is to choose the appropriate W to suit the data summary or their distributional characteristics or both.

The Weight Matrix, W

In Section 7.3 we noted that if the model of the data is correct in the population and the elements of S converge to those in Σ as the sample size increases, any fit function will give a consistent estimator of Θ, given a positive definite W. We also have noted that the usual way of choosing W in weighted least squares is to let any element of W, $w_{gh,ij}$, be a consistent estimate of the asymptotic covariance between s_{gh} and s_{ij}. If this is the case, we say that W^{-1} is a *correct weight matrix*. However, further assumptions must be made if one needs an asymptotically correct chi-squared measure of goodness-of-fit and asymptotically correct standard errors of parameter estimates.

"Classical" theory for covariance structures (see e.g., Browne, 1974, or Jöreskog, 1981), assumes that the variances and covariances of the elements of S are of the form

$$\mathrm{ACov}(s_{gh}, s_{ij}) = (1/N)(\sigma_{gi}\sigma_{hj} + \sigma_{gj}\sigma_{hi}) . \tag{7.14}$$

This holds, in particular, if the observed variables have a multivariate normal distribution, or if $\mathbf{S}$ has a Wishart distribution. The GLS and ML methods and their chi-square values and standard errors are based on (7.14). The GLS method corresponds to using a matrix $\mathbf{W}^{-1}$ in (7.1) whose general element is

$$w^{gh,ij} = N(2 - \delta_{gh})(2 - \delta_{ij})(s^{gi}s^{hj} + s^{gj}s^{hi}) , \tag{7.15}$$

where δ_{gh} and δ_{ij} are Kronecker deltas[1]. The fit function (7.11) for ML is not of the form (7.1) but may be shown to be equivalent to using a $\mathbf{W}^{-1}$ of the form (7.15), with s replaced by an estimate of σ which is updated in each iteration.

In recent fundamental work by Browne (1982, 1984), this classical theory for covariance structures has been generalized to any multivariate distribution (including non-normal distributions) for continuous variables satisfying very mild assumptions. This approach uses a $\mathbf{W}$ matrix with typical element

$$w_{gh,ij} = m_{ghij} - s_{gh}s_{ij} , \tag{7.16}$$

where

$$m_{ghij} = (1/N) \sum_{a=1}^{N} (z_{ag} - \bar{z}_g)(z_{ah} - \bar{z}_h)(z_{ai} - \bar{z}_i)(z_{aj} - \bar{z}_j) \tag{7.17}$$

are the fourth-order central moments. Using such a $\mathbf{W}$ in (7.1) gives what Browne calls "asymptotically distribution free (ADF)" estimators, for which correct asymptotic chi-squares and standard errors may be obtained. Browne has shown that this $\mathbf{W}$ matrix also may be used to compute correct asymptotic chi-squares and standard errors for estimates which have been obtained by the classical ML and GLS methods. WLS uses $\mathbf{W}$ as defined by (7.16), whereas GLS uses the $\mathbf{W}$ formulation in (7.15), which shows that WLS and GLS are different forms of weighted least squares: *WLS is asymptotically distribution free, while GLS is based on normal theory.*

The advantages of the WLS function include all those of ML and GLS, in addition to the advantage of postulating virtually no distributional assumptions. A considerable disadvantage is that very large sample sizes are required to arrive at a reliable estimate of $\mathbf{W}$. This means that the asymptotic characteristics of the distribution of the fitting function and covariance matrix of the estimates become trustworthy only when the sample size is large. A second drawback is the computational aspects of the function. We noted previously that the $\mathbf{W}$ matrix quickly becomes very large as the number of input variables (i.e., the order of the input covariance matrix) increases. If we have k variables to analyze, we have $q = \frac{1}{2}k(k+1)$ non-duplicate elements in $\mathbf{S}$ and $u = \frac{1}{2}q(q+1)$ non-duplicate elements in $\mathbf{W}$. Thus,

---

[1] The value of the Kronecker delta δ_{ij} is zero for $i \neq j$ and unity for $i = j$.

for example, analysis of $k = 20$ variables would yield a covariance matrix, $\mathbf{S}$, with $q = 210$ elements, and a weight matrix $\mathbf{W}$ with $u = 22155$ unique entries! A third drawback is that when there are missing observations in the data, different moments involved in (7.16) may be based on different numbers of cases unless listwise deletion is used. When pairwise deletion is used, it is not clear how to deal with this problem.

7.3.6 Additional Fitting Functions: Modified ML, DWLS, and Functions for Raw Data

Three further functions warrant a brief mention. First, there is a modified ML fitting function which yields correct overall χ^2 goodness-of-fit statistics and standard errors when the data are non-normally distributed and the assumption is made that the marginal distribution of the phenotypic variables are characterized by an identical kurtosis (the multivariate distribution is then called an "elliptical distribution"). When this hypothesis cannot be rejected, one can use the ML fitting function and correct the results (i.e., χ^2 goodness of fit index and standard errors) for the departure from normality (see Bollen, 1989; Browne, 1984). This method is very attractive, but the assumption of an elliptical distribution is rather restrictive.

The second fitting function is Diagonally Weighted Least Squares (DWLS; Jöreskog and Sörbom, 1989), which involves using only the diagonal elements of the $\mathbf{W}$ matrix when analyzing covariance matrices calculated from non-normal continuously varying variables. This function gives correct standard errors and χ^2 only under very limited circumstances. It is used when the WLS option is required, but the full $\mathbf{W}$ matrix does not fit in the computer memory; for example, in analyses of large correlation matrices. The DWLS function is considered to be a compromise between ULS and (ADF) WLS. It does not seem to have much to recommend it, although it is superior to ULS.

indexraw data Finally, we mention the possibility of fitting models to raw data. So far we have assumed that the phenotypic data are summarized in one or more dispersion matrices. This method of data summarization is very convenient but requires that each case (or "pedigree") has the same structure. When the data comprise cases of variable composition this convenient method of data summarization cannot be used for practical and statistical reasons and the model has to be fit directly to the raw data (Lange, *et al.*, 1976). A pedigree may vary in composition from a single individual to a complex pedigree comprising many different social and biological relationships. When the structure of the cases is highly variable (the pedigrees are said to be unbalanced), it is possible to use Maximum Likelihood by calculating the log-likelihood for each pedigree separately:

$$L_i = -\frac{1}{2}\log|\mathbf{\Sigma}_i| - \frac{1}{2}(\mathbf{x} - \mathcal{E}[\mathbf{x}])'\mathbf{\Sigma}_i^{-1}(\mathbf{x} - \mathcal{E}[\mathbf{x}]) + \text{constant}, \qquad (7.18)$$

where $\mathbf{\Sigma}_i$ is the expected covariance matrix for the ith pedigree, $\mathbf{x}$ is the vector of observed data within that pedigree, and $\mathcal{E}[\mathbf{x}]$ is a vector of expected means. The constant in this expression is $j\log(2\pi)$, where j is the number of variables being analyzed. This log-likelihood is maximized over all of the pedigrees $L = \sum_{i=1}^{k} L_i$, where k is the number of distinct pedigrees. This method is available in the package Mx (Neale, 1991). It is useful to recognize that when there are no missing data (the data are "balanced pedigrees") the sum of the k log-likelihoods in equation 7.18 can be expressed as (e.g., Mardia *et al.*, 1979, p. 97):

$$L_A = -\frac{k}{2}\log|\Sigma_i| - \frac{k}{2}tr(\Sigma^{-1}S) - \frac{k}{2}(\overline{x} - \mu)'\Sigma_i^{-1}(\overline{x} - \mu) + \text{constant}. \qquad (7.19)$$

In large populations, $\overline{x} = \mu$, so the term $(\overline{x} - \mu)'\Sigma_i^{-1}(\overline{x} - \mu)$ is zero, thus reducing to

$$L_A = -\frac{k}{2}\log|\Sigma_i| - \frac{k}{2}tr(\Sigma^{-1}S) + \text{constant}. \qquad (7.20)$$

For an explanation of the very close relationship between between the log-likelihood ratio function and the likelihood function, the reader is referred to Bollen (1989) or Lawley and Maxwell (1971). Neale *et al.*, (1989b) also have discussed this relationship in the context of genetic model-fitting.

Figure 7.1 serves as a partial summary of the preceding discussion of fitting functions and may be used as an aid in determining a suitable function when analyzing dispersion matrices.

7.3.7   Goodness of Fit and the Principle of Parsimony

indexgoodness-of-fit Each of the fit-functions described up to now measures the overall goodness of fit of a model. However, this really addresses only the first of the four aspects of model-fitting described in the introduction to this Chapter, namely whether or not the model fits the data. The mathematical consistency of the model is addressed by the use of path analysis and structural equations, but we have not considered how to judge whether or not a model is *simple*.

Quite often, simply adding more and more parameters to a model will allow it to explain (i.e., fit) the data perfectly. However, as we saw in Section 2.3.2, a model that has to fit perfectly does little more than transform the data. While it may prove useful for interpretation of data, it has the disadvantage of not being *falsifiable*. Thus a model that fits well is not necessarily useful; what counts is the ability to predict a wide range of phenomena with a smaller set of parameters. This is the principle of parsimony, recognized by the fourteenth-century philosopher, William of Occam, to whom we owe the term *Occam's razor*. For practical purposes, we can get an idea of the parsimony of a model by combining its goodness-of-fit χ^2 with its degrees of freedom. There are many such indices of fit (see, e.g., Browne and Cudeck, 1988; Marsh *et al.* 1988; Bollen 1989, Mulaik *et al* 1989; Kaplan, 1990) and the one we have selected here should not be considered to be necessarily the best, but for a variety of genetic models it seems to agree with expert opinion

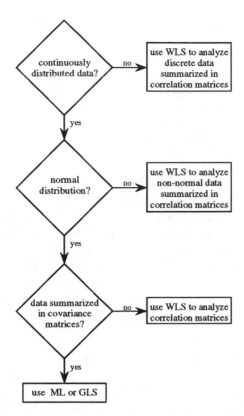

Figure 7.1: Flow chart to aid selection of a fitting function for the analysis of dispersion matrices.

most of the time. . We compute Akaike's Information Criterion for a model as

$$\chi^2 - 2\mathrm{df}$$

and the model with the lowest (i.e., largest negative) value of this index is said to fit best by AIC. Fitting best by this criterion is clearly *not* the same as fitting best by the χ^2 statistic; therefore we caution authors against the unqualified use of expressions such as 'model II fits best.'

7.4 Optimization

7.4.1 Introduction

We stated earlier that optimization is concerned with finding values for the unknown parameters, Θ_{fr}, that minimize a fitting function. Now we shall try to give some idea of how optimization works. We limit the discussion to a method known as the quasi-Newton algorithm. This and other methods are explained fully in Dennis and Schnabel (1983) and in Gill, Murray and Wright (1981).

As above, we have a fitting function F and a vector containing unknown parameters Θ. We estimate these parameters by finding values for them that minimize our chosen F. In general, minimization requires an iterative process because the parameter estimates that minimize the function cannot be solved in closed form. One well-known iterative method of minimizing a function is *Newton-Raphson*. We will consider this approach briefly in order to introduce the related quasi-Newton method and to introduce some terminology.

Consider the following simple optimization problem. The correlation for the personality trait "dominance" is .53 for MZ twins and .25 for DZ twins (Loehlin and Nichols, 1976). Suppose that we hypothesize that additive genetic effects are responsible for these correlations. This hypothesis leads to the pair of (slightly inconsistent) simultaneous equations: $.53 = a^2$ and $.25 = .5a^2$, which we will fit using the ULS function. As mentioned previously, in multiple group designs the loss function is the weighted sum of loss functions calculated in each group, $(1/N)\sum_{i=1}^{G} N_g F_g(\text{ULS})$, where N_g and F_g are respectively the sample size and function value for group g, and $N = \sum_{i=1}^{G} N_g$. So we have

$$F(\text{ULS}) = \frac{N_{MZ}}{N_{MZ} + N_{DZ}}(a^2 - .53)^2 + \frac{N_{DZ}}{N_{MZ} + N_{DZ}}(.5a^2 - .25)^2,$$

where N_{MZ} equals the number of MZ twin pairs ($N_{MZ} = 490$) and N_{DZ} equals the number of DZ twin pairs ($N_{DZ} = 317$). Then,

$$F(\text{ULS}) = .6072(a^2 - .53)^2 + .3928(.5a^2 - .25)^2.$$

To apply the Newton-Raphson minimization method, we require two sets of information. The first is the so-called first–order derivative of the function with respect to the unknown parameter a. This also is referred to as the *gradient*, and is represented by the m dimensional gradient vector g (m equals the number of unknown parameters). For example,

$$\frac{\partial F}{\partial a} = \frac{1}{N_{MZ} + N_{DZ}} a[a^2(4N_{MZ} + N_{DZ}) - (2.12N_{MZ} + .50N_{DZ})]$$

$$= 2.8216a^3 - 1.4837a$$

so $\text{g}' = [\frac{\partial F}{\partial a}]'$. Because in the present example we have only one parameter to estimate ($m = 1$), the vector g is one dimensional. The second piece of information is the matrix of second order partial derivatives. This ($m \times m$) symmetric matrix is called the *Hessian*, **H**, and is in the present example

$$\frac{\partial^2 F}{\partial a \partial a'} = \frac{1}{N_{MZ} + N_{DZ}} 3a^2(4N_{MZ} + N_{DZ}) -$$

$$(2.12N_{\mathrm{MZ}} + .50N_{\mathrm{DZ}})N_{\mathrm{MZ}} + N_{\mathrm{DZ}}$$
$$= 8.4648a^2 - 1.4837.$$

The Newton-Raphson algorithm is an iterative scheme that works as follows:

1. Choose a starting value for the vector Θ, the unknown parameters. Call this vector $\Theta^{(k)}$.

2. Calculate the function value, gradient vector, and Hessian matrix: $F^{(k)}$, $\mathbf{g}^{(k)}$, and $\mathbf{H}^{(k)}$.

3. Calculate the direction vector $\mathbf{d}^{(k)} = \mathbf{H}^{-1(k)}\mathbf{g}^{(k)}$.

4. Calculate $\Theta^{(k+1)} = \Theta^{(k)} - \mathbf{d}^{(k)}$; i.e., the estimates for iteration $k+1$.

5. Goto (2) replacing $\Theta^{(k)}$ by $\Theta^{(k+1)}$.

Given the starting values $\Theta^{(k)}$ this algorithm determines the direction in which to proceed by calculating the quantity $\mathbf{d}^{(k)}$. This continues until the difference between $F^{(k+1)}$ and $F^{(k)}$ is smaller than some predetermined constant, ϵ (e.g., $\epsilon = 0.0001$). Applying this algorithm to the example ULS fitting function starting at the point $a = 1.0$ yields the following results:

Iteration	a	F	$\mathbf{g}$	$\mathbf{H}$	$\mathbf{H}^{-1}\mathbf{g}$
1	1.0	.158681	1.3379360	6.981136	.1916502
2	.808350	1.156227E-02	.2910483	4.047485	7.190842E-02
3	.736441	2.686400E-04	3.433225E-02	3.107186	1.104931E-02
4	.725392	7.617289E-05	7.572186E-04	2.970459	2.549163E-04
5	.725137	7.607631E-05	3.625686E-07	2.967330	1.221868E-07
6	.725137	7.607632E-05	0	2.967328	0

Thus, the estimate $\hat{a} = .725$ is obtained from minimizing this fitting function. We note that $\mathbf{g}$ is zero at the minimum and that $\mathbf{H}$ is positive (2.96). These are necessary and sufficient conditions for the point $a = .725$ to be a true (local) minimum (Yamane, 1968). In the case that we have more than one unknown parameter these same conditions apply: the vector $\mathbf{g}$ should be a zero vector and the Hessian $\mathbf{H}$ should be positive definite.

Figure 7.2a depicts the function values given various values of the parameter a. The function can be seen to be approximately quadratic in the vicinity of the minimum ($a = .725$). Figure 7.2b demonstrates graphically the progression during the first two iterations of the Newton Raphson algorithm.

This algorithm generally works well given good starting values, but requires exact (analytic) expressions for both the first ($\mathbf{g}$) and the second order derivatives ($\mathbf{H}$). The latter can be time consuming and complicated to calculate for the fitting

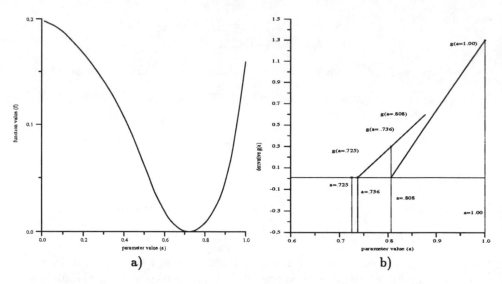

Figure 7.2: Graphic depiction of a) parameter space, and b) iterative progression of Newton-Raphson algorithm.

functions used in covariance structure analysis. The quasi-Newton method uses the same approach, but the exact Hessian is replaced by some approximation, $\mathbf{Y}$. Both $\mathbf{g}$ and $\mathbf{H}$ can be estimated by finite differences, but the Hessian can be approximated by a number of additional methods. The choice of the method, $\mathbf{Y}$, determines the optimization routine. The use of a matrix other than the exact Hessian complicates the Newton-Raphson algorithm in two respects:

1. A choice of $\mathbf{Y}$ has to be made. $\mathbf{Y}$ can be chosen to be fixed (unchanging throughout iteration) or can be updated during iteration (a new $\mathbf{Y}$ for each new set of estimates). The latter requires an additional algorithm for $\mathbf{Y}$.

2. An algorithm has to be determined at step (4) given above, because the calculation of $\Theta^{(k+1)} = \Theta^{(k)} - \mathbf{H}^{-1(k)}\mathbf{g}^{(k)}$ is replaced by $\Theta^{(k+1)} = \Theta^{(k)} - \alpha\mathbf{Y}^{-1(k)}\Theta^{(k)}$ where α is an unknown quantity called the *step length parameter* because it determines how much the current value of $\Theta^{(k+1)}$ will be changed using the information $\mathbf{Y}^{-1(k)}\mathbf{g}^{(k)}$.

7.4.2 Choice of Hessian approximation

It is mainly the choice of $\mathbf{Y}$ that determines the quasi-Newton optimization algorithm. The following gives an overview of possibilities:

Choice of $\mathbf{Y}$	Algorithm
$\mathbf{Y} = \mathbf{H}$. Exact Hessian	Newton-Raphson
$\mathbf{Y} \approx \mathbf{H}$. Finite Difference Approximation	Discrete Newton
Information Matrix	Gauss-Newton or Fisher's Scoring Method
$\mathbf{Y} = \mathbf{I}$. Identity matrix	Steepest Descent

LISREL 7 uses the Davidon-Fletcher-Powell (DFP) method as the default means of determining $\mathbf{Y}$. In this method, parameter estimates, gradients, and $\mathbf{Y}$ at iteration k, are used to obtain an approximation of $\mathbf{Y}$ for iteration $k + 1$ (see e.g., Lawley and Maxwell, 1971, for the relevant formulas). As iteration proceeds, the DFP update of $\mathbf{Y}$ converges on the matrix $\mathbf{H}$ (Gill, *et al.* 1981). Other options in LISREL 7 involve calculating the information matrix at each iteration. The information matrix is the Hessian calculated under the assumption that the true model is being fit $[\mathcal{E}(\mathbf{S}) = \mathbf{\Sigma}]$. Although this may seem like a very strong assumption, it practice it has been found to work well (Dolan and Molenaar, 1991). When one chooses the information matrix for $\mathbf{Y}$, the algorithm is called the Fisher-scoring method. Jöreskog (1988) points out that the Fisher scoring method and the Gauss-Newton algorithm are identical. Finally, one can choose a matrix $\mathbf{Y}$ that is fixed throughout iteration. For example, the steepest descent algorithm involves replacing $\mathbf{Y}$ with the identity matrix, $\mathbf{I}$.

7.5 Summary

In this chapter we have described and compared some of the commonly used fitting functions for structural equation modeling, including the group of weighted least squares and maximum likelihood functions for fitting to moment data matrices, and the maximum likelihood pedigree approach of Lange *et al.* (1976) for fitting to raw data. The ML moment matrix procedure is the most frequently used function for genetic analysis of twin data (it is also the default fit function in LISREL), due in large part to its desirable properties for estimators, standard errors, and relation to the chi-squared goodness-of-fit and likelihood ratio tests, and the fact that it has been reasonably well characterized in the literature. However, each of the fitting functions described here has unique advantages, which permits structural analysis of twin data in nearly any form or composition. Although not all of these functions are available in LISREL (most notably the raw data pedigree function), LISREL can handle a very wide range of input dispersion matrices, particularly when used in conjunction with PRELIS.

We also have presented a brief overview of optimization theory and practice, with emphasis upon the Newton-Raphson and quasi-Newton algorithms. Our description of these procedures has been kept simple, even superficial, in order to illustrate how parameters are estimated under a chosen model, yet not divert attention from our primary focus of genetic analysis of twin and family data. One of the chief advantages of using a commercial software package such as LISREL is that one need not be burdened by the intricacies of optimization, which are legion, but may, instead, concentrate on the characteristics of the data themselves. The remainder of this book is directed toward this task.

Chapter 8

Univariate Analysis

8.1 Introduction

In this chapter we take the univariate model for twin data, as described in Chapter 5, and apply it to twin data. We hope that this will enable the readers to apply the models to their own data, and deepen their understanding of both the scope and the limitations of the method. The first example concerns body mass index (BMI), a widely used measure of obesity, and Section 8.2 describes how we obtained and summarized these data. In Section 8.3 we develop and apply a model of additive genetic (A), dominance genetic (D), common environment (C), and random environment (E) effects, even though D and C are confounded when our data have been obtained from pairs of twins reared together. In Section 8.4 we start to fit this model to authentic data, using LISREL 7 in a path coefficients approach. To illustrate the univariate model fitted with variance components, we describe the use of LISREL 8 (in β-test version at the time of writing) in Section 8.5. This second treatment may be skipped without loss of continuity. The results of initial model-fitting to BMI data appear in Section 8.6 and two extensions to the model, the use of means and of unmatched twins, are described before drawing general conclusions about the BMI analyses in Section 8.9. The second example describes the collection and analysis of major depressive disorder in a sample of adult female twins (Section 8.10.1). This application serves to contrast the data summary and analysis required for an ordinal variable against those appropriate for a continuous variable. In most twin studies there is considerable heterogeneity of age between pairs. As we show in Section 8.11, such heterogeneity can give rise to inflated estimates of the effects of the shared environment. We, therefore, provide a method of incorporating age into the structural equation model to separate its effects from other shared environmental influences.

8.2   Body Mass Index in Twins

Table 8.1 summarizes twin correlations and other summary statistics (see Chapter 2) for untransformed BMI, defined as weight (in kilograms) divided by the square of height (in meters). BMI is an index of obesity which has been widely used in epidemiologic research (Bray, 1976; Jeffrey and Knauss, 1981), and has recently been the subject of a number of genetic studies (Stunkard et al., 1986; 1990; MacDonald and Stunkard, 1990; Grilo and Pogue-Guile, 1991; Longini et al., 1991; Price and Gottesman, 1991; Cardon and Fulker, 1992). Values between 20–25 are considered to fall in the normal range for this population, with BMI < 20 taken to indicate underweight, BMI > 25 overweight, and BMI > 28 obesity (Australian Bureau of Statistics, 1977). The data analyzed here come from a mailed questionnaire survey of volunteer twin pairs from the Australian NH&MRC twin register conducted in 1981 (Martin and Jardine, 1986; Jardine, 1985). Questionnaires were mailed to 5967 pairs age 18 years and over, with completed questionnaires returned by both members of 3808 (64%) pairs, and by one twin only from approximately 550 pairs, yielding an individual response rate of 68%.

The total sample has been subdivided into a young cohort, aged 18-30 years, and an older cohort aged 31 and above. This allows us to examine the consistency of evidence for environmental or genetic determination of BMI from early adulthood to maturity. For each cohort, twin pairs have been subdivided into five groups: monozygotic female pairs (MZF), monozygotic male pairs (MZM), dizygotic female pairs (DZF), dizygotic male pairs (DZM) and opposite-sex pairs (DZFM). We have avoided pooling MZ or like-sex DZ twin data across sex before computing summary statistics. Pooling across sexes is inappropriate unless it is known that there is no gender difference in mean, variance, or twin pair covariance, and no genotype × sex interaction; it should almost always be avoided. Among same-sex pairs, twins have been assigned as first or second members of a pair at random. In the case of opposite-sex twin pairs, data have been ordered so that the female is always the first member of the pair and the male the second.

In both sexes and both cohorts, MZ twin correlations are substantially higher than like-sex DZ correlations, suggesting that there may be a substantial genetic contribution to variation in BMI. In the young cohort, the like-sex DZ correlations are somewhat lower than one-half of the corresponding MZ correlations, but this finding does not hold up in the older cohort. In terms of additive genetic (V_A) and dominance genetic (V_D) variance components, the expected correlations between MZ and DZ pairs are respectively $r_{MZ} = V_A + V_D$ and $r_{DZ} = 0.5V_A + 0.25V_D$, respectively (see Chapters 3 and 6). Thus the fact that the like-sex DZ twin correlations are less than one-half the size of the MZ correlations in the young cohort suggests a contribution of genetic dominance, as well as additive genetic variance, to individual differences in BMI. Model-fitting analyses (e.g., Heath et al., 1989c) are needed to determine whether the data:

1. Are consistent with simple additive genetic effects

Table 8.1:

Twin correlations and summary statistics for untransformed Body Mass Index in twins concordant for participation in the Australian survey. BMI is calculated as kg/m^2. Notation used is N: sample size in pairs; r: correlation; $\bar{x}$: mean; σ^2: variance; skew: skewness; kurt: kurtosis. Groups consist of monozygotic (MZ) or dizygotic (DZ) twin pairs who are male (M) female (F) or opposite-sex (OS).

	N	r	First Twin[†]					Second Twin				
			$\bar{x}$	σ^2	skew	kurt	Min Max	$\bar{x}$	σ^2	skew	kurt	Min Max
MZF												
Young	534	.78	21.25	7.73	1.82	6.84	13.30 38.39	21.30	8.81	2.14	9.44	15.94 44.08
Older	637	.69	23.11	11.87	1.22	2.53	16.02 41.55	22.97	11.25	1.08	2.11	14.20 40.79
DZF												
Young	328	.30	21.58	8.56	1.75	6.04	15.05 37.50	21.64	9.84	2.38	12.23	15.59 46.25
Older	380	.32	22.77	10.93	1.40	4.03	16.01 32.69	22.95	12.63	1.26	2.43	16.60 38.95
MZM												
Young	251	.77	22.09	5.95	0.28	0.10	15.67 29.37	22.13	5.77	0.40	0.30	16.85 30.12
Older	281	.70	24.22	6.42	0.11	-0.05	17.63 31.18	24.30	7.85	0.43	0.63	17.31 35.43
DZM												
Young	184	.32	22.71	8.16	1.00	1.71	16.67 32.88	22.61	9.63	1.55	6.24	16.98 41.12
Older	137	.37	24.18	8.28	0.41	0.70	16.90 33.56	24.08	7.42	0.72	0.43	19.05 32.41
DZOS												
Young	464	.23	21.33	6.89	1.06	1.84	16.02 32.03	22.47	6.81	0.76	1.72	16.13 34.04
Older	373	.24	23.07	12.63	1.23	2.24	14.30 38.41	24.65	8.52	0.88	1.49	17.85 37.11

† Female twins are 'first twin' in opposite-sex pairs.

Table 8.2: Polynomial regression of absolute intra-pair difference in BMI ($|\text{BMI}_{T1}-\text{BMI}_{T2}|$) on pair sum ($\text{BMI}_{T1} + \text{BMI}_{T2}$), sum^2, and sum^3. The multiple regression on these three quantities is shown for raw and log-transformed BMI scores.

Sample	Raw BMI R^2	Log BMI R^2
Young MZF	0.11***	0.04***
Older MZF	0.16***	0.06***
Young MZM	0.10***	0.04*
Older MZM	0.09***	0.03*
Young DZF	0.34***	0.15***
Older DZF	0.27***	0.12***
Young DZM	0.15***	0.06*
Older DZM	0.03	0.01

***$p < .001$; *$p < .05$.

2. Provide evidence for significant dominance genetic effects

3. Enable us to reject a purely environmental model

4. Indicate significant genotype × age-cohort interaction.

Skewness and kurtosis measures in Table 8.1 indicate substantial non-normality of the marginal distributions for raw BMI. We have also computed the polynomial regression of absolute intra-pair difference in BMI values on pair sum[1] separately for each like-sex twin group. These are summarized in Table 8.2. If the joint distribution of twin pairs for BMI is bivariate normal, these regressions should be non-significant. Here, however, we observe a highly significant regression: on average, pairs with high BMI values also exhibit larger intra-pair differences in BMI. This is likely to be an artefact of scale, since using a log-transformation substantially reduces the magnitude of the polynomial regression (as well as reducing marginal measures of skewness and kurtosis).

In general, variance-covariance matrices, not correlations, should be used for model-fitting analyses with continuously distributed variables such as Body Mass

---

[1]i.e. the unsigned difference between twin 1 and twin 2 of each pair, $|\text{BMI}_{\text{twin 1}} - \text{BMI}_{\text{twin 2}}|$ with $\text{BMI}_{\text{twin 1}} + \text{BMI}_{\text{twin 2}}$

Index. The simple genetic models we fit here predict no difference in variance between like-sex MZ and DZ twin pairs, but *the presence of such variance differences may indicate that the assumptions of the genetic model are violated.* This is an important point which we must consider it in some detail. To many researchers the opportunity to expose an assumption as false may seem like something to be avoided if possible. Why shouldn't we use a technique that will hide any such failure? For sure, if we fitted models to correlation matrices, variance differences would never be observed, but to do so would be like, in physics, breaking the thermometer if a temperature difference did not agree with the theory. Rather, we should look at failures of assumptions as opportunities in disguise; the opportunity can be to statistically control for the assumption, or to detect a novel effect. Further opportunities to develop new methods may also present themselves as 'problems' in data analysis.

To return to the task in hand, we present summary twin pair covariance matrices in Table 8.3. These statistics have been computed for 7 ln (BMI), and means have been computed as (7ln (BMI) − 21), to yield summary statistics with magnitudes of approximately unity. Rescaling the data in this way will often improve the efficiency of the optimization routines used in model-fitting analyses (Gill *et al.*, 1981).

8.3 Basic Genetic Model

Derivations of the expected variances and covariances of relatives under a simple univariate genetic model have been reviewed briefly in the chapters on biometrical genetics and path analysis (Chapters 3 and 5). In brief, from biometrical genetic theory we can write structural equations relating the phenotypes, P, of relatives i and j (e.g., BMI values of first and second members of twin pairs) to their underlying genotypes and environments which are latent variables whose influence we must infer. We may decompose the total genetic effect on a phenotype into contributions of:

- Additive effects of alleles at multiple loci (A),

- Dominance effects at multiple loci (D),

- Higher-order epistatic interactions between pairs of loci (additive × additive, additive × dominance, dominance × dominance: AA, AD, DD), and so on.

In practice even additive × dominance and dominance × dominance epistasis are confounded with dominance in studies of humans, and the power of resolving genetic dominance and additive × additive epistasis is very low. We shall therefore limit our consideration to additive and dominance genetic effects.

Similarly, we may decompose the total environmental effect into that due to environmental influences shared by twins or sibling pairs reared in the same family

Table 8.3: Covariances of Twin Pairs for Body Mass Index: 1981 Australian Survey. BMI $= 7 \times \ln(\text{kg}/(\text{m}^2))$.

	Young Cohort (< 30)		
	Covariance Matrix		Means[a]
	Twin 1	Twin 2	$\bar{x}'$
MZ female pairs	(N=534 pairs)		
Twin 1	0.7247	0.5891	0.3408
Twin 2	0.5891	0.7915	0.3510
DZ female pairs	(N=328 pairs)		
Twin 1	0.7786	0.2461	0.4444
Twin 2	0.2461	0.8365	0.4587
MZ male pairs	(N=251 pairs)		
Twin 1	0.5971	0.4475	0.6248
Twin 2	0.4475	0.5692	0.6378
DZ male pairs	(N=184 pairs)		
Twin 1	0.7191	0.2447	0.8079
Twin 2	0.2447	0.8179	0.7690
Opposite-sex pairs	(N=464 pairs)		
Female twin	0.6830	0.1533	0.3716
Male twin	0.1533	0.6631	0.7402

	Older Cohort (≥ 30)		
	Covariance Matrix		Means[a]
	Twin 1	Twin 2	$\bar{x}'$
MZ female pairs	(N=637 pairs)		
Twin 1	0.9759	0.6656	0.9087
Twin 2	0.6656	0.9544	0.8685
DZ female pairs	(N=380 pairs)		
Twin 1	0.9150	0.3124	0.8102
Twin 2	0.3124	1.0420	0.8576
MZ male pairs	(N=281 pairs)		
Twin 1	0.5445	0.4128	1.2707
Twin 2	0.4128	0.6431	1.2884
DZ male pairs	(N=137 pairs)		
Twin 1	0.6885	0.2378	1.2502
Twin 2	0.2378	0.5967	1.2281
Opposite-sex pairs	(N=373 pairs)		
Female twin	1.0363	0.1955	0.8922
Male twin	0.1955	0.6463	1.3860

[a] $\bar{x}' = \bar{x} - 21$.

(*shared, common,* or *between-family* environmental (C) effects), and that due to environmental effects which make family members differ from one another (*within-family, specific,* or *random environmental* (E) effects). Thus, the observed phenotypes, P_i and P_j, will be linear functions of the underlying additive genetic deviations (A_i and A_j), dominance genetic deviations (D_i and D_j), shared environmental deviations (C_i and C_j), and random environmental deviations (E_i and E_j). Assuming all variables are scaled as deviations from zero, we have

$$P_1 = e_1 E_1 + c_1 C_1 + a_1 A_1 + d_1 D_1$$
$$P_2 = e_2 E_2 + c_2 C_2 + a_2 A_2 + d_2 D_2 \qquad (8.1)$$

In most models we do not expect the magnitude of genetic effects, or the environmental effects, to differ between first and second twins, so we set $e_1 = e_2 = e, c_1 = c_2 = c, a_1 = a_2 = a, d_1 = d_2 = d$. Likewise, we do not expect the values of $e, c, a,$ and d to vary as a function of relationship. In other words, the effects of genotype and environment on the phenotype are the same regardless of whether one is an MZ twin, a DZ twin, or not a twin at all. In matrix form, we may write

$$
\begin{pmatrix} P_1 \\ P_2 \end{pmatrix} = \begin{pmatrix} a & c & e & d & 0 & 0 & 0 & 0 \\ 0 & 0 & 0 & 0 & a & c & e & d \end{pmatrix} \begin{pmatrix} A_1 \\ C_1 \\ E_1 \\ D_1 \\ A_2 \\ C_2 \\ E_2 \\ D_2 \end{pmatrix}
$$

which we can represent in the usual LISREL form as

$$\eta = \Gamma \xi .$$

Unless two or more waves of measurement are used, or several variables index the phenotype under study, residual effects (such as measurement error) will form part of the random environmental component, and are not explicitly included in the model.

To obtain estimates for the genetic and environmental effects in this model, we must also specify PHI (Φ), which is the matrix of variances and covariances among the latent genetic and environmental factors. Two alternative parameterizations are possible: 1) the variance components approach (Chapter 3), or 2) the path coefficients model (Chapter 5). The variance components approach becomes cumbersome for designs involving more complex pedigree structures than pairs of relatives, but it does have some numerical advantages (see Chapter 6, p. 122).

In the *variance components approach* we estimate variances of the latent non-shared and shared environmental and additive and dominance genetic variables, $V_E, V_C, V_A,$ or V_D, and fix $a = c = e = d = 1$. Thus, the phenotypic variance is simply the sum of the four variance components. In the *path coefficients approach* we standardize the variances of the latent variables to unity ($V_E = V_C = V_A = V_D =1$) and estimate a combination of $a, c, e,$ and d as free parameters. Thus, the phenotypic variance is a weighted sum of standardized variables. In this volume we refer often to models having various combinations of free parameters in the general path coefficients model. Specifically, we refer to an ACE model as one having only additive genetic, common environment, and random environment effects; an ADE model as one having additive genetic, dominance, and random environment effects; an AE model as one having additive genetic and random environment effects, and so on.

Figures 5.4a and 5.4b in Chapter 5 represent path diagrams for the two alternative parameterizations of the full basic genetic model, illustrated for the case of pairs of monozygotic twins (MZ) or dizygotic twins (DZ), who may be reared together (MZT, DZT) or reared apart (MZA, DZA). For simplicity, we make certain strong assumptions in this chapter, which are implied by the way we have drawn the path diagrams in Figure 5.4:

1. No genotype-environment correlation, i.e., latent genetic variables A are uncorrelated with latent environmental variables C and E;

2. No genotype × environment interaction, so that the observed phenotypes are a linear function of the underlying genetic and environmental variables;

3. Random mating, i.e., no tendency for like to marry like, an assumption which is implied by fixing the covariance of the additive genetic deviations of DZ twins or full sibs to $0.5V_A$;

4. Random placement of adoptees, so that the rearing environments of separated twin pairs are uncorrelated.

We discuss ways in which these assumptions may be relaxed in subsequent chapters, particularly Chapter 11 and Chapter 17.

8.4   LISREL 7 Example: Path Coefficients Model

With the introduction from the previous Sections and Chapters, we are now in a position to set up a simple genetic model using LISREL 7. The script in Appendix C.1 fits a simple univariate genetic model, estimating path coefficients, to covariance matrices for two like-sex twin groups: MZ twin pairs reared together, and DZ twin pairs reared together. The script is written to ignore information on means. The full path diagram is given in Figure 8.1 We have drawn this figure to correspond to the variables in the LISREL model. The latent genetic and environmental variables A, C, E and D are ξ variables that cause the η variables P_1 and P_2. In turn these are the only cause of the observed phenotypes Y_1 and Y_2. The script is written to fit a model with free parameters $e, a,$ and d, and fixing c to zero

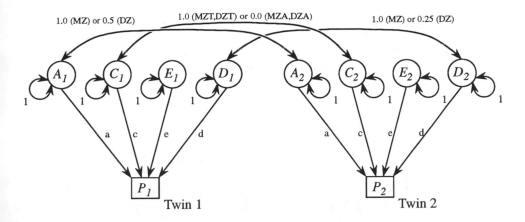

Figure 8.1: Univariate model for data from monozygotic (MZ) or dizygotic (DZ) twins reared together (T) or apart (A). Genetic and environmental latent variables cause the phenotypes P_1 and P_2, which in turn cause the observed variables Y_1 and Y_2

— implying that there are no effects of shared environment on Body Mass Index. The script is extensively documented using the comment facility in LISREL 7: any line beginning with a semi-colon is interpreted as a comment. We shall consider this first example LISREL script in detail. Please note that reading this section is *not* a substitute for reading in detail the LISREL 7 manual (Jöreskog and Sörbom, 1989), but merely a quick introduction to the essentials of a LISREL script for genetic applications.

8.4.1 Building a LISREL 7 script

Each new control statement in a script begins on a new line. For each twin group, we will have the following sequence of control lines:

1. Title — as many as 79 characters (or more than one record if the 80th column is not blank)

2. Data-parameters line

3. Input data control lines

4. Model control lines

5. Output control line

Control statements can be abbreviated to the first two letters (e.g., DA, MO, OU). Any record beginning with a semi-colon is interpreted by LISREL 7 as a comment line. In addition to allowing documentation of the script, the semi-colon permits us to include expressions for alternative models (e.g., with or without additive genetic effects) in the same script. We shall now examine the control lines in greater detail, focusing on our BMI model.

- *Title line*

  `Analysis of Australian BMI data-young female MZ twins pairs`

  A new title line must be given at the start of each twin group. If the 80th column of the record is not blank, LISREL expects the next record to contain a continuation of the title.

- *Data-parameter line*

  `DA NG=2 NI=2 NO=534 MA=CM`

  where:

  1. NG is number of groups. The default is 1; this parameter is specified for the first group only

  2. NI is number of input variables, i.e., $2n$, if there are n variables assessed for each member of a twin pair

  3. NO is number of observations or sample size, i.e., number of pairs used to compute the data matrix in the first group

  4. MA is the type of matrix to be used for data analysis, e.g.,
     (a) MA=CM — covariance matrix (default)
     (b) MA=KM — correlation matrix (product-moment correlation)
     (c) MA=PM — matrix including polychoric and polyserial correlations.

- *Input data control lines — variable names*

  `LA`
  `BMI-Tw1 BMI-Tw2`

  LISREL allows the user the option of reading a list of names for the observed variables (y-variables, and x-variables if any). This is *very* useful for clarification of the LISREL output.

- *Input control lines — reading covariance or correlation matrices*
  LISREL will read a covariance matrix (CM), a correlation matrix (KM), or a moment matrix (MM). The matrix may be read as a full matrix (FU), or as a lower triangle (SY – new line for each row), or as a lower triangle in free format (the default). It will also read means (ME) and standard deviations (SD) when these are needed. The matrix which LISREL reads need not be the same as the matrix which is analyzed (determined by the DA line). Summary statistics can be read from within the LISREL script, for example,

```
CM SY
0.7247
0.5891 0.7915
```

Alternatively, the data matrices can be read from separate files, e.g.,

```
CM SY FI=ozbmimzf.mat
```

- *Model control lines — Specifying the number of variables*

  - NY – gives the number of y-variables ($2n$ in most univariate models)
  - NE – gives the number of Eta, η, or endogenous (dEpendent) variables, again $2n$ in most simple cases
  - NK – gives the number of ksI, ξ, or exogenous (Independent) variables
  - NX – gives the number of x-variables, which is zero in most simple applications to twin data

  x–variables are used to simplify specification in certain applications such as those involving twins and parents (see Chapter 17).

  Thus, for the model illustrated in Figure 8.1, we have:

```
MO NY=2 NX=0 NE=2 NK=8 . . .
```

- *Model control lines - latent variable names* It is useful to label the latent variables in the model, as well as the observed. This can be done with the LE (label eta) and LK (label ksi) commands.

- *Model control lines - the PHI matrix*

  The PHi (Φ) matrix is an NK × NK symmetric matrix (SY) which is used to specify the covariances and variances of our exogenous variables (or correlations, in the case of standardized variables). We have already shown these quantities in our path diagram [remembering that the variances of the exogenous variables in Figure 8.1 are unity, so all unidirectional loops (two-headed arrows from a variable to itself) have been omitted]. LISREL allows the elements of the Φ matrix to be either fixed values (e.g., 1 or .5 for the correlation between the additive genotypes of MZ or DZ pairs; or 0) or free parameters whose values are to be estimated. In our applications most of the elements of Φ are fixed (FI), so we set this to be the default on the model line for each twin group:

        MO NY=2 NX=0 NE=2 NK=6 PH=SY,FI . . .

By default, LISREL assumes all fixed values are zero. Later in the LISREL script we give the fixed values for the Φ matrix for MZ pairs (lower triangle only, since the matrix is symmetric) using

MA PH
1.00
0.00 1.00
etc.

The same process is repeated for the second, DZ twin group — the diagonal elements of the Φ matrix are the same, but whereas the off-diagonal elements $\phi(6,2)$, $\phi(7,3)$, and $\phi(8,4)$ [corresponding to the covariances of shared environment effects (C1 and C2), additive genetic effects (A1 and A2) and dominance genetic effects (D1 and D2)] are all unity in MZ pairs, in DZ pairs they are 1.0, 0.5, and 0.25, respectively.

- *Model control lines: Setting up the GAMMA matrix*

The GAmma matrix (Γ) is an NE $\times$ NK matrix which is used to represent paths from the Independent (ksI) variables to the dEpendent (Eta) variables. Most of the model parameters that we wish to estimate are contained in this matrix. In example 1, we have designated this a full matrix of fixed parameters (GA=FU,FI) on the model line, as this is usually most convenient. For the first group, on the model statement, we will have:

MO NY=2 NX=0 NE=2 NK=8 PH=SY,FI GA=FU,FI. . .

The ij^{th} element of Γ gives the path coefficient from the jth independent variable to the ith dependent variables. Thus, from Figure 8.1, the elements of Γ for the first group that we wish to estimate are:

$$\begin{array}{cccccccc} a & c & e & d & 0 & 0 & 0 & 0 \\ 0 & 0 & 0 & 0 & a & c & e & d \end{array}$$

We use a PAttern statement to tell LISREL which of these parameters we wish to estimate — a, d, and e in the present application — (indicated by 1s), and which we wish to be fixed (indicated by 0s):

```
PA GA
1 0 1 1 0 0 0 0
0 0 0 0 1 0 1 1
```

We have commented out pattern statements for other models, so that one can fit alternative models simply by placing a ';' at the beginning of the pattern statements for the "ADE model", and removing the ';' at the beginning of the pattern statement for another model. Path coefficients a, c, e, and d are expected to be the same in first and second twins from like-sex pairs. Therefore, we include in the script, after the pattern statement, a series of EQuality statements to equate the appropriate elements of the GAmma matrix for all models:

```
EQ GA(1,1) GA(2,5)
EQ GA(1,2) GA(2,6)
EQ GA(1,3) GA(2,7)
EQ GA(1,4) GA(2,8)
```

Path coefficients also should be the same in MZ and DZ twin groups — the only difference between the path diagrams for MZ and DZ pairs in Figure 8.1 are the different covariances of the additive and dominance genetic deviations. To specify this similarity in our model, we set the GAmma matrix for the second group (DZ pairs) to be INvariant, i.e., equal to the GAmma matrix for the first group:

```
MO NY=2 NX=0 NE=2 NK=8 PH=SY,FI GA=IN
```

In the simple example of Figure 8.1 we make all the matrices for the second group invariant *except* the Φ matrix.

- *Model control lines: Setting up the BETA matrix and other matrices*

  The BEta (B) matrix is an NE × NE matrix which is used to represent paths between dependent variables. The ij^{th} element of B is used to represent the path from the jth dependent variable to the ith dependent variable. In the model of Figure 8.1 there is no direct path from P1 to P2, or from P2 to P1. Thus, all the elements of B will be zero, which we can tell LISREL with the keyword BE=ZE (this is the default setting). If this were not the case, we could declare it a full, fixed matrix (BE=FU,FI) and use a pattern statement and equality statements to free the appropriate elements of the matrix in the same way as in the case of the GAmma (Γ) matrix. Likewise, the PSi (Ψ) matrix and TE (theta-epsilon; Θ_ϵ) matrices are zero; since we have only a single measurement on each twin, it is not possible to separate out measurement error effects from random environmental effects. The one-to-one mapping of η variables onto y variables is represented by setting lambda-Y (Λ_y) to an identity matrix (LY=ID). Thus, our full model line for the simple univariate genetic model is:

```
MO NY=2 NX=0 NE=2 NK=6 PH=SY,FI GA=FU,FR LY=ID PS=ZE TE=ZE BE=ZE
```

Because we have fixed the number of x variables to zero, matrices LX (lambda-x; Λ_x) and TD (theta-delta; Θ_δ) also default to zero. We have specified no mean vectors on the model line, so these all default to zero as well.

- *Model control statements: Assignment of starting values to free parameters*

In genetic problems, we must assign starting values to parameters. In the present case, the only parameters to be estimated are in the Γ matrix. We can do this by using a MA GA command followed by the matrix of values for the Γ matrix (just as we did to assign fixed values to the Φ matrix); or, more conveniently, we can assign the same starting value to all the free parameters:

```
START .6 GA(1,1)-GA(2,8)
```

In choosing starting values for twin data, a useful rule of thumb is to assume that the total variance is divided equally between the parameters that are to be estimated. In this case the predicted total variance is $3 \times .6^2 = 1.08$ which is close to the observed total variance in these data. For other data, other starting values may be required. Good starting values can save a significant amount of computer time, whereas bad starting values may cause any optimizer to fail to find a global minimum, or to hit a maximum number of iterations before converging.

- *Output control statements*

The OUtput statement controls the type of estimation procedure that is used and the amount of information that LISREL prints when it has found a solution. Usually, the choice of estimation procedure will be either maximum likelihood (ME=ML is the default) if covariance matrices are being analyzed, or weighted least squares (ME=WLS or ME=DWLS) if matrices of polychoric, polyserial, or product-moment correlations are being analyzed. The parameter NS forces LISREL to use the user-defined values as starting values, rather than computing its own initial estimates. LISREL's automatic starting values don't work for multiple group genetic problems in which the number of ξ variables (NK) is greater than the number of observed variables (NY + NX). The instruction AD=OFF instructs LISREL not to perform an admissibility test which assesses whether the Φ matrix is positive-definite: in genetic models such as Figure 8.1 it is not expected to be! It is critical that AD=OFF is included — otherwise LISREL will terminate model-fitting before it has found a solution. By default, LISREL prints the

1. User's input script
2. Parameter specifications
3. Matrix or matrices to be analyzed
4. Starting values (LISREL 7 only)
5. Estimates at the solution
6. Measures of overall goodness-of-fit.

Other useful output can be requested by additional parameters on the OU line, including:

- SE – print standard errors
- TV – print t-values
- PC – print correlations of estimates
- RS – print expected covariance matrix and matrix of residuals
- SC – print completely standardized solution (LISREL 7.16 and higher)
- EF – print total effects and indirect effects (this is needed only when we are also estimating some of the elements of the beta matrix as free parameters, e.g., in models incorporating sibling effects, where we wish to examine whether the 'stability index' is less than unity, as will be discussed later)
- TM=xx – set time limit of xx seconds for problem (default: $xx = 1200$ seconds)
- ND=x – set number of decimals in printed output ($0 < x < 8$, default: $x = 3$) — useful for simulation work.
- IT=xx – set maximum number of iterations for problem (default: $xx = 3 \times$ the number of free parameters).

The LISREL 7 manual should be consulted for a full description of the output options. For now we keep the OU line relatively simple, since the volume of output can become quite overwhelming when many options are invoked.

```
OU NS SE IT=500 AD=OFF
```

8.4.2   Interpreting LISREL 7 Output

We can run the example of Appendix C.1 on a personal computer with LISREL 7 installed by typing:

```
lisrel7 univar.l7 univar.ou7
```

where univar.l7 is the name of the script file, and univar.ou7 is the name of the output file. We recommend l7 and ou7 as file extensions to make LISREL 7 input and output distinct from input and output of other programs such as PRELIS or LISREL 8. This example fits a model allowing for random environmental effects, additive genetic effects, and dominance genetic effects, to the young female like-sex MZ and DZ covariance matrices for log-transformed BMI. The LISREL 7 output includes:

1. Listing of the LISREL script.

2. Numbers of variables, sample size, and observed covariance matrix for each group.

3. Parameter specification matrices for each group, indicating the parameters to be estimated, e.g.,

GAMMA

	A1	C1	E1	D1	A2	C2
P1	1	0	2	3	0	0
P2	0	0	0	0	1	0

GAMMA

	E2	D2
P1	0	0
P2	2	3

where 1 identifies the first free parameter to be estimated (a), 2 identifies parameter e, and 3 identifies parameter d. It is important to check these to confirm that parameters have been correctly constrained to be equal between first and second twins from MZ and DZ twin groups, and that the total number of estimated parameters corresponds to the number of free parameters in the model to be fitted.

4. Starting values of parameters for each group.

5. Under the heading LISREL ESTIMATES for the first group (i.e., MZ twin pairs in our case) the parameter estimates obtained at the solution are printed, together with a warning message if model fitting has not converged. In the case of Appendix C.1, for example, we obtain

GAMMA

	A1	C1	E1	D1	A2	C2
P1	0.56207	0.00000	0.41193	0.54409	0.00000	0.0000

```
P2      0.00000   0.00000   0.00000   0.00000   0.56207   0.0000
GAMMA
               E2        D2

           --------  --------
P1      0.00000   0.00000
P2      0.41193   0.54409
```

In other words, our maximum-likelihood parameter estimates are $a = 0.56$, $d = 0.54$, and $e = 0.41$ for these data.

6. If we put the keyword RS on the OUtput line, the expected ('fitted') covariance matrix and residuals appear; standard errors appear if we include the keyword SE. Comparison of models should normally be based on likelihood-ratio chi-squared tests, since significance tests based on standard errors will be misleading for this example (Neale *et al.*, 1989b). However, extremely large standard errors may indicate an attempt to fit an underidentified model.

7. Whichever options are requested in the first group are automatically included for every group, so parameter estimates, their standard errors, t-values are repeated for the second (DZ) group, although in this analysis they are constrained to be the same as for the MZ group. Likewise, the observed and expected covariance matrix and residuals are given for this group; these, however, usually differ from those of the first group.

8. The goodness-of-fit chi-squared is reported. In this example, $\chi_3^2 = 3.71, p = 0.29$, indicating that the model gives a good fit to the data.

9. If we have requested PC on the output line, the correlations between parameter estimates are reported. In this example, the correlations between our estimates of e and a (0.09) and between e and d (-0.14) are quite modest, but there is a substantial negative correlation between our estimates of additive and dominance genetic effects (-0.98). This confirms the relatively poor power of twin data for resolving additive and nonadditive genetic effects.

10. Finally, standardized parameter estimates are reported for each group:

```
GAMMA
           A1        C1        E1        D1        A2        C2

       --------  --------  --------  --------  --------  --------
P1      0.63575   0.00000   0.46593   0.61541   0.00000   0.00000
P2      0.00000   0.00000   0.00000   0.00000   0.63575   0.00000
GAMMA
               E2        D2

           --------  --------
P1      0.00000   0.00000
P2      0.46593   0.61541
```

These give parameter estimates restandardized to give a total phenotypic variance of unity: $a = 0.64$, $e = 0.47$, and $d = 0.62$. Squaring these numbers gives the proportion of the total variance in BMI which is accounted for by by additive genetic effects (40.4%), random environmental effects (21.7%), and by dominance genetic effects (37.9%). These analyses suggest that in young women age 30 and under, additive and non-additive genetic factors account for approximately 78% of the variance in Body Mass Index.

Discussion of these results continues in Section 8.6.

8.5   LISREL 8 Example: The Variance Components Model

We include the variance components parameterization of the basic structural equation model for completeness. It will not be developed and applied in as great detail as the path coefficients parameterization because (i) it is difficult to generalize to more complex pedigree structures or multivariate problems, and (ii) doing so would contribute much by weight but little by insight to this volume. Readers seeking an easy introduction to twin models in LISREL may skip this section and focus their attention on Section 8.4, the path coefficients parameterization.

For MZ and DZ twin pairs reared in the same family, elements of the Φ matrix in the variance components parameterization (Figure 5.4a) will be:

$$\Phi_{MZ} = \begin{bmatrix} V_E & 0 & 0 & 0 & 0 & 0 & 0 & 0 \\ 0 & V_C & 0 & 0 & 0 & V_C & 0 & 0 \\ 0 & 0 & V_A & 0 & 0 & 0 & V_A & 0 \\ 0 & 0 & 0 & V_D & 0 & 0 & 0 & V_D \\ 0 & 0 & 0 & 0 & V_E & 0 & 0 & 0 \\ 0 & V_C & 0 & 0 & 0 & V_C & 0 & 0 \\ 0 & 0 & V_A & 0 & 0 & 0 & V_A & 0 \\ 0 & 0 & 0 & V_D & 0 & 0 & 0 & V_D \end{bmatrix} \tag{8.2}$$

and

$$\Phi_{DZ} = \begin{bmatrix} V_E & 0 & 0 & 0 & 0 & 0 & 0 & 0 \\ 0 & V_C & 0 & 0 & 0 & V_C & 0 & 0 \\ 0 & 0 & V_A & 0 & 0 & 0 & .5V_A & 0 \\ 0 & 0 & 0 & V_D & 0 & 0 & 0 & .25V_D \\ 0 & 0 & 0 & 0 & V_E & 0 & 0 & 0 \\ 0 & V_C & 0 & 0 & 0 & V_C & 0 & 0 \\ 0 & 0 & .5V_A & 0 & 0 & 0 & V_A & 0 \\ 0 & 0 & 0 & .25V_D & 0 & 0 & 0 & V_D \end{bmatrix} \tag{8.3}$$

Corresponding Φ matrices for the standardized case can be derived from these by fixing $V_E + V_C + V_A + V_D = 1$. When we have only cross-sectional univariate twin data, no information is available about measurement error, so we specify Λ_y as an identity matrix and the Θ_ϵ matrix as a zero matrix. We can derive the expected covariance matrix for the ith group of relatives as $\Lambda_y \Gamma \Phi \Gamma' \Lambda_y'$. Under the simplifying assumptions of the present chapter, the 2×2 expected covariance matrix of twin pairs (Σ) will be, in terms of variance components,

$$\left[\begin{array}{cc} V_E + V_C + V_A + V_D & \omega_i V_C + \alpha_i V_A + \delta_i V_D \\ \omega_i V_C + \alpha_i V_A + \delta_i V_D & V_E + V_C + V_A + V_D \end{array} \right]$$

where ω_i is 1 for twins, full sibs or adoptees reared in the same household, but 0 for separated twins or other biological relatives reared apart; α_i is 1 for MZ twin pairs, 0.5 for DZ pairs, full sibs, or parents and offspring, and 0 for genetically unrelated individuals; and δ_i is 1 for MZ pairs, 0.25 for DZ pairs or full sibs, and 0 for most other relationships. In terms of path coefficients, we need only substitute $V_E = e^2$, $V_C = c^2$, $V_A = h^2$, and $V_D = d^2$.

In data on twin pairs reared together the effects of shared environment and genetic dominance are confounded. If both additive genetic effects and shared environmental effects contribute to variation in a trait, the covariance of DZ twin pairs will be less than the MZ covariance, but greater than one-half the MZ covariance. If both additive genetic effects and dominance genetic effects contribute to variation in a trait, the covariance of DZ pairs will be less than one-half the MZ covariance. In terms of variance components, therefore, a substantial dominance genetic effect will lead to a negative estimate of the shared environmental variance component, if a model allowing for additive genetic and shared environmental variance components is fitted; while conversely a substantial shared environmental effect will lead to a negative estimate of the dominance genetic variance component, if a model allowing for additive and dominance genetic variance components is fitted (Martin *et al.*, 1978). In terms of path coefficients, however, since we are estimating parameters c or d, c^2 or d^2 can never take negative values, and so we will obtain an estimate of $c = 0$ in the presence of dominance, or $d = 0$ in the presence of shared environmental effects. Additional data on separated twin pairs (Jinks and Fulker, 1970) or on the parents or other relatives of twins (Fulker, 1982; Heath, 1983) are needed to resolve the effects of shared environment and genetic dominance when both are present.

8.5.1 Building a LISREL 8 Script

Appendix C.2 illustrates an example script for fitting a variance components model to twin pair covariance matrices for two like-sex twin pair groups. In this example, we fix elements of the Γ matrix $e = c = a = d = 1$, and estimate additive genetic, dominance genetic and random environmental variance components in the Φ matrix. The model line is the same as for the path model example, but we now use a MAtrix statement to assign fixed values to the Γ matrix

MA GA

```
1 1 1 1 0 0 0 0
0 0 0 0 1 1 1 1
```

and use a PAttern statement to identify free parameters in the Φ matrix:

```
PA PH
2
0 0
0 0 3
0 0 0 4
0 0 0 0 2
0 0 0 0 0 0
0 0 3 0 0 0 3
0 0 0 4 0 0 0 4
```

A new feature is that we identify free parameters by number (1 is still used in its traditional LISREL sense of identifying any free parameter, and so cannot be used here), making much simpler the task of equating parameters between first and second twins[2]. In this example, parameter '2' corresponds to the random environmental variance component, parameter '3' to the additive genetic variance component, and parameter '4' to the dominance genetic variance component. In the DZ twin group, we must constrain elements $\phi(7,3) = 0.5V_A$ and element $\phi(8,4) = 0.25V_D$. This cannot be achieved directly in LISREL 7, but LISREL 8 will handle constraints of this form[3]:

```
CO PH(7,3)=0.5*PH(1,7,3)
CO PH(8,4)=0.25*PH(1,8,4)
```

Finally, it should be noted that we set the Φ matrix to be invariant for the DZ group, and then override this for certain elements of the Φ matrix using EQuality and COnstraint statements.

8.5.2 Interpreting LISREL 8 Output

If a personal computer has LISREL 8 installed, we can run the example variance components script of Appendix C.2, by typing

```
LISREL8 varcomp.18 varcomp.ou8
```

where the example script has been copied to the file varcomp.18. This model fits to the covariance matrices for young male like-sex MZ and DZ twin pairs a model estimating random environmental, additive genetic, and dominance genetic variance components. LISREL 8 output follows basically the same format as for LISREL 7, with a few exceptions:

---

[2] This option is not available in LISREL 7 or earlier versions.

[3] See Chapter 17 for a description of constraint specification in LISREL 8.

1. Under the PARAMETER SPECIFICATIONS output, some parameters may now be constrained and are listed as such, e.g., for the second DZ group we have:

PARAMETER SPECIFICATIONS

PHI

	E1	C1	A1	D1	E2	C2
E1	1					
C1	0	0				
A1	0	0	2			
D1	0	0	0	3		
E2	0	0	0	0	1	
C2	0	0	0	0	0	
A2	0	0	Constr'd	0	0	0
D2	0	0	0	Constr'd	0	0

PHI

	A2	D2
A2	2	
D2	0	3

2. By default, starting values are not printed

3. Parameter estimates and their standard errors and t-values are output together. In our example, the estimated parameter values are contained in the Φ matrix (of which we reproduce only the first few rows):

PHI

	E1	C1	A1	D1
E1	.13810			
	(.01231)			
	11.21747			
C1	.00000	.00000		
A1	.00000	.00000	.24780	
			(.18280)	
			1.35561	
D1	.00000	.00000	.00000	.29450
				(.17877)
				1.64738

For the young male like-sex pairs, we estimate $V_E = 0.14$, $V_A = 0.25$, and $V_D = 0.29$. We must compute standardized variance components by hand, as $V_E^* = V_E/V_P$, $V_A^* = V_A/V_P$, and $V_D^* = V_D/V_P$, where $V_P = V_E + V_A + V_D = 0.6804$ (which can be read directly from the variance in the expected covariance matrix). In this example, random environmental effects account for 20.3% of the variance, additive genetic effects for 36.4% of the variance, and dominance genetic effects for 43.3% of the variance of Body Mass Index in young adult males. As before, we caution that standard errors should not be used to test the significance of individual variance components.

4. A much broader range of goodness-of-fit statistics are reported. By chi-squared test of goodness-of-fit, our model gives only a marginally acceptable fit to the data ($\chi_3^2 = 7.28, p = 0.06$).

8.6   Interpreting Results of Model-fitting

In model-fitting to univariate twin data, whether we use a variance components or a path coefficients model, we are essentially testing the following hypotheses:

1. No family resemblance ("E" model: $e > 0$, $a = c = d = 0$)

2. Family resemblance solely due to additive genetic effects ("AE" model: $a > 0, e > 0, c = d = 0$)

3. Family resemblance solely due to shared environmental effects ("CE" model: $e > 0, c > 0, a = d = 0$)

4. Family resemblance due to additive genetic plus dominance genetic effects ("ADE" model: $a > 0, d > 0, e > 0, c = 0$)

5. Family resemblance due to additive genetic plus shared environmental effects ("ACE" model: $a > 0, c > 0, e > 0, d = 0$).

Note that we never fit a model that excludes random environmental effects, because it predicts perfect MZ twin pair correlations, which in turn generate a singular expected covariance matrix[4]. From inspection of the twin pair correlations for BMI, we noted that they were most consistent with a model allowing for additive genetic, dominance genetic, and random environmental effects. Model-fitting gives three important advantages at this stage:

1. An overall test of the goodness of fit of the model

2. A test of the relative goodness of fit of different models, as assessed by likelihood-ratio χ^2. For example, we can test whether the fit is significantly worse if we omit genetic dominance for BMI

---

[4] A singular matrix cannot be inverted (see Chapter 4) and, therefore, the maximum likelihood loss function (see Chapter 7) cannot be computed.

Table 8.4: Results of fitting models to twin pairs covariance matrices for Body Mass Index: Two-group analyses, complete pairs only.

	Females				Males			
	Young		Older		Young		Older	
Model (d.f.)	χ^2	p	χ^2	p	χ^2	p	χ^2	p
CE (4)	160.72	<.001	87.36	<.001	97.20	<.001	37.14	<.001
AE (4)	8.06	.09	2.38	.67	10.88	.03	5.03	.28
ACE (3)	8.06	<.05	2.38	.50	10.88	.01	5.03	.17
ADE (3)	3.71	.29	1.97	.58	7.28	.06	5.03	.17

3. Maximum-likelihood parameter estimates under the best-fitting model.

Table 8.4 tabulates goodness-of-fit chi-squares obtained in four separate analyses of the data from younger or older, female or male like-sex twin pairs. Let us consider the results for young females first. The non-genetic model (CE) yields a chi-squared of 160.72 for 4 degrees of freedom[5], which is highly significant and implies a very poor fit to the data indeed. In stark contrast, the alternative model of additive genes and random environment (AE) is not rejected by the data, but fits moderately well ($p = .09$). Adding common environmental effects (the ACE model) does not improve the fit whatsoever, but the loss of a degree of freedom makes the χ^2 significant at the .05 level. Finally, the ADE model which substitutes genetic dominance for common environmental effects, fits the best according to the probability level. We can test whether the dominance variation is significant by using the likelihood ratio test. The difference between the χ^2 of a general model (χ_G^2) and the that of a submodel (χ_S^2) is itself a χ^2 and has $df_S - df_G$ degrees of freedom (where subscripts S and G respectively refer to the submodel and general model. In this case, comparing the AE and the ADE model gives a likelihood ratio χ^2 of $8.06 - 3.71 = 4.35$ with $4 - 3 = 1df$. This is significant at the .05 level, so we say that there is significant deterioration in the fit of the model when the parameter d is fixed to zero, or simply that the parameter d is significant.

Now we are in a position to compare the results of model-fitting in females and males, and in young and older. In each case, a non-genetic (CE) model yields a significant chi-squared, implying a very poor fit to the data: the deviations of the observed covariance matrices from the expected covariance matrices under the maximum-likelihood parameter estimates are highly significant. In all groups, a

---

[5] The degrees of freedom associated with this test are calculated as the difference between the number of observed statistics (n_s) and the number of estimated parameters (n_p) in the model. Our data consist of two variances and a covariance for each of the MZ and DZ groups, giving $n_s = 6$ in total. The CE model has two parameters c and e, so $n_s - n_p = 6 - 2 = 4df$.

Table 8.5: Standardized parameter estimates under best-fitting model. Two-group analyses, complete pairs only.

	Estimate			
	a^2	c^2	e^2	d^2
Young females	0.40	0	0.22	0.38
Older females	0.69	0	0.31	0
Young males	0.36	0	0.20	0.44
Older males	0.70	0	0.30	0

full model allowing for additive plus dominance genetic effects and random environmental effects (ADE) gives an acceptable fit to the data, although in the case of young males the fit is somewhat marginal. In the two older cohorts, however, a model which allows for only additive genetic plus random environmental effects (AE) does *not* give a significantly worse fit than the full (ADE) model, by likelihood-ratio χ^2 test. In older females, for example, the likelihood-ratio chi-square is $2.38 - 1.97 = 0.41$, with degrees of freedom equal to $4 - 3 = 1$, i.e., $\chi_1^2 = 0.41$ with probability $p = 0.52$; while in older males we have $\chi_1^2 = 0.00, p = 1.00$. For the older cohorts, therefore, we find no significant evidence for genetic dominance. In young adults, however, significant dominance is observed in females (as noted above) and the dominance genetic effect is almost significant in males ($\chi_1^2 = 3.6, p = 0.06$).

Table 8.5 summarizes variance component estimates under the best-fitting models. We note that random environment accounts for a relatively modest proportion of the total variation in BMI, but appears to be having a larger effect in older than in younger individuals (30-31% versus 20-22%). Although the estimate of the narrow heritability (i.e., proportion of the total variance accounted for by additive genetic factors) is higher in the older cohort (69-70% vs 36-40%), the broad heritability (additive plus non-additive genetic variance) is higher in the young twins (78-80%).

8.7   Testing the Equality of Means

Applications of structural equation modeling to twin and other family data typically tend to ignore means. That is, observed measures are treated as deviations from the phenotypic mean (and are thus termed *deviation phenotypes*)[6], and likewise genotypic and environmental latent variables are expressed as deviations from

---

[6]Except where explicitly noted, all models presented in this text treat observed variables as deviation phenotypes.

their means, which usually are assumed to be 0. Most simple genetic models predict the same mean for different groups of relatives, so, for example, MZ twins, DZ twins, males from opposite-sex twin pairs, and males from like-sex twin pairs should have (within sampling error) equal means. Where significant mean differences are found, they may indicate sampling problems with respect to the variable under study or other violations of the assumptions of the basic genetic model. Testing for mean differences also may be important in follow-up studies, where we are concerned about the bias introduced by sample attrition, but can compare mean scores at baseline for those relatives who remain in a study with those who drop out. Fortunately, LISREL facilitates tests for mean differences between groups.

LISREL defines four parameter vectors for means: α, τ_x, τ_y, for η, x, and y variables (which we have already encountered in Chapter 5); plus κ, the vector of means for the ξ variables. These vectors are fixed to zero by default, but can be included explicitly by naming them on the LISREL MOdel statement. The predicted mean of η may be derived (Jöreskog and Sörbom, 1989) as

$$\mathcal{E}(\eta) = (\mathbf{I} - \mathbf{B})^{-1}(\alpha + \boldsymbol{\Gamma}\kappa)$$

with corresponding predicted means for the x and y variables

$$\mathcal{E}(\mathbf{x}) = \tau_x + \boldsymbol{\Lambda}_x\kappa$$

and

$$\mathcal{E}(\mathbf{y}) = \tau_y + \boldsymbol{\Lambda}_y(\mathbf{I} - \mathbf{B})^{-1}(\alpha + \boldsymbol{\Gamma}\kappa),$$

where $\mathcal{E}(\mathbf{y})$ means the *expected value* of y. In simple univariate problems where we wish to test equality of means between twin groups, we shall use τ_y for this purpose, fixing the other mean vectors to zero.

Appendix C.3 contains a LISREL 7 script for fitting a univariate genetic model which also estimates the means of first and second twins from MZ and DZ pairs. The first change we make is to feed LISREL the observed means in our sample, which we do with the ME command:

```
ME
0.9087 0.8685
```

Second, we revise the model statement:

```
MO NY=2 NE=2 NK=8 GA=FI LY=ID PH=FI PS=ZE TE=ZE TY=FI AL=ZE KA=ZE
```

with the MZ twin means declared as free parameters and equated between first and second twins

```
FR TY(1,1) TY(2,2)
EQ TY(1,1) TY(2,2)
```

Table 8.6: Results of fitting models to twin pair covariance matrices and twin means for Body Mass index: Two-group analyses, complete pairs only.

| | | Female | | | | Male | | | |
| | | Young | | Older | | Young | | Older | |
Model	df	χ^2	p	χ^2	p	χ^2	p	χ^2	p
1. No heterogeneity									
of means	6	7.84	.25	5.74	.57	12.81	.05	5.69	.58
2. Heterogeneity									
MZ vs DZ	5	3.93	.56	4.75	.58	7.72	.17	5.36	.50
3. Heterogeneity									
MZ/DZ & T1/T2	3	3.71	.29	2.38	.67	7.28	.06	5.03	.17
Genetic Model		ADE		AE*		ADE		AE*	

* AE models have one more degree of freedom than shown in the df column

In the DZ group we also supply the observed means, and adjust the model statement. We can then either (i) equate the mean for MZ twins to that for DZ twins using the EQ command:

EQ TY(1,1,1) TY(1,1) TY(2,2)

to fit a *no heterogeneity* model; or (ii) equate DZ twin 1 and DZ twin 2 means but allow them to differ from the MZ means:

EQ TY(1,1,1) TY(1,1) TY(2,2)

to fit a zygosity dependent means model ($\overline{MZ} \neq \overline{DZ}$); or (iii) estimate four means, i.e., first and second twins in each of the MZ and DZ groups. This third option gives a perfect fit to the data with regard to mean structure, so that the only contribution to the fit function comes from the covariance structure. Hence the four means model gives the same goodness-of-fit χ^2 as in the analyses ignoring means.

   Table 8.6 reports the results of fitting models incorporating means to the like-sex twin pair data on BMI. In each analysis, we have considered only the best-fitting genetic model identified in the analyses ignoring means. Again we subtract the χ^2 of a more general model from the χ^2 of a more restricted model to get a likelihood ratio test of the difference in fit between the two. For the two older cohorts we find no evidence for mean differences either between zygosity groups or between first and second twins. That is, the model that assumes no heterogeneity of means (model 1) does not give a significantly worse fit than either (i) estimating separate MZ and DZ means (model 2), or (ii) estimating 4 means. For older females, likelihood-ratio chi-squares are $\chi_1^2 = 0.99, p = 0.32$ and $\chi_3^2 = 3.36, p = 0.34$; and for older males,

$\chi_1^2 = 0.36, p = 0.55$ and $\chi_3^2 = 0.43, p = 0.33$. Maximum-likelihood estimates of mean log BMI in the older cohort are, respectively, 21.87 and 22.26 for females and males; estimates of genetic and environmental parameters are unchanged from those obtained in the analyses ignoring means. In the younger cohorts, however, we do find significant mean differences between zygosity groups, both in females ($\chi_1^2 = 3.91, p < 0.05$) and in males ($\chi_1^2 = 5.09, p < 0.02$). In both sexes, mean log BMI values are lower in MZ pairs (21.35 for females, 21.63 for males) than for DZ pairs (21.45 for females, 21.79 for males). As these data are not age-corrected, it is possible that BMI values are still changing in this age-group, and that the zygosity difference reflects a slight mean difference in age. We shall return to this question in Section 8.9.

8.8   Incorporating Data from Singleton Twins

In most twin studies, there are many twin pairs in which only one twin agrees to cooperate. We call these pairs *discordant-participant* as opposed to *concordant-participant* pairs, in which data are collected from both members of the pair. Sadly, data from discordant-participant pairs are often just thrown away. This is unfortunate not only because of the wasted effort on the part of the twins, researchers, and data entry personnel, but also because they provide valuable information about the representativeness of the sample for the variable under study. If sampling is satisfactory, then we would expect to find the same mean and variance in concordant-participant pairs as in discordant-participant pairs. Thus, the presence of mean differences or variance differences between these groups is an indication that biased sampling may have occurred with respect to the variable under investigation. To take a concrete example, suppose that overweight twins are less likely to respond to a mailed questionnaire survey. Given the strong twin pair resemblance for BMI demonstrated in previous sections, we might expect to find that individuals from discordant-participant pairs are on average heavier than individuals from concordant-participant pairs. Such sampling biases will have differential effects on the covariances of MZ and DZ twin pairs, and thus may lead to biased estimates of genetic and environmental parameters (Lykken *et al.*, 1987; Neale *et al.*, 1989b).

Table 8.7 reports means and variances for transformed BMI from individuals from discordant-participant pairs in the 1981 Australian survey. Zygosity assignment for MZ twins must be regarded as somewhat tentative, since most algorithms for zygosity diagnosis based on questionnaire data require reports from both members of a twin pair to confirm monozygosity (e.g., Eaves *et al.*, 1989b). In most groups, comparing Table 8.7 to Table 8.3, we observe both higher means and higher variances in the discordant-participant pairs. It is clearly important to test whether these differences are statistically significant.

To fit a model simultaneously to the means, variances, and covariances of concordant-participant pairs and the means and variances of discordant-participant pairs, requires that we analyze data where there are different numbers of observed

Table 8.7: Means and variances for Body Mass Index of twins whose cotwin did not cooperate in the 1981 Australian survey.

Group	Young Cohort ($<=30$)			Older Cohort (>30)		
	N	$\bar{x}'$	σ^2	N	$\bar{x}'$	σ^2
MZ Female Twins	33	0.1795	1.0640	44	0.6852	1.1461
DZ Female Twins	55	0.5836	0.8983	62	1.0168	1.7357
MZ Male Twins	24	1.3266	1.2477	36	1.3585	1.1036
DZ Male Twins	47	1.2705	1.5309	48	1.0379	1.6716
Opp-Sex Pair Females	65	0.6551	1.4390	81	0.9756	1.2690
Opp-Sex Pair Males	28	0.8724	0.9754	27	1.7149	1.0019

variables per group. Although, in principle, there is no problem with fitting models to such data by maximum-likelihood (see e.g., Bentler's EQS or Neale's Mx program, described in Chapter 18), the LISREL program requires that each group has the same number of variables. We circumvent this obstacle by using dummy variables (see Jöreskog and Sörbom, 1989, p. 259). Appendix C.4 presents a LIS-REL script for testing for differences in mean or variance using this technique. For MZ discordant-participant pairs we are going to pretend that we have data from the non-participant cotwin. To do this, we set up dummy data with zero mean, unit variance, and zero covariance with BMI in the participant twin:

```
LA
BMI-tw1 Dummy
CM SY
1.1461
0.0     1.0
ME
0.6852 0.0
```

(twin 2 is the dummy here). We do the same thing for DZ discordant-participant twins. For both these groups we set all elements of the Φ matrix to zero, except for the genetic and environmental variances of the first twin (which we leave at unity). The elements of the Γ matrix are constrained to be the same as in previous groups. We estimate two types of dummy parameters: (i) residual variance for the non-responding twin (which should be estimated at unity to match the dummy data); and (ii) a mean for the non-responding cotwin (which should estimated to be zero). These dummy parameters are estimated separately for for MZ 'pairs' and for DZ 'pairs', which ensures that our chi-squared is based on the correct number of degrees of freedom. Finally, we constrain the means of the responding twin in groups three (MZ discordant-participant) and four (DZ discordant-participant) to equal those of twins from the concordant-participant pairs. Our test for significant difference in means between the concordant-participant and discordant-participant groups is the improvement in goodness-of-fit obtained when we allow these latter, discordant-participant pairs, to take their own mean value.

Table 8.8 summarizes the results of model-fitting. For these analyses, we considered only the best-fitting genetic model based on the results of the analyses ignoring means, and allowed for zygosity differences in mean only if these were found to be significant in the analyses of the previous Section (i.e., in the younger twin pairs; young female pairs are the *only* group in which we find no difference between concordant-participant pairs and discordant-participant pairs). In the two older cohorts a model allowing for heterogeneity of means (Model 3) gives a substantially better fit than one that assumes no heterogeneity of means or variances (Model 1: older females: $\chi_2^2 = 12.86, p < 0.001$; older males: $\chi_2^2 = 30.87, p < 0.001$). Specifying heterogeneity of variances in addition to heterogeneity of means does not produce a further improvement in fit (older females: $\chi_2^2 = 2.02, p = 0.36$; older males: $\chi_2^2 = 1.99, p = 0.37$). Such a result is not atypical because the power to detect differences in mean is much greater than that to detect a difference in variance.

When considering these results, we must bear in mind several possibilities. Numbers of twins from the discordant-participant groups are small, and estimates of mean and variance in these groups will be particularly vulnerable to outlier-effects; that is, to inflation by one or two individuals of very high BMI. Further outlier analyses (e.g., Bollen, 1989) would be needed to determine whether this is an explanation of the variance difference. In the young males, it is also possible that age differences between concordant-participant pairs and discordant-participant pairs could generate the observed mean differences.

8.9 Conclusions: Genetic Analyses of BMI Data

The analyses of Australian BMI data which we have presented indicate a significant and substantial contribution of genetic factors to variation in BMI, consistent with other twin studies referred to at the beginning of Section 8.2. In the young cohort like-sex pairs, we find significant evidence for genetic dominance (or other genetic nonadditivity), in addition to additive genetic effects, but in the older cohort non-additive genetic effects are non-significant. Further analyses are needed to determine whether genetic and environmental parameters are significantly different across cohorts, or indeed between males and females (see Chapter 11).

We have discovered unexpected mean differences between zygosity groups (in the young cohort), and between twins whose cotwin refused to participate in the 1981 survey, and twins from concordant-participant pairs. It is possible that these differences reflect only outlier effects caused by a handful of observations. In this case, if we recode BMI as an ordinal variable, we might expect to find no significant

Table 8.8: Results of fitting models to twin pair covariance matrices and twin means for Body Mass Index: Two like-sex twin groups, plus data from twins from incomplete pairs. Models test for heterogeneity of means or variances between twins from pairs concordant vs discordant for cooperation in 1981 survey.

| | | Female | | | | Male | | | |
| | | Young | | Older | | Young | | Older | |
Model	df	χ^2	p	χ^2	p	χ^2	p	χ^2	p
1. No heterogen.[†] of means or variances	11	8.16	.70	20.62	.08	54.97	.001*	48.55	.001*
2. Heterogeneity[†] of means	9	6.03	.74	17.84	.09	29.22	.001*	44.58	.001*
3. Heterogeneity[†] of variances	9	5.70	.77	7.76	.74	22.76	.01	7.68	.74
4. Heterogeneity of means and variances	7	3.93	.79	5.74	.77	7.72	.36	5.69	.77
Genetic Model		ADE		AE#		ADE		AE#	
Means Model		$\overline{MZ} \neq \overline{DZ}$		$\overline{MZ} = \overline{DZ}$		$\overline{MZ} \neq \overline{DZ}$		$\overline{MZ} = \overline{DZ}$	

[†]Between concordant-participant versus discordant-participant twins.
* $p < .001$.
# AE models have two more degrees of freedom than shown in the df column

differences in the proportions of twins falling into each category[7]. Alternatively, it is possible that there is an overall shift in the distribution of BMI, in which case we must be concerned about the undersampling of obese individuals. If the latter finding were confirmed, further work would be needed to explore the degree to which genetic and environmental parameters might be biased (cf. Lykken et al., 1987; Neale *et al.*, 1989a; Neale and Eaves, 1992).

8.10   Fitting Genetic Models to Binary Data

It is very important to realize that binary or ordinal data do not preclude model-fitting. A large number of applications, from item analysis (e.g., Neale, *et al*, 1986; Kendler *et al.*, 1987) to psychiatric or physical illness (e.g., Kendler *et al*, 1992b,c) do not have measures on a quantitative scale but are limited to discontinuous forms

---

[7]Excessive contributions to the χ^2 by a small number of outliers could also be detected by fitting models directly to the raw data using Mx. Though a more powerful method of assessing the impact of outliers, it is beyond the scope of this volume.

of assessment. In Chapter 2 we discussed how ordinal data from twins could be summarized as contingency tables from which polychoric correlations and their asymptotic variances could be computed. Fitting models to this type of summary statistic involves a number of additional wrinkles, which we illustrate here with data on major depressive disorder. Although details of the sample and measures used have been provided in several published articles (Kendler *et al.*, 1991a,b; 1992a), we briefly reiterate the methods to emphasize some of the practical issues involved with an interview study of twins.

8.10.1 Major Depressive Disorder in Twins

Data for this example come from a study of genetic and environmental risk factors for common psychiatric disorders in Caucasian female same-sex twin pairs sampled from the Virginia Twin Registry. The Virginia Twin Registry is a population-based register formed from a systematic review of all birth certificates in the Commonwealth of Virginia. Twins were eligible to participate in the study if they were born between 1934 and 1971 and if both members of the pair had previously responded to a mailed questionnaire, to which the individual response rate was approximately 64%. The cooperation rate was almost certainly higher than this, as an unknown number of twins did not receive their questionnaire due to faulty addresses, improper forwarding of mail, and so on. Of the total 1176 eligible pairs, neither twin was interviewed in 46, one twin was interviewed and the other refused in 97, and both twins were interviewed in 1033 pairs. Of the completed interviews, 89.3% were completed face to face, nearly all in the twins' home, and 10.7% (mostly twins living outside Virginia) were interviewed by telephone. The mean age ($\pm$SD) of the sample at interview was 30.1 (7.6) and ranged from 17 to 55.

Zygosity determination was based on a combination of review of responses to questions about physical similarity and frequency of confusion as children — which alone have proved capable of determining zygosity with over 95% accuracy (Eaves *et al.*, 1989b) — and, in over 80% of cases, photographs of both twins. From this information, twins were classified as either: definitely MZ, definitely DZ, probably MZ, probably DZ, or uncertain. For 118 of the 186 pairs in the final three categories, blood was taken and eight highly informative DNA polymorphisms were used to resolve zygosity. If all probes are identical then there is a .9997 probability that the pair is MZ (Spence *et al.*, 1988). Final zygosity determination, using blood samples where available, yielded 590 MZ pairs, 440 DZ pairs and 3 pairs classified as uncertain. The DNA methods validated the questionnaire- and photograph-based 'probable' diagnoses in 84 out of 104 pairs; all 26 of 26 pairs in the definite categories were confirmed as having an accurate diagnosis. The error rate in zygosity assignment is probably well under 2%.

Lifetime psychiatric illness was diagnosed using an adapted version of the Structured Clinical Interview for DSM-III-R Diagnosis (Spitzer *et al.*, 1987) an instrument with demonstrable reliability in the diagnosis of depression (Riskind *et al.*,

Table 8.9: Contingency tables of twin pair diagnosis of lifetime major depressive illness.

		MZ Twin 1		DZ Twin 1	
		Normal	Depressed	Normal	Depressed
Twin 2	Normal	329	83	201	94
	Depressed	95	83	82	63

1987). Interviewers were initially trained for 80 hours and received bimonthly review sessions during the course of the study. Each member of a twin pair was invariably interviewed by a different interviewer. DSM-III-R criteria were applied by a blind review of the interview by K.S. Kendler, an experienced psychiatric diagnostician. Diagnosis of depression was not given when the symptoms were judged to be the result of uncomplicated bereavement, medical illness, or medication. Inter-rater reliability was assessed in 53 jointly conducted interviews. Chance corrected agreement (kappa) was .96, though this is likely to be a substantial overestimate of the value that would be obtained from independent assessments[8].

Contingency tables of MZ and DZ twin pair diagnoses are shown in Table 8.9. PRELIS estimates of the correlation in liability to depression are .435 for MZ and .186 for DZ pairs. Details of using PRELIS to derive these statistics and associated estimates of their asymptotic variances are given in Chapter 2, Section 2.3. The PM command is used to read in the tetrachoric correlation matrix, and the AC command reads the asymptotic weight matrices. In both cases we use the FI keyword in order to read these data from files. Therefore our univariate input script for LISREL 7 is unchanged from that shown in Appendix C.1 on page 383, except that the first four command lines are now

```
Major depressive disorder in adult female MZ twins
DA NG=2 NI=2 NO=590 MA=PM
PM FI=MZdep.cov
AC FI=MZdep.asy
```

in the MZ group, with the same commands for the DZ group except for NO=440 and a global replacement of DZ for MZ. For clarity, the comments at the beginning also should be changed.

Results of fitting the ACE and ADE models and submodels are summarized in Table 8.10. First, note that the degrees of freedom for fitting to correlation

---

[8]Such independent assessments would risk retest effects if they were close together in time. Conversely, assessments separated by a long interval would risk actual phenotypic change from

Table 8.10: Major depressive disorder in Virginia adult female twins. Parameter estimates and goodness-of-fit statistics for models and submodels including additive genetic (A), common environment (C), random environment (E), and dominance genetic (D) effects.

Model	Parameter Estimates				Fit statistics		
	a	c	e	d	χ^2	df	p
E	—	—	1.000	—	56.40	2	.00
CE	—	0.58	0.81	—	6.40	1	.01
AE	0.65	—	0.76	—	.15	1	.70
ACE	0.65	—	0.76	—	.15	0	—
ADE	.56	—	0.75	0.36	.00	0	—

matrices are fewer than when fitting to covariance matrices. Although we provide LISREL with two correlation matrices, each consisting of 1's on the diagonal and a correlation on the off-diagonal, the 1's on the diagonal cannot be considered unique. In fact, only one of them conveys information which effectively 'scales' the covariance. There is no information in the remaining three 1's on the diagonals of the MZ and DZ correlation matrices, *but LISREL does not make this distinction*. Therefore, we must adjust the degrees of freedom by putting DF=-3 on the OU line. Another way of looking at this is that the diagonal 1's convey no information whatsoever, but that we use one parameter to estimate the diagonal elements (e; it appears only in the expected variances, not the expected covariances). Thus, there are 4 imaginary variances and 1 parameter to estimate them — giving 3 statistics too many.

Second, the substantive interpretation of the results is that the model with just random environment fails, indicating significant familial aggregation for diagnoses of major depressive disorder. The environmental explanation of familial covariance also fails ($\chi_1^2 = 6.40$) but a model of additive genetic and random environment effects fits well ($\chi_1^2 = .15$). There is no possible room for significant improvement with the addition of any other parameter, since there are only .15 χ^2 units left. Nevertheless, we fitted both ACE and ADE models and found that dominance genetic effects could account for the remaining variability whereas shared environmental effects could not. This finding is in agreement with the observation that the MZ correlation is slightly greater than twice the DZ correlation. The heritability of liability to major depressive disorder is moderate but significant at 42%, with the remaining variability associated with random environmental sources including error of measurement. These results are not compatible with the view that shared

one occasion to the next. For a methodological review of the area, see Helzer (1977)

family experiences such as parental rearing, social class, or parental loss are key factors in the etiology of major depression. More modest effects of these factors may be detected by including them in multivariate model fitting (Kendler *et al.*, 1992a; Neale *et al.*, 1992).

Of course, every study has its limitations, and here the primary limitations are that: (i) the results only apply to females; (ii) the twin population is not likely to be perfectly representative of the general population, as it lacks twins who moved out of or into the state, or failed to respond to initial questionnaire surveys; (iii) a small number of the twins diagnosed as having major depression may have had bipolar disorder (manic depression), which may be etiologically distinct; (iv) the reliance on retrospective reporting of lifetime mental illness may be subject to bias by either currently well or currently ill subjects or both; (v) MZ twins may be treated more similarly as children than DZ twins; and (vi) not all twins were past the age at risk of first onset of major depression. Consideration of the first five of these factors is given in Kendler *et al.* (1992c). Of particular note is that a test of limitation (v), the 'equal environments' assumption, was performed by logistic regression of absolute pair difference of diagnosis (scored 0 for normal and 1 for affected) on a quasi-continuous measure of similarity of childhood treatment. Although MZ twins were on average treated more similarly than DZ twins, this regression was found to be non-significant. General methods to handle the effects of zygosity differences in environmental treatment form part of the class of data-specific models to be discussed in Section 18.2.3. Overall there was no marked regression of age on liability to disease in these data, indicating that correction for the contribution of age to the common environment is not necessary (see the next section). Variable age at onset has been considered by Neale *et al.* (1989) but a full treatment of this problem is beyond the scope of this volume. Such methods incorporate not only censoring of the risk period, but also the genetic architecture of factors involved in age at onset and their relationship to factors relevant in the etiology of liability to disease. Note, however, that this problem, like the problem of measured shared environmental effect, may also be considered as part of the class of data-specific models.

8.11   Model for Age-Correction of Twin Data

We now turn to a slightly more elaborate example of univariate analysis, using data from the Australian twin sample that was used in the BMI example earlier, but in this case data on social attitudes. Factor analysis of the item responses revealed a major dimension with low scores indicating radical attitudes and high scores attitudes commonly labelled as "conservative." Our *a priori* expectation is that variation in this dimension will be largely shaped by social environment and that genetic factors will be of little or no importance. This expectation is based on the differences between the MZ and DZ correlations; $r_{MZ} = .0.68$ and $r_{DZ} = 0.59$, indicating little, if any, genetic influence on social attitudes. We also might expect

Table 8.11: Conservatism in Australian females: standardized parameter estimates for additive genotype (A), common environment (C), random environment (E) and dominance genotype (D).

Model	Parameter Estimates				Fit statistics		
	a	c	e	d	χ^2	df	p
E	—	—	1.000	—	823.76	5	.000
CE	—	0.804	0.595	—	19.41	4	.001
AE	0.836	—	0.549	—	56.87	4	.000
ACE	0.464	0.687	0.559	—	3.07	3	.380
ADE	0.836	—	0.549	0.000	56.87	3	.000

*parameter on lower bound. This gives the diagnostic:
WARNING: GA(1,2) MAY NOT BE IDENTIFIED.

that Conservatism scores are affected by age. We can use the LISREL script in Appendix C.5 to examine the age effects , reading in the age of each twin pair and the Conservatism scores for twin 1 (CON1) and twin 2 (CON2). Since in this specification we have data on age, Conservatism for twin 1, and Conservatism for twin 2, we have 3 indicator variables, or NI=3. If we initially ignore age, as an exploratory analysis, we can select (SE) only the conservatism scores for analysis (note that the list of variables selected must end with a forward slash '/').

The script we use fits the ACE model, so that in contrast to the ADE model fitted in the first example, element $\phi(5,2)$ which represents the correlation for the second parameter, is the same in both twin groups. The results of this model are presented in the fourth line of the standardized results (obtained by placing SC on the OU line), which shows that the squares of parameters estimated from the model sum to one, because these correspond to the proportions of variance associated with each source (A, C, and E). These results are found in the output file under the section labeled WITHIN GROUP COMPLETELY STANDARDIZED SOLUTION.

The significance of common environmental contributions to variance in Conservatism may be tested by dropping c (AE model) but this leads to a worsening of χ^2 by 53.8 for 1 d.f., confirming its importance. Similarly, the poor fit of the CE model confirms that genetic factors also contribute to individual differences (significance of a is $19.41 - 3.07 = 16.34$ for 1 df, which is highly significant). The e model, which hypothesizes that there is no family resemblance for Conservatism, is overwhelmingly rejected, giving some indication of the great power of this data set to discriminate between competing hypotheses. For interest, we also present the results of the ADE model. Since we have already noted that r_{DZ} is appreciably greater than half the MZ correlation, it is clear that this model is inappropriate. Symmetric with the results of fitting an ACE model to the BMI data (where $2r_{DZ}$

was still less than r_{MZ}, indicating dominance), we now find that the estimate of d gets "stuck" on a lower bound of zero and generates a LISREL diagnostic. The BMI and Conservatism examples illustrate in a practical way the perfect reciprocal dependence of c and d in the classical twin design. Only one may be estimated, and the consequences of choosing the wrong one are severe in this LISREL formulation of the model! The issue of the reciprocal confounding of shared environment and genetic nonadditivity (dominance or epistasis) in the classical twin design is discussed in detail in papers by Martin *et al.*, (1978), Grayson (1989), and Hewitt (1989).

It is clear from the results above that there are major influences of the shared environment on Conservatism. One aspect of the environment that is shared with perfect correlation by cotwins is their age. If a variable is strongly related to age and if a twin sample is drawn from a broad age range, as opposed to a cohort sample covering a narrow range of birth years, then differences between twin pairs in age will contribute to estimated common environment variance. This is the case for the twins in the Australian sample, who range from 18 to 88 years old. It is clearly of interest to try to separate this variance due to age differences from genuine cultural differences contributing to the estimate of c.

Fortunately, LISREL provides a very easy way of allowing for the effects of age regression while simultaneously estimating the genetic and environmental effects (Neale and Martin, 1989). Figure 8.2 illustrates the method with a path diagram, in which the regression of CON1 and CON2 on Age is s (for senescence), and this is specified in the script excerpt below.

We now work with the full 3×3 covariance matrices (so the SE line is dropped from the previous job), declare age as the third y and η variable (NY=3 NE=3), and declare an additional factor AGE_L (NK=7) which loads on both the η variable AGE and on the η variables corresponding to the two measures of Conservatism.

```
MO NY=3 NE=3 NK=7 GA=FU,FI LY=ID PH=SY,FI TE=ZE PS=ZE
LE
age con1 con2
LK
AGE A1 C1 E1 A2 C2 E2
PA GA
1 0 0 0 0 0 0
1 1 1 1 0 0 0
1 0 0 0 1 1 1
EQ GA(2,2) GA(3,5)
EQ GA(2,3) GA(3,6)
EQ GA(2,4) GA(3,7)
EQ GA(2,1) GA(3,1)
MA PH
1.
0. 1.
```

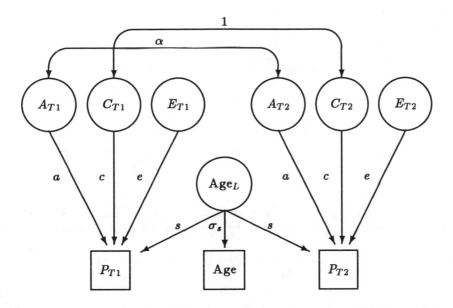

Figure 8.2: Path model for additive genetic (A), shared environment (C) and specific environment (E) effects on phenotypes (P) of pairs of twins (T1 and T2). α is fixed at 1 for MZ twins and at .5 for DZ twins. The effects of age are modelled as a standardized latent variable, Age_L, which is the sole cause of variance in observed Age.

```
0. 0. 1.
0. 0. 0. 1.
0. 1. 0. 0. 1.
0. 0. 1. 0. 0. 1.
0. 0. 0. 0. 0. 0. 1.
```

Results of fitting the ACE model with age correction are in the first row of Table 8.11. Standardized results are presented, from which we see that the standardized regression of Conservatism on age (constrained equal in twins 1 and 2) is 0.422. In the unstandardized solution, the first loading on the age factor is the standard deviation of the sample for age, in this case 13.2 years. The latter is an estimated parameter, making five free parameters in total. In each group we have NY(NY+1)/2 statistics so there are 2× NY ((NY+1)/2-5=7 degrees of free-

Table 8.12: Age correction of Conservatism in Australian females: standardized parameter estimates for models of additive genetic (A), common environment (C), random environment (E), and senescence or age (S).

Model	Parameter Estimates				Fit statistics		
	a	c	e	s	χ^2	df	p
$ACES$	0.474	0.534	0.558	0.422	7.41	7	.388
AES	0.720	—	0.547	0.426	31.56	8	.000
CES	—	0.685	0.595	0.421	25.49	8	.001
ACE	0.464	0.687	0.559	—	370.17	8	.000

dom. Dropping either c or a still causes significant worsening of the fit, and it also is very clear that one cannot omit the age regression itself (final ACE model; $\chi^2_8 = 370.17, p = .000$).

It is interesting to compare the results of the ACE model in Table 8.11 with those of the ACES model in Table 8.12. We see that the estimates of e and a are identical in the two tables, accounting for $0.559^2 = 31\%$ and $0.464^2 = 22\%$ of the total variance, respectively. However, in the first table the estimate of $c = 0.687$, accounting for 47% of the variance. In the analysis with age however, $c = 0.534$ and accounts for 29% of variance, and age accounts for $0.422^2 = 18\%$. Thus, we have partitioned our original estimate of 47% due to shared environment into 18% due to age regression and the remaining 29% due to 'genuine' cultural differences. If we choose, we may recalculate the proportions of variance due to a, c, and e, as if we were estimating them from a sample of uniform age — assuming of course that the causes of variation do not vary with age (see Chapter 11). Thus, genetic variance now accounts for $22/(100 - 18) = 27\%$ and shared environment variance is estimated to be $29/82 = 35\%$.

Our analysis suggests that cultural differences are indeed important in determining individual differences in social attitudes. However, before accepting this result too readily, we should reflect that estimates of shared environment may not only be inflated by age regression, but also by the effects of assortative mating — the tendency of like to marry like. Since there is known to be considerable assortative mating for Conservatism (spouse correlations are typically greater than 0.6), it is possible that a substantial part of our estimate of c^2 may arise from this source (Martin et al., 1986). This issue will be discussed in greater detail in Chapter 17.

Age is a somewhat unusual variable since it is perfectly correlated in both MZ and DZ twins (so long as we measure the members of a pair at the same time). There are relatively few variables that can be handled in the same way, partly because we have assumed a strong model that age causes variability in the observed phenotype. Thus, for example, it would be inappropriate to model length of time spent living together as a cause of cancer, even though cohabitation may lead to greater similarity between twins. In this case a more suitable model would be one in which the shared environment components are more highly correlated the longer the twins have been living together. Such a model would predict greater twin similarity, but would not predict correlation between cohabitation and cancer. Some further discussion of this type of model is given in Section 18.2.3 in the context of data-specific models. One group of variables that may be treated in a similar way to the present treatment of age consists of maternal gestation factors. Vlietinck *et al.* (1989) fitted a model in which both gestational age and maternal age predicted birthweight in twins.

Finally we note that at a technical level, age and similar putative causal agents might most appropriately be treated as x-variables in a multiple regression model. Thus the observed covariance of the x-variables is incorporated directly into the expected matrix, so that the analysis of the remaining y-variables is conditional on the covariance of the x-variables. This type of approach is free of distributional assumptions for the x-variables, and is analogous to the analysis of covariance. However, when we fit a model that estimates a single parameter for the variance of age in each group, the estimated and observed variances are generally equal, so the same results are obtained.

Chapter 9

Power and Sample Size

In this chapter we discuss the power of the twin study to detect variance components in behavioral characters. Our discussion is not in any way intended to be an exhaustive description of the power of the twin study under all possible combinations of causal factors and model parameters. Such a description is in large part available for the continuous case (Martin *et al.*, 1978) and there is an extensive comparison of the power of various designs to detect cultural transmission (Heath *et al.*, 1985). As we move out of the framework of the univariate classical twin study to consider multivariate hypotheses and data from additional classes of relatives, a comprehensive treatment rapidly becomes unmanageably large. Fortunately, it seems rather unnecessary because the prospective researcher usually has certain specific aims of a study in mind, and often has a reasonable idea about the values of some of the parameters in the model. This information can be used to prune the prodigious tree of possible scenarios to manageable proportions. All that is required is an understanding of the principles involved, which we aim to provide in Section 9.2. We illustrate these methods with a limited range of examples for continuous and categorical twin data.

9.1 Factors Contributing to Power

One of the greatest advantages of the model-fitting approach is that it allows us to conduct tests of significance of alternative hypotheses. We can ask, for example, whether a given data set really supports our assertion that shared environmental effects contribute to variation in one trait or another (i.e., is $c^2 > 0$?).

Our ability to show that a specific effect is important obviously depends on a number of factors. These include:

1. The effect under consideration, for example, a^2 or c^2;

2. The actual size of the effect in the population being studied — larger values are detected more easily than small values;

3. The probability level adopted as the conventional criterion for rejection of the null-hypothesis that the effect is zero — rejection at higher significance levels will be less likely to occur for a given size of effect;

4. The actual size of the sample chosen for study — larger samples can detect smaller effects;

5. The actual composition of the sample with respect to the relative frequencies of the different biological and social relationships selected for study;

6. The level of measurement used — categorical, ordinal, or continuous.

All of these considerations lead us to the important question of *power*. If we are trying to get a sense of what we are likely to be able to infer from our own data set, or if we are considering a new study, we must ask either "What inferences can we hope to be able to make with our data set?" or "What kind of data set and sample sizes is it likely we will need to answer a particular set of questions?" In the next Section we show how to answer these questions in relation to simple hypotheses with twin studies and suggest briefly how these issues may be explored for more complex designs and hypotheses.

9.2 Steps in Power Analysis

The basic approach to power analysis is to imagine that we are doing an identical study many times. For example, we pretend that we are trying to estimate a, c, and e for a given population by taking samples of a given number of MZ and DZ twins. Each sample would give somewhat different estimates of the parameters, depending on how many twins we study, and how big a, c, and e are in the study population. Suppose we did a very large number of studies and tabulated all the estimates of the shared environmental component, c^2. In some of the studies, even though there was some shared environment in the population, we would find estimates of c^2 that were not significant. In these cases we would commit "type II errors." That is, we would not find a significant effect of the shared environment even though the value of c^2 in the population was truly greater than zero. Assuming we were using a χ^2 test for 1 d.f. to test the significance of the shared environment, and we had decided to use the conventional 5% significance level, the probability of Type II error would be the expected proportion of samples in which we mistakenly decided in favor of the null hypothesis that $c^2 = 0$. These cases would be those in which the observed value of χ^2 was less than 3.84, the 5% critical value for 1 d.f. The other samples in which χ^2 was greater than 3.84 are those in which we would decide, correctly, that there was a significant shared environmental effect in the population. The expected proportion of samples in which we decide correctly against the null hypothesis is the *power of the test*.

Designing a genetic study boils down to deciding on the numbers and types of relationships needed to achieve a given power for the test of potentially important genetic and environmental factors. There is no general solution to the problem of power. The answers will depend on the specific values we contemplate for all the factors listed above. Before doing any power study, therefore, we have to decide the following questions in each specific case:

1. What kinds of relationships are to be considered?

2. What significance level is to be used in hypothesis testing?

3. What values are we assuming for the various effects of interest in the population being studied?

4. What power do we want to strive for in designing the study?

When we have answered these questions exactly, then we can conduct a power analysis for the specified set of conditions by following some basic steps:

1. Obtain expected covariance matrices for each set of relationships by substituting the assumed values of the population parameters in the model for each relationship.

2. Assign some initial arbitrary sample sizes to each separate group of relatives.

3. Use LISREL to analyze the expected covariance matrices just as we would to analyze real data and obtain the χ^2 value for testing the specific hypothesis of interest.

4. Find out (from statistical tables) how big that χ^2 has to be to guarantee the power we need.

5. Use a simple formula (given below) to multiply our assumed sample size and solve for the sample size we need.

It is essential to remember that the sample size we obtain in step five only applies to the particular effect, design, sample sizes, and even to the distribution of sample sizes among the different types of relationship assumed in a specific power calculation. To explore the question of power fully, it often will be necessary to consider a number, sometimes a large number, of different designs and population values for the relevant effects of genes and environment.

9.2.1   Example: The Power of the Classical Twin Study to Detect the Shared Environment

A common question in genetic research concerns the ability of a study of twins reared together to detect the effects of the shared environment. Let us investigate this issue using LISREL. Following the steps outlined above, we start by stipulating that we are going to explore the power of a classical twin study — that is, one in which we measure MZ and DZ twins reared together. We shall assume that 50% of the variation in the population is due to the unique environmental experiences of individuals $(e^2 = 0.5)$. The expected MZ twin correlation is therefore 0.50. This intermediate value is chosen to be typical of many of the less-familial traits. Anthropometric traits, and many cognitive traits, tend to have higher MZ correlations than this, so the power calculations should be conservative as far as such variables are concerned. We assume further that the additive genetic component explains 30% of the total variation $(a^2 = 0.30)$ and that the shared family environment accounts for the remaining 20% $(c^2 = 0.20)$. We now substitute these parameter values into the algebraic expectations for the variances and covariances of MZ and DZ twins:

Total variance	$= a^2 + c^2 + e^2$	$= 0.30 + 0.2 + 0.5$	$= 1.00$
MZ covariance	$= a^2 + c^2$	$= 0.30 + 0.2$	$= 0.50$
DZ covariance	$= .5a^2 + c^2$	$= 0.15 + 0.2$	$= 0.35$

In Appendix D.1 we show a version of the LISREL code for fitting the ACE model to the simulated covariance matrices. In addition to the expected covariances we must assign an arbitrary sample size and structure. Initially, we shall assume the study involves equal numbers, 1000 each, of MZ and DZ pairs. In order to conduct the power calculations for the c^2 component, we can run the job for the full (ACE) model first and then the AE model, obtaining the expected difference in χ^2 under the full and reduced models just as we did earlier for testing the significance of the shared environment in real data.

Notice that fitting the full ACE model yields a goodness-of-fit χ^2 of zero. This should always be the case when we use LISREL to solve for all the parameters of the model we used to generate the expected covariance matrices because, since there is no sampling error attached to the simulated covariance matrices, there is perfect agreement between the matrices supplied as "data" and the expected values under the model. In addition, the parameter estimates obtained should agree precisely with those used to simulate the data; if they are not, but the fit is still perfect, it suggests that the model is not identified (see Section 5.7) Therefore, as long as we are confident that we have specified the structural model correctly and that the full model is identified, there is really no need to fit the full model to the simulated covariances matrices since we know in advance that the "χ^2" is expected to be zero. In practice it is often helpful to recover this known result to increase our confidence that both we and the software are doing the right thing.

Table 9.1: Non-centrality parameter, λ, of non-central χ^2 distribution for 1 d.f. required to give selected values of the power of the test at the 5% significance level (selected from Pearson and Hartley, 1972).

Desired Power	λ
0.25	1.65
0.50	3.84
0.75	6.94
0.80	7.85
0.90	10.51
0.95	13.00

For our specific case, with samples of 1000 MZ and DZ pairs, we obtain a goodness-of-fit χ_4^2 of 11.35 for the AE model. Since the full model yields a perfect fit ($\chi_3^2 = 0$), the expected difference in χ^2 for 1 d.f. — testing for the effect of the shared environment — is 11.35. Such a value is well in excess of the 3.84 necessary to conclude that c^2 is significant at the 5% level. However, this is only the value expected in the ideal situation. With real data, individual χ^2 values will vary greatly as a function of sampling variance. We need to choose the sample sizes to give an expected value of χ^2 such that observed values exceed 3.84 in a specified proportion of cases corresponding to the desired power of the test.

It turns out that such problems are very familiar to statisticians and that the expected values of χ^2 needed to give different values of the power at specified significance levels for a given d.f. have been tabulated extensively (see Pearson and Hartley, 1972). The expected χ^2 is known as the *centrality parameter* (λ) of the non-central χ^2 distribution (i.e., when the null-hypothesis is false). Selected values of the non-centrality parameter are given in Table 9.1 for a χ^2 test with 1 d.f. and a significance level of 0.05.

With 1000 pairs of MZ and DZ twins, we find a non-centrality parameter of 11.35 when we use the χ^2 test to detect c^2 which explains 20% of the variation in our hypothetical population. This corresponds to a power somewhere between 90% ($\lambda = 10.51$) and 95% ($\lambda = 13.00$). That is, 1000 pairs each of MZ and DZ twins would allow us to detect, at the 5% significance level, a significant shared environmental effect when the true value of c^2 was 0.20 in about 90-95% of all possible samples of this size and composition. Conversely, we would only fail to detect this much shared environment in about 5-10% of all possible studies.

Suppose now that we want to figure out the sample size needed to give a power of 80%. Let this sample size be N^*. Let N_0 be the sample size assumed in the initial power analysis (2000 pairs, in our case). Let the expected χ^2 for the particular test being explored with this sample size be χ_E^2 (11.35, in this example). From

Table 9.1, we see that the non-centrality parameter, λ, needs to be 7.85 to give a power of 0.80. Since the value of χ^2 is expected to increase linearly as a function of sample size we can obtain the sample size necessary to give 80% power by solving:

$$N^* = \frac{\lambda}{\chi_E^2} N_0 \qquad (9.1)$$

$$= \frac{7.85}{11.35} \times 2000$$

$$= 1383$$

That is, in a sample comprising 50% MZ and 50% DZ pairs reared together, we would require 1,383 pairs in total, or approximately 692 pairs of each type to be 80% certain of detecting a shared environmental effect explaining 20% of the total variance, when a further 30% is due to additive genetic factors.

It must be emphasized again that this particular sample size is specific to the study design, sample structure, parameter values and significance level assumed in the simulation. Smaller samples will be needed to detect larger effects. Greater power requires larger samples. Larger studies can detect smaller effects, and finally, some parameters of the model may be easier to detect than others.

9.3 Loss of Power with Ordinal Data

An important factor which affects power but is often overlooked is the form of measurement used. So far we have considered only continuous, normally distributed variables, but of course, these are not always available in the biosocial sciences. An exhaustive treatment of the power of the ordinal classical twin study is beyond the scope of this text, but we shall simply illustrate the loss of power incurred when we use more crude scales of measurement. Consider the example above, but suppose this time that we wish to detect the presence of additive genetic effects, a^2, in the data. For the continuous case this is a trivial modification of the input file to fit a model with just c and e parameters. The chi-squared from running this program is 19.91, and following the algebra above (equation 9.1) we see that we would require $2000 \times 7.85/19.91 = 788$ pairs in total to be 80% certain of rejecting the hypothesis that additive genes do not affect variation when in the true world they account for 30%, with shared environment accounting for a further 20%. Suppose now that rather than measuring on a continuous scale, we have a dichotomous scale which bisects the population; for example, an item on which 50% say 'yes' and 50% say no. The data for this case may be summarized as a contingency table, and we wish to generate tables that: (i) have a total sample size of 1000; (ii) reflect a correlation in liability of .5 for MZ and .35 for DZ twins; and (iii) reflect our threshold value of 0 to give 50% either side of the threshold. Any routine that will compute the bivariate normal integral for given thresholds and correlation is suitable to generate the expected proportions in each cell. In this case we use a short Mx script (Neale,

1991) to generate the data for PRELIS. We can use the weight variable option in PRELIS to indicate the cell counts for our contingency tables. Thus, the PRELIS script might be:

```
Power calculation MZ twins
DA NI=3 NO=0
LA; SIM1 SIM2 FREQ
RA FI=expectmz.frq
WE FREQ
OR sim1 sim2
OU MA=PM SM=SIMMZ.COV SA=SIMMZ.ASY PA
```

with the file expectmz.frq looking like this:

```
0 0 333.333
0 1 166.667
1 0 166.667
1 1 333.333
```

A similar approach with the DZ correlation and thresholds gives expected frequencies which can be used to compute the asymptotic variance of the tetrachoric correlation for this second group. The simulated DZ frequency data might appear as

```
0 0 306.9092
0 1 193.0908
1 0 193.0908
1 1 306.9092
```

The cells display considerable symmetry — there are as many concordant 'no' pairs as there are concordant 'yes' pairs because the threshold is at zero. Running PRELIS generates output files, and we can see immediately that the correlations for MZ and DZ twins remain the desired .5 and .35 assumed in the population. The next step is to feed the correlation matrix and the weight matrix (which only contains one element, the asymptotic variance of the correlation between twins) into LISREL, in place of the covariance matrix that we supplied for the continuous case. This can be achieved by changing just three lines in each group of our LISREL power script:

```
DA NG=2 NI=2 NO=1000 MA=PM
PM File=SIMMZ.COV
AC File=SIMMZ.ASY
```

with corresponding filenames for the DZ group, of course. When we fit the model to these summary statistics we observe a much smaller χ^2 than we did for the continuous case; the χ^2 is only 6.08, which corresponds to a requirement of 2,582 pairs in total for 80% power at the .05 level. That is, *we need more than three times as many pairs to get the same information about a binary item than we need for a continuous variable.* The situation further deteriorates as we move the threshold to one side of the distribution. Simulating contingency tables, computing tetrachorics and weight matrices, and fitting the false model when the threshold is one standard deviation (SD) to the right (giving 15.9% in one category and 84.1% in the other), the χ^2 is a mere 3.29, corresponding a total sample size of 4,772 total pairs. More extreme thresholds further reduce power, so that for an item (or a disease) with a 95:5% split we would require 13,534 total pairs. Only in the largest studies could such sample sizes be attained, and they are quite unrealistic for data that could be collected by personal interview or laboratory measurement. On the positive side, it seems unlikely that given the advantages of the clinical interview or laboratory setting, our only measure could be made at the crude 'yes or no' binary response level. If we are able to order our data into more than two categories, some of the lost power can be regained. Following the procedure outlined above, and assuming that there are two thresholds, one at -1 SD and one at $+1$ SD, then the χ^2 obtained is 8.16, corresponding to 'only' 1,924 pairs for 80% chance of finding additive variance significant at the .05 level. If one threshold is 0 and the other at 1 SD then this rises slightly to a χ^2 of 9.07, or 1,730 pairs. Further improvement can be made if we increase the measurements to comprise four categories. For example, with thresholds at -1, 0, and 1 SD the χ^2 is 12.46, corresponding to a sample size of 1,240 twin pairs.

While estimating tetrachoric correlations from a random sample of the population has considerable advantages, it is not always the method of choice for studies focused on a single outcome, such as schizophrenia. In cases where the base rates are so low (e.g., 1%) then it becomes inefficient to sample randomly, and an ascertainment scheme in which we select cases and examine their relatives is a practical and powerful alternative, if we have good information on the base rate in the population studied. Discussion of these methods is beyond the scope of this book, and beyond the scope of the current versions of PRELIS and LISREL. Still, an outline of the methods can be found in Section 18.2.1 of this volume. The necessary power calculations can be performed using the computer packages LISCOMP (Muthen, 1987) or Mx (Neale, 1991).

9.4   Exercises

1. Change the example program to obtain the expected χ^2 for the test for additive genetic effects. Find out how many pairs are needed to obtain significant estimates of a^2 in 80% of all possible samples.

2. Explore the effect of power of a particular test of altering the proportion of MZ and DZ twins in the sample.

3. Show that the change in expected χ^2 is proportional to the change in sample size.

4. Obtain and tabulate the sample sizes necessary to detect a significant a^2 when the population parameter values are as follows:

a^2	c^2
0.10	0.00
0.30	0.00
0.60	0.00
0.90	0.00

In what way do these values change if there are shared environmental effects?

5. Show that with small sample sizes for the number of pairs in each group, some bias in the chi-squared is introduced. Consider whether or not this may be due to the $n-1$ part of the maximum likelihood loss function (Equation 7.11 on page 138).

Chapter 10

Social Interaction

10.1   Introduction to Recursive Models

This chapter introduces a technique for specifying and estimating paths between dependent variables, i.e., η variables in the LISREL model. Uses of this technique include: modeling social interactions, for example, sibling competition and cooperation; testing for direction of causation in bivariate data, e.g., whether life events cause depression or vice versa; and developmental models for longitudinal or repeated measurements.

Models for sibling interaction have been popular in genetics for some time (Eaves, 1976b), and the reader should see Carey (1986b) for a thorough treatment of the problem in the context of variable family size. Here we provide an introductory outline and application for the restricted case of pairs of twins, and we assume no effects of other siblings in the family. We further confine our treatment to sibling interactions *within variables*. Although multivariate sibling interactions (such as aggression in one twin causing depression in the cotwin) may in the long run prove to be more important than those within variables, they are beyond the scope of this introductory text.

10.2   Background

Up to this point, we have been concerned primarily with decomposing observed phenotypic variation into its genetic and environmental components. This has been accomplished by estimating the paths from latent or independent variables, specified as ξ variables in the LISREL model, to dependent variables, specified as η variables in the LISREL model. These dependent variables are observed as y variables, allowing us to specify that the dependent variable is observed with error if we so choose. A basic univariate path diagram involving the three types of

199

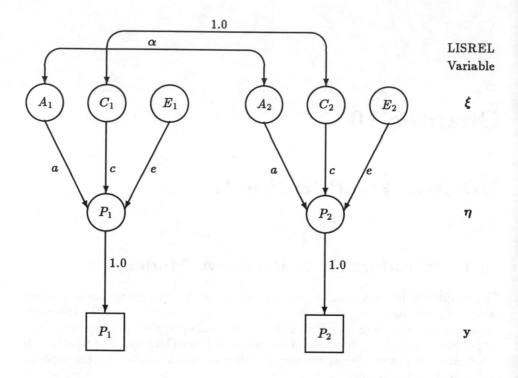

Figure 10.1: Basic path diagram for univariate twin data, including ξ, η, and y variables.

variables — ξ, η, and y — is set out in Figure 10.1. This path diagram shows the deviation phenotypes P_1 and P_2, of a pair of twins. Here we refer to the phenotypes as *deviation phenotypes* to emphasize the point that the model assumes variables to be measured as deviations from the means, which is the case whenever we fit models to covariance matrices and do not include means. The deviation phenotypes P_1 and P_2 result from their respective additive genetic deviations, A_1 and A_2, their shared environment deviations, C_1 and C_2, and their non-shared environmental deviations, E_1 and E_2. The linear model corresponding to the path diagram is:

$$\begin{aligned} Y_1 &= P_1 &= aA_1 + cC_1 + eE_1 \\ Y_2 &= P_2 &= aA_2 + cC_2 + eE_2 \end{aligned}$$

In matrix form we can write:

$$\begin{pmatrix} Y_1 \\ Y_2 \end{pmatrix} = \begin{pmatrix} 1 & 0 \\ 0 & 1 \end{pmatrix} \begin{pmatrix} P_1 \\ P_2 \end{pmatrix}$$

or

$$y = \Lambda_y \eta$$

where $\Lambda_y = I$. We also have

$$\begin{pmatrix} P_1 \\ P_2 \end{pmatrix} = \begin{pmatrix} a & c & e & 0 & 0 & 0 \\ 0 & 0 & 0 & a & c & e \end{pmatrix} \begin{pmatrix} A_1 \\ C_1 \\ E_1 \\ A_2 \\ C_2 \\ E_2 \end{pmatrix}$$

or as a matrix expression

$$\eta = \Gamma\xi .$$

For this linear model we also specify the Φ matrix of correlations between the six ξ variables. Details of specifying and estimating this basic univariate model are given in Chapter 8. One of the interesting assumptions of this basic ACE model is that the siblings' or twins' phenotypes have no influence on each other. This assumption may well be true of height or finger print ridge count, but is it necessarily true for a behavior like smoking, a psychiatric condition like depression, delinquent behavior in children or even an anthropometric measure like the body mass index? We should not, in general, assume *a priori* that a source of variation is absent, especially when an empirical test of the assumption may be readily performed. However, we may as well recognize from the onset that evidence for social interactions or sibling effects is pretty scarce. The fact is that usually one form or another of the basic univariate model adequately describes a twin or family data set, within the power of the study. This tells us that there will not be evidence of significant social interactions since, were such effects substantial, they would lead to failure of basic univariate models (as we shall see). Nevertheless, this extension of the basic models is of considerable theoretical interest and studying its outcome on the expectations derived from the models can provide insight into the nature and results of social influences. The applications to bivariate and multivariate causal modeling are perhaps even more intriguing and will be taken up in the next chapter.

10.3 Sibling Interaction Model

Suppose that we are considering a phenotype like number of cigarettes smoked. For the sake of exposition we will set aside questions about the appropriate scale of measurement, what to do about non-smokers and so on, and assume that there is a well-behaved quantitative variable, which we can call 'smoking' for short. What we want to specify is the influence of one sibling's (twin's) smoking on the other sibling's (cotwin's) smoking. Figure 10.2 shows a path diagram which extends the

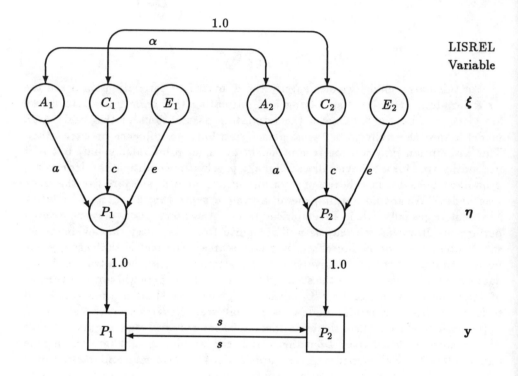

Figure 10.2: Path diagram for univariate twin data, incorporating sibling interaction.

basic univariate model for twins to include a path of magnitude s from each twin's smoking to the cotwin. If the path s is positive then the sibling interaction is essentially cooperative, i.e., the more (less) one twin smokes the more (less) the cotwin will smoke as a consequence of this direct influence. We can easily conceive of a highly plausible mechanism for this kind of influence when twins are cohabiting; as a twin lights up she offers her cotwin a cigarette. If the path s is negative then the sibling interaction is essentially competitive. The more (less) one twin smokes the less (more) the cotwin smokes. We must note that although such competition contributes negatively to the covariance between twins, it may well not override the positive covariance resulting from shared familial factors. Thus, even in the presence of competition the observed phenotypic covariation may still be positive. If interactions are cooperative in some situations and competitive in others, our analyses will reveal the predominant mode. But before considering the detail of our expectations, let us look more closely at how the model is specified. The linear model for the η variables is now:

$$P_1 = sP_2 + aA_1 + cC_1 + eE_1 \tag{10.1}$$
$$P_2 = sP_1 + aA_2 + cC_2 + eE_2 \tag{10.2}$$

In matrix form we have $\eta = \Gamma \xi$ as before, and then:

$$\begin{pmatrix} P_1 \\ P_2 \end{pmatrix} = \begin{pmatrix} 0 & s \\ s & 0 \end{pmatrix} \begin{pmatrix} P_1 \\ P_2 \end{pmatrix} + \begin{pmatrix} a & c & e & 0 & 0 & 0 \\ 0 & 0 & 0 & a & c & e \end{pmatrix} \begin{pmatrix} A_1 \\ C_1 \\ E_1 \\ A_2 \\ C_2 \\ E_2 \end{pmatrix}$$

or

$$\eta = \mathbf{B}\eta + \mathbf{\Gamma}\xi \ .$$

In this form the $\mathbf{B}$ matrix is an NE $\times$ NE matrix (where NE is the number of dependent (η) variables). The leading diagonal of the $\mathbf{B}$ matrix contains zeros. The element in row i and column j represents the path from the jth dependent variable to the ith dependent variable. To specify the full model in LISREL, in addition to the $\mathbf{B}$, $\mathbf{\Gamma}$, and $\mathbf{\Lambda}_y$ matrices we need to specify the $\mathbf{\Phi}$ matrix of correlations between the ξ variables as before (see Chapters 6 to 8, especially p. 160).

10.4   Application to CBC Data

By way of illustration we shall analyze data collected using the Achenbach Child Behavior Checklist (CBC; Achenbach & Edelbrock, 1983) on juvenile twins aged 8 through 16 years living in Virginia. Mothers were asked the extent to which a series of problem behaviors were characteristic of each of their twin children over the last six months. The 118 problem behaviors that were rated can be categorized, on the basis of empirical clustering, into two broad dimensions of *internalizing* and *externalizing* problems. The former are typified by fears, psychosomatic complaints, and symptoms of anxiety and depression. Externalizing behaviors are characterized by "acting out" — delinquent and aggressive behaviors. The factor patterns vary somewhat with the age and sex of the child but there are core items which load on the broad factors in both boys and girls at younger (6-11 years) and older (12-16 year) ages. The 24 core items for the externalizing dimension analyzed by Silberg *et al.* (1992) and Hewitt *et al.* (1992) include among other things: arguing a lot, destructive behavior, disobedience, fighting, hanging around with children who get into trouble, running away from home, stealing, and bad language. For such behaviors we might suspect that siblings will influence each other in a cooperative manner through imitation or mutual reinforcement. The LISREL script in Appendix F.1 specifies the model for sibling interactions shown in Figure 10.2 and also allows for the choice of dominance effects (D) instead of shared environmental influences (C).

By varying the script, the standard E, AE, CE, and ACE models may be fitted to the data to obtain the results shown in Table 10.1. Clearly the variation and

Table 10.1: Preliminary results of model fitting to externalizing behavior problems of boys from larger families.

	Fit statistics			Parameter Estimates		
Model	df	χ^2	AIC	a	c	e
AE	4	32.57	24.6	.78	—	.33
CE	4	29.80	21.8	—	.78	.43
ACE	3	4.95	-1.0	.50	.64	.34

co-aggregation of boys' behaviors problems cannot be explained either by a model which allows only for additive genetic effects (along with non-shared environmental influences), nor by a model which excludes genetic influences altogether. The ACE model fits very well ($p = .18$) and suggests a heritability of 33% with shared environmental factors accounting for 52% of the variance[1]. But is the ACE model the best in this case? We observe that the pooled individual phenotypic variances of the MZ twins (0.915) are greater than those of the DZ twins (0.689) and, although this discrepancy is apparently not statistically significant with our sample sizes (171 MZ pairs and 194 DZ pairs), we might be motivated to consider sibling interactions.

---

[1] The reader might like to consider what the components of this shared variance might include in these data obtained from the mothers of the twins and think forward to our treatment of rating data in Chapter 16.

Fitting the model shown in Figure 10.2 yields results given in Table 10.2. Our

Table 10.2: Parameter estimates and goodness of fit statistics from fitting models of sibling interaction to CBC data on MZ and DZ twins.

	Fit statistics			Parameter estimates			
Model	d.f.	χ^2	AIC	a	c	e	s
E+s	4	29.80	21.8	—	—	*	*
AE+s	3	1.80	-4.2	.611	—	.419	.230
CE+s	3	29.80	21.8	—	.882	.282	-.101
ACE+s	2	1.80	-2.2	.611	.000[1]	.419	.230

* Indicates parameters out of bounds.
[1]This parameter is fixed on the lower bound (0.0) by LISREL.

general conclusion is that while the evidence for social interactions is not unequivocal, a model including additive genetic effects, non-shared environments, and reciprocal sibling cooperation provides the best account of these data.

10.5 Consequences for Variation and Covariation

In this section we will work through the matrix algebra to derive expected variance and covariance components for a simplified model of sibling interaction. We then show how this model can be adapted to handle the specific cases of additive and dominant genetic, and shared and non-shared environmental effects. Numerical examples of strong competition and cooperation will be used to illustrate their effects on the variances and covariances of twins and unrelated individuals reared in the same home.

10.5.1 Derivation of Expected Covariances

To understand what it is about the observed statistics that suggests sibling interactions in our twin data we must follow through a little algebra. We shall try to keep this as simple as possible by considering the path model in Figure 10.3, which depicts the influence of an arbitrary latent variable, X, on the phenotype P. As long as our latent variables — A, C, E, etc. — are independent of each other, their effects can be considered one at a time and then summed, even in the presence of social interactions. The linear model corresponding to this path diagram is

$$P_1 = sP_2 + xX_1 \qquad (10.3)$$
$$P_2 = sP_1 + xX_2 \qquad (10.4)$$

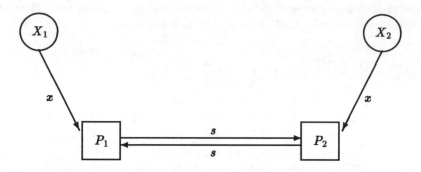

Figure 10.3: Path diagram showing influence of arbitrary exogenous variable X on phenotype P in a pair of relatives (for univariate twin data, incorporating sibling interaction).

Or, in matrices:

$$\begin{pmatrix} P_1 \\ P_2 \end{pmatrix} = \begin{pmatrix} 0 & s \\ s & 0 \end{pmatrix} \begin{pmatrix} P_1 \\ P_2 \end{pmatrix} + \begin{pmatrix} x & 0 \\ 0 & x \end{pmatrix} \begin{pmatrix} X_1 \\ X_2 \end{pmatrix}$$

which in turn we can write more economically as

$$\eta = \mathbf{B}\eta + \mathbf{\Gamma}\xi \ .$$

Following the rules for matrix algebra set out in Chapters 4 and 6, we can rearrange this equation:

$$\begin{aligned} \eta - \mathbf{B}\eta &= \mathbf{\Gamma}\xi & (10.5) \\ \mathbf{I}\eta - \mathbf{B}\eta &= \mathbf{\Gamma}\xi & (10.6) \\ (\mathbf{I} - \mathbf{B})\eta &= \mathbf{\Gamma}\xi \ , & (10.7) \end{aligned}$$

and then, multiplying both sides of this equation by the inverse of $(\mathbf{I} - \mathbf{B})$, we have

$$\eta = (\mathbf{I} - \mathbf{B})^{-1}\mathbf{\Gamma}\xi \ . \tag{10.8}$$

In this case, the matrix $(\mathbf{I} - \mathbf{B})$ is simply

$$\begin{pmatrix} 1 & -s \\ -s & 1 \end{pmatrix} ,$$

which has determinant $1 - s^2$, so $(\mathbf{I} - \mathbf{B})^{-1}$ is

$$\frac{1}{1-s^2} \otimes \begin{pmatrix} 1 & s \\ s & 1 \end{pmatrix} .$$

The symbol $\otimes$ is used to represent the kronecker product, which in this case simply means that each element in the matrix is to be multiplied by the constant $\frac{1}{1-s^2}$.

We have a vector of phenotypes on the left hand side of equation 10.8. In the chapter on matrix algebra (p. 82) we showed how the covariance matrix could be computed from the raw data matrix $\mathbf{T}$ by expressing the observed data as deviations from the mean to form matrix $\mathbf{U}$, and computing the matrix product $\mathbf{UU}'$. The same principle is applied here to the vector of phenotypes, which has an expected mean of $\mathbf{0}$ and is thus already expressed in mean deviate form. So to find the expected variance-covariance matrix of the phenotypes P_1 and P_2, we multiply by the transpose:

$$\mathcal{E}\{\boldsymbol{\eta}\boldsymbol{\eta}'\} = \{(\mathbf{I} - \mathbf{B})^{-1}\boldsymbol{\Gamma}\boldsymbol{\xi}\}\{(\mathbf{I} - \mathbf{B})^{-1}\boldsymbol{\Gamma}\boldsymbol{\xi}\}' \tag{10.9}$$

$$= (\mathbf{I} - \mathbf{B})^{-1}\boldsymbol{\Gamma}\boldsymbol{\xi}\boldsymbol{\xi}'\boldsymbol{\Gamma}'(\mathbf{I} - \mathbf{B})^{-1'} . \tag{10.10}$$

Now in the middle of this equation we have the matrix product $\boldsymbol{\xi}\boldsymbol{\xi}'$. We have noted earlier that this matrix product, the covariance matrix of the $\boldsymbol{\xi}$ variables, is defined as $\boldsymbol{\Phi}$ in LISREL (see Chapter 6). Therefore, we have

$$\mathcal{E}\{\boldsymbol{\eta}\boldsymbol{\eta}'\} = (\mathbf{I} - \mathbf{B})^{-1}\boldsymbol{\Gamma}\boldsymbol{\Phi}\boldsymbol{\Gamma}'(\mathbf{I} - \mathbf{B})^{-1'} \tag{10.11}$$

and this expectation forms a reduced part of the full LISREL model for y variables (submodel 2; see p. 118). In the LISREL model, the only variables that may mutually cause each other in this way are the η variables, so we always have to use the $\mathbf{B}$ matrix to define 'feedback' relations of this type. Naturally, the $\mathbf{B}$ matrix may be used to define ordinary (non-feedback) relations, and is essential for complex models with long (over 3 variables) causal chains. For our particular example, we want two standardized variables, X_1 and X_2 to have unit variance and correlation r so the $\boldsymbol{\Phi}$ matrix is:

$$\begin{pmatrix} 1 & r \\ r & 1 \end{pmatrix} .$$

We now have all the pieces required to compute the covariance matrix, recalling that for this case,

$$\boldsymbol{\Gamma} = \begin{pmatrix} x & 0 \\ 0 & x \end{pmatrix} \tag{10.12}$$

$$(\mathbf{I} - \mathbf{B})^{-1} = \frac{1}{1-s^2} \otimes \begin{pmatrix} 1 & s \\ s & 1 \end{pmatrix} \tag{10.13}$$

$$\boldsymbol{\Phi} = \begin{pmatrix} 1 & r \\ r & 1 \end{pmatrix} . \tag{10.14}$$

The reader may wish to show as an exercise that by substituting the right hand sides of equations 10.12 to 10.14 into equation 10.11, and carrying out the multiplication, we obtain:

$$\mathcal{E}\{\eta\eta'\} = \frac{x^2}{(1-s^2)^2} \otimes \begin{pmatrix} 1+2sr+s^2 & r+2s+rs^2 \\ r+2s+rs^2 & 1+2sr+s^2 \end{pmatrix} \quad (10.15)$$

We can use this result to derive the effects of sibling interaction on the variance and covariance due to a variety of sources of individual differences. For example, when considering:

1. additive genetic influences, $x^2 = a^2$ and $r = \alpha$, where α is 1.0 for MZ twins and 0.5 for DZ twins;

2. shared environment influences, $x^2 = c^2$ and $r = 1$;

3. non-shared environmental influences, $x^2 = e^2$ and $r = 0$;

4. genetic dominance, $x^2 = d^2$ and $r = \delta$, where $\delta = 1.0$ for MZ twins and $\delta = 0.25$ for DZ twins.

These results are summarized in Table 10.3.

Table 10.3: The effects of sibling interaction(s) on variance and covariance components between pairs of relatives.

Source	Variance	Covariance
Additive genetic	$\omega(1+2s+s^2)a^2$	$\omega(\alpha+2s+\alpha s^2)a^2$
Dominance genetic	$\omega(1+2s+s^2)d^2$	$\omega(\delta+2s+\delta s^2)d^2$
Shared environment	$\omega(1+2s+s^2)c^2$	$\omega(1+2s+s^2)c^2$
Non-shared environment	$\omega(1+s^2)e^2$	$\omega 2se^2$

ω represents the scalar $\frac{1}{(1-s^2)^2}$ obtained from equation 10.15.

10.5.2 Numerical Illustration

To illustrate these effects numerically, let us consider a simplified situation in which $a^2 = .5, d^2 = 0, c^2 = 0, e^2 = .5$ in the absence of social interaction (i.e., $s = 0$); in the presence of strong cooperation, $s = .5$; and in the presence of strong competition, $s = -.5$. Table 10.4 gives the numerical values for MZ and DZ twins and unrelated pairs of individuals reared together (e.g., adoptive siblings). In terms of correlations, phenotypic cooperation mimics the effects of shared environment while phenotypic competition may mimic the effects of non-additive genetic variance. However, the effects can be distinguished because social interactions result in

Table 10.4: Effects of strong sibling interaction on the variance and covariance between MZ, DZ, and unrelated individuals reared together. The interaction parameter s takes the values 0, .5, and $-.5$ for no sibling interaction, cooperation, and competition, respectively.

Interaction	MZ twins			DZ twins			Unrelated		
	Var	Cov	r	Var	Cov	r	Var	Cov	r
None	1.00	.50	.50	1.00	.25	.25	1.00	.00	.00
Cooperation	3.11	2.89	.93	2.67	2.33	.88	2.22	1.78	.80
Competition	1.33	.44	.33	1.78	-.67	-.38	2.22	-1.78	-.80

different total phenotypic variances for differently related pairs of individuals. All of the other kinds of models we have considered predict that the population variance of individuals is not affected by the presence or absence of relatives. However, cooperative interactions increase the variance of more closely related individuals the most, while competitive interactions increase them the least and under some circumstances may decrease them. Thus, in twin data, cooperation is distinguished from shared environmental effects because cooperation results in greater total phenotypic variance in MZ than in DZ twins. Competition is distinguished from non-additive genetic effects because it results in lower total phenotypic variance in MZ than in DZ twins. This is the bottom line: social interactions cause the variance of a phenotype to depend on the degree of relationship of the social actors.

There are three observations we should make about this result. First, a test of the contrary assumption, i.e., that the total observed variance is independent of zygosity in twins, was set out by Jinks and Fulker (1970) as a preliminary requirement of their analyses and, as has been noted, is implicitly provided whenever we fit models without social interactions to covariance matrices. For I.Q., educational attainment, psychometric assessments of personality, social attitudes, body mass index, heart rate reactivity, and so on, the behavior genetic literature is replete with evidence for the *absence* of the effects of social interaction. Second, analyses of family correlations (rather than variances and covariances) effectively standardize the variances of different groups of individuals and throw away the very information we need to distinguish social interactions from other influences. Third, if we are working with categorical data and adopting a threshold model (see Chapter 2), we can make predictions about the standardized thresholds in different groups. Higher quantitative variances lead to smaller (i.e., less deviant) thresholds and therefore higher prevalence for the extreme categories. Thus, for example, if abstinence vs. drinking status is influenced by sibling cooperation on a latent underlying phenotype, and abstinence has a frequency of 10% in DZ twins, we should expect a higher frequency of abstinence in MZ twins. It is not possible to fit such models in LISREL 7, but they are relatively simple to implement in Mx (Neale, 1991).

Chapter 11

Sex-limitation and G × E Interaction

11.1 Introduction

As described in Chapter 8, the basic univariate ACE model allows us to estimate genetic and environmental components of phenotypic variance from like-sex MZ and DZ twin data. When data are available from both male and female twin pairs, an investigator may be interested in asking whether the variance profile of a trait is similar across the sexes or whether the magnitude of genetic and environmental influences are sex-dependent. To address this issue, the ACE model may be fitted independently to data from male and female twins, and the parameter estimates compared by inspection. This approach, however, has three severe limitations: (1) it does not test whether the heterogeneity observed across the sexes is significant; (2) it does not attempt to explain the sex differences by fitting a particular sex-limitation model; and (3) it discards potentially useful information by excluding dizygotic opposite-sex twin pairs from the analysis. In the first part of this chapter (section 11.2), we outline three models for exploring sex differences in genetic and environmental effects (i.e., models for sex-limitation) and provide an example of each by analyzing twin data on body mass index (BMI).

Just as the magnitude of genetic and environmental influences may differ according to sex, they also may vary under disparate environmental conditions. If differences in genetic variance across environmental exposure groups result in differential heritability estimates for these groups, a genotype × environment interaction is said to exist. Historically, genotype × environment (G × E) interactions have been noted in plant and animal species (Mather and Jinks, 1982); however, there is increasing evidence that they play an important role in human variability as well (Heath and Martin, 1986; Heath *et al.*, 1989b). A simple method for detecting

G × E interactions is to estimate components of phenotypic variance conditional on environmental exposure (Eaves, 1982). In the second part of this chapter (section 11.4), we illustrate how this method may be employed by suitably modifying models for sex-limitation. We then apply the models to depression scores of female twins and estimate components of variance conditional on a putative buffering environment, marital status.

11.2   Sex-limitation Models

11.2.1   General Model for Sex-limitation

Overview

The general sex-limitation model allows us to (1) estimate the *magnitude* of genetic and environmental effects on male and female phenotypes and (2) determine whether or not it is the *same set* of genes or shared environmental experiences that influence a trait in males and females. Although the first task may be achieved with data from like-sex twin pairs only, the second task requires that we have data from opposite-sex pairs (Eaves *et al.*, 1978). Thus, the LISREL 7 script we describe will include model specifications for all 5 zygosity groups (MZ–male, MZ–female, DZ–male, DZ–female, DZ–opposite-sex).

To introduce the general sex-limitation model, we consider a path diagram for opposite-sex pairs, shown in Figure 11.1. Included among the ultimate variables in the diagram are female and male additive genetic (A_f and A_m), dominant genetic (D_f and D_m), and unique environmental (E_f and E_m) effects, which influence the latent phenotype of the female (P_f) or male (P_m) twin. The additive and dominant genetic effects are correlated within twin pairs ($\alpha = 0.50$ for additive effects, and $\beta = 0.25$ for dominant effects) as they are for DZ like-sex pairs in the simple univariate ACE model. This correlational structure implies that the genetic effects represent *common* sets of genes which influence the trait in both males and females; however, since a_m and a_f or d_m and d_f are not constrained to be equal, the common effects need not have the same *magnitude* across the sexes.

Figure 11.1 also includes ultimate variables for the male member of the opposite-sex twin pair (A'_m and D'_m) which do not correlate with genetic effects on the female phenotype. For this reason, we refer to A'_m and D'_m as sex-specific variables. Significant estimates of their effects indicate that the set of genes which influences a trait in males is not identical to that which influences a trait in females. To determine the extent of male-female genetic similarity, one can calculate the male-female genetic correlation (r_g). As usual (see Chapter 2) the correlation is computed as the covariance of the two variables divided by the product of their respective standard deviations. Thus, for additive genetic effects we have

$$r_g = \frac{a_m a_f}{\sqrt{a_f^2(a_m^2 + a'^2_m)}}$$

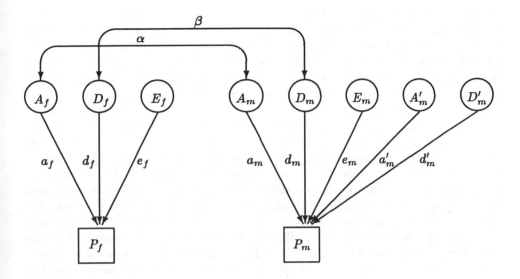

Figure 11.1: The general genotype × sex interaction model for twin data. Path diagram is shown for DZ opposite-sex twin pairs. $\alpha = 0.5$ and $\beta = 0.25$.

Alternatively, a similar estimate may be obtained for dominant genetic effects. However, the information available from twin pairs reared together precludes the estimation of *both* sex-specific parameters, a'_m and d'_m and, consequently, both additive and dominance genetic correlations. Instead, models including A'_m or D'_m may be fit to the data, and their fits compared using appropriate goodness-of-fit indices, such as Akaike's Information Criteria (AIC; Akaike, 1987; see Section 7.3.7). This criterion may be used to compare the fit of an *ACE* model to the fit of an *ADE* model. AIC is one member of a class of indices that reflect both the goodness of fit of a model and its parsimony, or ability to account for the observed data with few parameters.

To generalize the model specified in Figure 11.1 to other zygosity groups, the parameters associated with the female phenotype are equated to similar effects on the phenotypes of female same-sex MZ and DZ twin pairs. In the same manner, all parameters associated with the male phenotype (reflecting effects which are common to both sexes as well as those specific to males) are equated to effects on both members of male same-sex MZ and DZ pairs. As a result, the model predicts that variances will be equal for all female twins, and all male twins, regardless of zygosity group or twin status (i.e., twin 1 vs. twin 2). The model does not necessarily predict equality of variances *across* the sexes.

LISREL 7 Specification

In theory, the same approach that was used to specify the simple univariate ACE model (Chapter 8) in LISREL 7 could be used for the general sex-limitation model. That is, genetic and environmental parameters could be estimated in the Γ matrix while fixing Λ_y to an identity matrix. However, because one is unable to directly impose boundary constraints in LISREL 7, this specification often leads to *negative* parameter estimates for one sex, especially when the DZ opposite-sex correlation is low, as compared to DZ like-sex correlations. Such negative parameter estimates result in a negative genetic (or common environmental) covariation between the sexes. Although a negative covariation is plausible, it seems quite unlikely that the *same* genes or common environmental influences would have *opposite* effects across the sexes. For this reason, we consider an alternative parameterization of the general sex-limitation model which constrains the male-female covariance components to be non-negative. Rindskopf (1984) describes how programs like LISREL can be 'tricked' into imposing linear and non-linear equality or inequality constraints on parameters; some of these methods were used by Neale and Martin (1989) and are adopted here. Figure 11.2 illustrates the approach taken to impose these constraints; again, the path diagram for DZ opposite-sex pairs is used to introduce the concept. Variables to be specified in the LISREL 7 script are provided in the margin.

As can be seen in Figure 11.2, the eight ξ variables do not influence two phenotypes, but rather a corresponding number of η variables. Each of these eight η variables, in turn, influences a latent phenotype (LP_f or LP_m) which is also an η variable. The paths from the ξ to the η variables (specified in the Γ matrix), as well as those between η variables (specified in the **B** matrix), are equal to the square root of the genetic or environmental path coefficients shown in Figure 11.1. By estimating the square root of a_m, d_m, a_f, and d_f, rather than the coefficients themselves, the male-female genetic covariance is constrained to be non-negative. Although it is not *necessary* to impose the same non-negative constraint on path coefficients representing effects which are *not* shared by males and females (e.g., e_m, e_f, a'_m, and d'_m), we do so anyway to maintain consistency in the model.

In writing the LISREL 7 specification for the general G × E model, it is necessary to remember that the model results in a total of ten ξ variables (A_m, D_m, E_m, A'_m, and D'_m for twin 1 and twin 2) for *like-sex male twin pairs*. This is the greatest number of ξ variables required for any zygosity group; however, since LISREL 7 does not allow the user to change the value of NK within a given job, NK must be equal to 10 for all five groups. For those groups without the sex-specific effects, the extra ξ variables will be essentially dummy variables (see Jöreskog and Sörbom, 1989, p. 259 for general use of dummy variables in LISREL). Keeping this in mind, we show below the matrices used for DZ opposite-sex pairs in the LISREL 7 analysis. The dummy ξ variables, X_1 and X_2, have been included. Note that the Λ_y matrix is no longer an identity matrix as it was in the simple univariate ACE

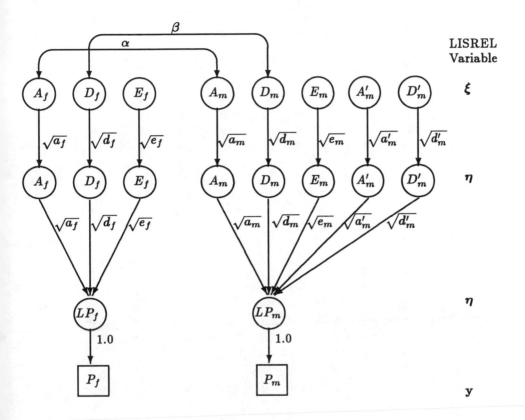

Figure 11.2: The general genotype × sex interaction model for twin data with the square root of path coefficients estimated. Path diagram is shown for DZ opposite-sex twin pairs. $\alpha = 0.5$ and $\beta = 0.25$. The corresponding LISREL variables are given along the right-hand column.

model. In the Φ matrix, $\alpha = 0.5$ and $\beta = 0.25$.

$$
\mathbf{\Gamma} =
\begin{array}{c}
\\ A_f \\ D_f \\ E_f \\ X1 \\ X2 \\ A_m \\ D_m \\ E_m \\ A'_m \\ D'_m \\ P_f \\ P_m
\end{array}
\begin{array}{c}
\begin{array}{cccccccccc}
A_f & D_f & E_f & X1 & X2 & A_m & D_m & E_m & A'_m & D'_m
\end{array} \\
\left[
\begin{array}{cccccccccc}
\sqrt{a_f} & 0 & 0 & 0 & 0 & 0 & 0 & 0 & 0 & 0 \\
0 & \sqrt{d_f} & 0 & 0 & 0 & 0 & 0 & 0 & 0 & 0 \\
0 & 0 & \sqrt{e_f} & 0 & 0 & 0 & 0 & 0 & 0 & 0 \\
0 & 0 & 0 & 0 & 0 & 0 & 0 & 0 & 0 & 0 \\
0 & 0 & 0 & 0 & 0 & 0 & 0 & 0 & 0 & 0 \\
0 & 0 & 0 & 0 & 0 & \sqrt{a_m} & 0 & 0 & 0 & 0 \\
0 & 0 & 0 & 0 & 0 & 0 & \sqrt{d_m} & 0 & 0 & 0 \\
0 & 0 & 0 & 0 & 0 & 0 & 0 & \sqrt{e_m} & 0 & 0 \\
0 & 0 & 0 & 0 & 0 & 0 & 0 & 0 & \sqrt{a'_m} & 0 \\
0 & 0 & 0 & 0 & 0 & 0 & 0 & 0 & 0 & \sqrt{d'_m} \\
0 & 0 & 0 & 0 & 0 & 0 & 0 & 0 & 0 & 0 \\
0 & 0 & 0 & 0 & 0 & 0 & 0 & 0 & 0 & 0
\end{array}
\right]
\end{array}
$$

$$
\mathbf{B} =
\begin{array}{c}
\\ A_f \\ D_f \\ E_f \\ X1 \\ X2 \\ A_m \\ D_m \\ E_m \\ A'_m \\ D'_m \\ P_f \\ P_m
\end{array}
\begin{array}{c}
\begin{array}{cccccccccc}
A_f & D_f & E_f & X1 & X2 & A_m & D_m & E_m & A'_m & D'_m
\end{array} \\
\left[
\begin{array}{cccccccccc}
0 & 0 & 0 & 0 & 0 & 0 & 0 & 0 & 0 & 0 \\
0 & 0 & 0 & 0 & 0 & 0 & 0 & 0 & 0 & 0 \\
0 & 0 & 0 & 0 & 0 & 0 & 0 & 0 & 0 & 0 \\
0 & 0 & 0 & 0 & 0 & 0 & 0 & 0 & 0 & 0 \\
0 & 0 & 0 & 0 & 0 & 0 & 0 & 0 & 0 & 0 \\
0 & 0 & 0 & 0 & 0 & 0 & 0 & 0 & 0 & 0 \\
0 & 0 & 0 & 0 & 0 & 0 & 0 & 0 & 0 & 0 \\
0 & 0 & 0 & 0 & 0 & 0 & 0 & 0 & 0 & 0 \\
0 & 0 & 0 & 0 & 0 & 0 & 0 & 0 & 0 & 0 \\
0 & 0 & 0 & 0 & 0 & 0 & 0 & 0 & 0 & 0 \\
\sqrt{a_f} & \sqrt{d_m} & \sqrt{e_m} & 0 & 0 & 0 & 0 & 0 & 0 & 0 \\
0 & 0 & 0 & 0 & 0 & \sqrt{a_m} & \sqrt{d_m} & \sqrt{e_m} & \sqrt{a'_m} & \sqrt{d'_m}
\end{array}
\right]
\end{array}
$$

$$
\begin{array}{c}
\\ A_f \\ D_f \\ E_f \\ X1 \\ X2 \\ A_m \\ D_m \\ E_m \\ A'_m \\ D'_m \\ P_f \\ P_m
\end{array}
\begin{array}{c}
\begin{array}{cc}
P_f & P_m
\end{array} \\
\left[
\begin{array}{cc}
0 & 0 \\
0 & 0 \\
0 & 0 \\
0 & 0 \\
0 & 0 \\
0 & 0 \\
0 & 0 \\
0 & 0 \\
0 & 0 \\
0 & 0 \\
0 & 0 \\
0 & 0
\end{array}
\right]
\end{array}
$$

$$
\Lambda_y = \begin{array}{c} \\ P_f \\ P_m \end{array}
\begin{array}{c} \begin{array}{cccccccccccc} A_f & D_f & E_f & X1 & X2 & A_m & D_m & E_m & A'_m & D'_m & P_f & P_m \end{array} \\
\left[\begin{array}{cccccccccccc}
0 & 0 & 0 & 0 & 0 & 0 & 0 & 0 & 0 & 0 & 1 & 0 \\
0 & 0 & 0 & 0 & 0 & 0 & 0 & 0 & 0 & 0 & 0 & 1
\end{array} \right]
\end{array}
$$

$$
\Phi = \begin{array}{c} \\ A_f \\ D_f \\ E_f \\ X1 \\ X2 \\ A_m \\ D_m \\ E_m \\ A'_m \\ D'_m \end{array}
\begin{array}{c} \begin{array}{cccccccccc} A_f & D_f & E_f & X1 & X2 & A_m & D_m & E_m & A'_m & D'_m \end{array} \\
\left[\begin{array}{cccccccccc}
1 & 0 & 0 & 0 & 0 & \alpha & 0 & 0 & 0 & 0 \\
0 & 1 & 0 & 0 & 0 & 0 & \beta & 0 & 0 & 0 \\
0 & 0 & 1 & 0 & 0 & 0 & 0 & 0 & 0 & 0 \\
0 & 0 & 0 & 1 & 0 & 0 & 0 & 0 & 0 & 0 \\
0 & 0 & 0 & 0 & 1 & 0 & 0 & 0 & 0 & 0 \\
\alpha & 0 & 0 & 0 & 0 & 1 & 0 & 0 & 0 & 0 \\
0 & \beta & 0 & 0 & 0 & 0 & 1 & 0 & 0 & 0 \\
0 & 0 & 0 & 0 & 0 & 0 & 0 & 1 & 0 & 0 \\
0 & 0 & 0 & 0 & 0 & 0 & 0 & 0 & 1 & 0 \\
0 & 0 & 0 & 0 & 0 & 0 & 0 & 0 & 0 & 1
\end{array} \right]
\end{array}
$$

The full LISREL 7 specification for the general sex-limitation model is provided in Appendix G.1. In this example, we estimate sex-specific additive genetic effects (and fix the sex-specific dominance effects to zero). The data are log-transformed indices of body mass index (BMI) obtained from twins belonging to the Virginia and American Association of Retired Persons twin registries. A detailed description of these data will be provided in section 11.3, in the discussion of the model-fitting results.

11.2.2 Restricted Models for Sex-limitation

In this section, we describe two restricted models for sex-limitation. The first we refer to as the *common effects sex-limitation model*, and the second, the *scalar sex-limitation model*. Both are sub-models of the general sex-limitation model and therefore can be compared to the more general model using likelihood-ratio χ^2 difference tests.

Common Effects Sex-limitation Model

The common effects sex-limitation model is simply one in which the primed pathways in Figures 11.1 or 11.2 (a'_m or d'_m) are fixed to zero. As a result, only the genetic effects which are *common* to both males and females account for phenotype variance and covariance. Although the genes may be the same, the magnitude of their effect is still allowed to differ across the sexes. This restricted model may be compared to the general sex-limitation model using a χ^2 difference test with a single degree of freedom.

Information to discern between the general sex-limitation model and the common effects model comes from the covariance of DZ opposite-sex twin pairs. Specifically, if this covariance is significantly less than that predicted from genetic effects which are *common* to both sexes (i.e., less than $[(a_m \times a_f) + (d_m \times d_f)]$), then there is evidence for sex-specific effects. Otherwise, the restricted model without these effects should not fit significantly worse than the general model. Mere inspection of the *correlations* from DZ like-sex and opposite-sex pairs may alert one to the fact that sex-specific effects are playing a role in trait variation, if it is found that the opposite sex-correlation is markedly less than the like-sex DZ correlations.

Scalar Effects Sex-limitation Model

The scalar sex-limitation model is a sub-model of both the general model and the common effects model. In the scalar model, not only are the sex-specific effects removed, but the variance components for females are all constrained to be equal to a *scalar* multiple (k^2) of the male variance components, such that $a_f^2 = k^2 a_m^2$, $d_f^2 = k^2 d_m^2$, and $e_f^2 = k^2 e_m^2$. As a result, the standardized variance components (e.g., heritability estimates) are equal across sexes, even though the unstandardized components differ.

Figure 11.3 shows a path diagram for DZ opposite-sex under the scalar sex-limitation model, and Appendix G.2 provides the LISREL 7 specification. Unlike the model in Figure 11.2, the scalar model does not include separate parameters for genetic and environmental effects on males and females — instead, these effects are equated across the sexes. Because of this equality, negative estimates of male-female genetic covariance cannot result, and the scalar model may be directly parameterized in terms of a, d, and e, rather than their square roots. To introduce a scaling factor for the male variance components, elements of the $\mathbf{B}$ and $\mathbf{\Lambda}_y$ matrices are employed. Specifically, the element corresponding to the path from a latent non-scaled male phenotype ($L1_m$ – an η variable) to a second latent non-scaled phenotype ($L2_m$ – also an η variable) is set free and equated to the path from $L2_m$ to the observed phenotype (a y-variable). As a result, the estimate of both paths will be equal to $\sqrt{k}$. By estimating $\sqrt{k}$ rather than k itself, one again avoids obtaining a negative estimate of the male-female covariance.

The full scalar sex-limitation model may be compared to the full common effects model using a χ^2 difference test with 2 degrees of freedom. Similarly, the scalar sex-limitation model may be compared to the model with no sex differences (that is, one which fixes $\sqrt{k}$ to 1.0) using a χ^2 difference test with a single degree of freedom.

Comments

The restricted sex-limitation models described in this section are not an exhaustive list of the sub-models of the general sex-limitation model. Within either of these restricted models (as within the general model), one can test hypotheses regarding

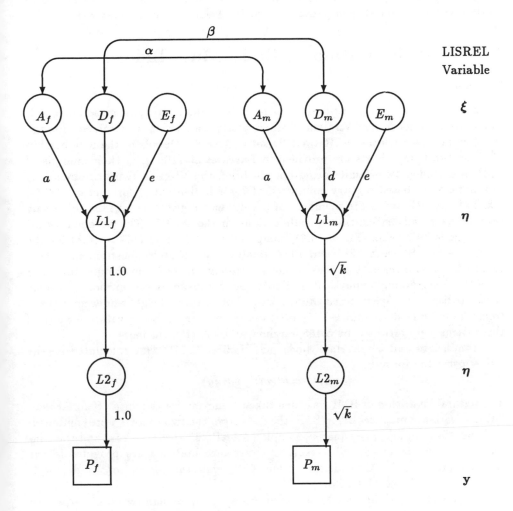

Figure 11.3: The scalar genotype × sex interaction model for twin data. Path diagram is shown for DZ opposite-sex twin pairs. The $\alpha = 0.5$ and $\beta = 0.25$. The corresponding LISREL variables are given along the right-hand column.

the significance of genetic or environmental effects. Also, within the common effects sex-limitation model, one may test whether *specific* components of variance are equal across the sexes (e.g., a_m may be equated to a_f, or e_m to e_f). Again, submodels may be compared to more saturated ones through χ^2 difference tests, or to models with same number of parameters with Akaike's Information Criteria.

11.3   Sex-limitation in Body Mass Index

The sample

In this section, we apply sex-limitation models to data on body mass index collected from twins in the Virginia Twin Registry and twins ascertained through the American Association of Retired Persons (AARP). Details of the membership of these two twin cohorts are provided in Eaves *et al.* (1991), in their analysis of BMI in extended twin-family pedigrees. In brief, the Virginia twins are members of a population based registry comprised of 7,458 individuals (Corey *et al.*, 1986), while the AARP twins are members of a volunteer registry of 12,118 individuals responding to advertisements in publications of the AARP. The Virginia twins' mean age is 39.7 years (SD = 14.3), compared to 54.5 years (SD = 16.8) for the AARP twins. Between 1985 and 1987, Health and Lifestyle questionnaires were mailed to twins from both of these cohorts. Among the items on the questionnaire were those pertaining to physical similarity and confusion in recognition by others (used to diagnose zygosity) and those asking about current height and weight (used to compute body mass indices). Questionnaires with no missing values for any of these items were returned by 5,465 Virginia and AARP twin pairs.

From height and weight data, body mass indices (BMI) were calculated for the twins, using the formula:

$$\text{BMI} = ht(m)^2/wt(kg)$$

The natural logarithm of BMI was then taken to normalize the data. Before calculating covariance matrices of log BMI, the data from the two cohorts were combined, and the effects of age, age squared, sample (AARP vs. Virginia), sex, and their interactions were removed. The resulting covariance matrices are provided in the LISREL programs in Appendices G.1 and G.2, while the correlations and sample sizes appear in Table 11.1 below.

We note that both like-sex MZ correlations are greater than twice the respective DZ correlations; thus, models with dominant genetic effects, rather than common environmental effects, were fit to the data.

Model-fitting Results

In Table 11.2, we provide selected results from fitting the following models: general sex-limitation (I); common effects sex-limitation (II-IV); and scalar sex-limitation (V). We first note that the general sex-limitation model provides a good fit to the

Table 11.1: Sample sizes and correlations for BMI twin data.

Zygosity Group	N	r
MZF	1802	0.744
DZF	1142	0.352
MZM	750	0.700
DZM	553	0.309
DZO	1341	0.251

data, with $p = 0.32$. The estimate of a'_m under this model is fairly small, and when set to zero in model II, found to be non-significant ($\chi^2_1 = 2.54$, $p > 0.05$). Thus, there is no evidence for sex-specific additive genetic effects, and the common effects sex-limitation model (model II) is favored over the general model. As an exercise, the reader may wish to verify that the same conclusion is reached if the general sex-limitation model with sex-specific dominant genetic effects is compared to the common effects model with d'_m removed.

Note that under model II the dominant genetic parameter for females is quite small; thus, when this parameter is fixed to zero in model III, there is not a significant worsening of fit, and model III becomes the most favored model. In model IV, we consider whether the dominant genetic effect for males can also be fixed to zero. The goodness-of-fit statistics indicate that this model fits the data poorly ($p < 0.01$) and provides a significantly worse fit than model III ($\chi^2_1 = 26.73$, $p < 0.01$). Model IV is therefore rejected and model III remains the favored one.

Finally, we consider the scalar sex-limitation model. Since there is evidence for dominant genetic effects in males and not in females, it seems unlikely that this model, which constrains the variance components of females to be scalar multiples of the male variance components, will provide a good fit to the data, unless the additive genetic variance in females is also much smaller than the male additive genetic variance. The model-fitting results support this contention: the model provides a marginal fit to the data ($p = 0.05$), and is significantly worse than model II ($\chi^2_2 = 7.82$, $p < 0.05$). We thus conclude from Table 11.2 that III is the best fitting model. This conclusion would also be reached if AIC was used to assess goodness-of-fit.

Using the parameter estimates under model III, the expected variance of log BMI (residuals) in males and females can be calculated. A little arithmetic reveals that the phenotypic variance of males is markedly lower than that of females (0.17 vs. 0.28). Inspection of the parameter estimates indicates that the sex difference in phenotypic variance is due to increased *genetic* and *environmental* variance in females. However, the increase in genetic variance in females is proportionately greater than the increase in environmental variance, and this difference results in a

Table 11.2: Parameter estimates obtained by fitting genotype × sex interaction models to Virginia and AARP body mass index (BMI) twin data.

Parameter	MODEL				
	I	II	III	IV	V
a_f	0.449	0.454	0.454	0.454	0.346
d_f	0.172	0.000	–	–	0.288
e_f	0.264	0.265	0.265	0.267	0.267
a_m	0.210	0.240	0.240	0.342	–
d_m	0.184	0.245	0.245	–	–
e_m	0.213	0.213	0.213	0.220	–
a'_m	0.198	–	–	–	–
k	–	–	–	–	0.778
χ^2	9.26	11.80	11.80	38.53	19.62
$d.f.$	8	9	10	11	11
p	0.32	0.23	0.30	0.00	0.05
AIC	-6.74	-6.20	-8.20	16.53	-2.38

somewhat larger broad sense (i.e., $a^2 + d^2$) heritability estimate for females (75%) than for males (69%).

Comments

The detection of sex-differences in environmental and genetic effects on BMI leads to questions regarding the nature of these differences. Speculation might suggest that the somewhat lower male heritability estimate may be due to the fact that males are less accurate in their self-report of height and weight than are females. With additional information, such as test-retest data, this hypothesis could be rigorously tested. The sex-dependency of genetic dominance is similarly curious. It may be that the common environment in females exerts a greater influence on BMI than in males, and, consequently, masks a genetic dominance effect. Alternatively, the genetic architecture may indeed be different across the sexes, resulting from sex differences in selective pressures during human evolution. Again, additional data, such as that from reared together adopted siblings, could be used to explore these alternative hypotheses.

One sex-limitation model that we have not considered, but which is biologically reasonable, is that the across-sex correlation between additive genetic effects is the same as the across-sex correlation between the dominance genetic effects[1]. Fitting

---

[1] The reasoning goes like this: (e.g.) males have a elevated level of a chemical that prevents *any* gene expression from certain loci, at random with respect to the phenotype under study. Thus,

a model of this type involves a constraint that is very tricky to implement within LISREL 7. At the time of writing, problems with the beta version of LISREL 8 prevent its use for this application. However, we expect that future versions will resolve this difficulty. In any case, these models are very easy to fit with Mx (Neale, 1991).

11.4 Genotype × Environment Interaction

As stated in the introduction of this chapter, genotype × environment (G × E) interactions can be detected by estimating components of phenotypic variance *conditional* on environmental exposures. To do so, MZ and DZ covariance matrices are computed for twins concordant for exposure, concordant for non-exposure , and discordant for exposure, and structural equation models are fitted to the resulting six zygosity groups. The LISREL 7 specifications for alternative G × E interaction models are quite similar to those used in a sex-limitation analysis; however, there are important differences between the two. In a G × E interaction analysis, the presence of a sixth group provides the information for an additional parameter to be estimated. Further, the nature of alternative hypotheses used to explain heterogeneity across groups differs from those invoked in a sex-limitation analysis. In section 11.4.1 we detail these differences, and in section 11.5 we illustrate the method with an application to data on marital status and depression.

11.4.1 Models for G × E Interactions

Testable Assumptions

The LISREL models described in this section are appropriate for analyzing G × E interaction when genes and environment are acting independently. However, if there is genotype – environment correlation, then more sophisticated statistical procedures are necessary for the analysis. One way of detecting a G – E correlation is to compute the cross-correlations between one twin's environment and the trait of interest in the cotwin (Heath *et al.*, 1989b). If the cross-correlation is not significant, there is no evidence for a G – E correlation, and the G × E analysis may proceed using the methods described below.

General G × E Interaction Model

First we consider the general G × E interaction model, similar to the general sex-limitation model discussed in section 11.2.2. This model not only allows the magnitude of genetic and environmental effects to vary across environmental conditions,

---

both additive and dominant genetic effects would be reduced in males vs females, and hence the same genetic correlation between the sexes would apply to both.

but also, by using information from twin pairs discordant for environmental exposure, enables us to determine whether it is the same set of genes or environmental features that are expressed in the two environments. Just as we used twins who were discordant for sex (i.e., DZO pairs) to illustrate the sex-limitation model, we use twins discordant for environmental exposure to portray the general G × E interaction model. Before modeling genetic and environmental effects on these individuals, one must order the twins so that the first of the pair has not been exposed to the putative modifying environment, while the second has (or *vice versa*, as long as the order is consistent across families and across groups). The path model for the discordant DZ pairs is then identical to that used for the dizygotic opposite-sex pairs in the sex-limitation model; for the discordant MZ pairs, it differs only from the DZ model in the correlation structure of the ultimate genetic variables (see Figure 11.4).

Among the ultimate variables in Figure 11.4 are genetic effects that are correlated between the unexposed and exposed twins and those that influence only the latter (i.e., environment-specific effects). For the concordant unexposed and concordant exposed MZ and DZ pairs, path models are comparable to those used for female-female and male-male MZ and DZ pairs in the sex-limitation analysis, with environment-specific effects (instead of sex-specific effects) operating on the exposed twins (instead of the male twins). As a result, the model predicts equal variances *within* an exposure class, across zygosity groups.

In specifying the general G × E interaction model in LISREL 7, one must again estimate the square root of genetic and environmental path coefficients, rather than the coefficients themselves, in order to avoid negative covariance estimates for the pairs discordant for exposure. Appendix G.3 contains a LISREL script which uses this technique.

Unlike the general sex-limitation analysis, there is enough information in a G × E analysis to estimate two environment-specific effects. Thus, the magnitude of environment-specific additive and dominant genetic *or* additive genetic and common environmental effects can be determined. It still is not possible to simultaneously estimate the magnitude of common environmental and dominant genetic effects.

Common Effects G × E Interaction Model

A *common effects G × E model* can also be fitted to covariance matrices computed conditionally on environmental exposure by simply fixing the environment-specific effects of the general model to zero, and comparing the two using a χ^2 difference test. The information from pairs discordant for environmental exposure allows for this comparison.

A critical sub-model of the common effects G × E model is one which tests the hypothesis that exposure group heterogeneity is *solely due to heteroscedasticity*, or *group differences in random environmental variance*, rather than *group differences*

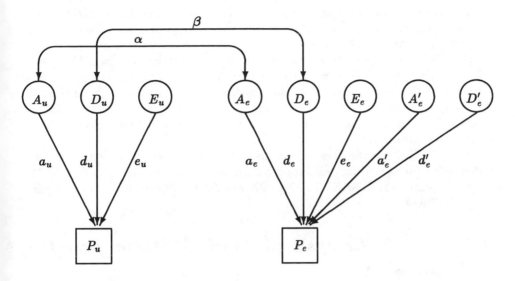

Figure 11.4: The general genotype × environment interaction model for twin data. Path diagram is for MZ and DZ twins discordant for environmental exposure. For MZ pairs, $\alpha = 1.0$ and $\beta = 1.0$; for DZ pairs, $\alpha = 0.5$ and $\beta = 0.25$. The subscripts u and e identify variables and parameters and unexposed and exposed twins, respectively.

in genetic variance. To fit this model, the genetic parameters are simply equated across groups, while allowing the random environmental effects to take on different values. If this model does not fit worse than the full common effects model, then there is evidence for heteroscedasticity.

A second sub-model of the common effects G × E interaction model is one which constrains the *environmental* parameters to be equal across exposure groups, while allowing the genetic variance components to differ. If this model is not significantly worse than the full common effects model, then there is evidence to suggest that the environmental interaction only involves a differential expression of genetic, but not environmental, influences.

Scalar Effects G × E Interaction Model

As with the scalar sex-limitation model, the *scalar G × E interaction model* equates genetic and environmental effects on exposed twins to be a scalar multiple of similar effects on twins who have not been exposed to a modifying environment. As a consequence, the heritability of a trait remains constant across exposure groups, and there is *no* evidence for a genotype × environment interaction. This situation may arise if there is a mean-variance relationship, and an increase in trait mean under a particular environmental condition is accompanied by an increase in phenotypic variation. When this is the case, the ratio of the genetic variance component and environmental variance component is expected to remain the same in different environments.

The LISREL 7 specification for the scalar G × E interaction model is identical to that used for the scalar sex-limitation model, except for the addition of MZ discordant pairs. The LISREL 7 script in Appendix G.4 illustrates how these pairs may be included.

11.5   G × E Analysis of Marital Status and Depression

In this section, we determine whether the heritability of self-report depression scores varies according to the marital status of female twins. Our hypothesis is that marriage, or a marriage-type relationship, serves as a buffer to decrease an individual's inherited liability to depression, consequently decreasing the heritability of the trait.

The Data

The data were collected from twins enrolled in the Australian National Health and Medical Research Council Twin register. In this sample, mailed questionnaires were sent to the 5,967 pairs of twins on the register between November 1980 and March 1982 (see also Chapter 12). Among the items on the questionnaire were those from the state depression scale of the Delusions-Symptoms States Inventory (DSSI; Bedford *et al.*, 1976) and a single item regarding marital status. The analyses performed here focus on the like-sex MZ and DZ female pairs who returned completed questionnaires. The ages of the respondents ranged from 18 to 88 years; however, due to possible differences in variance components across age cohorts, we have limited our analysis to those twins who were age 30 or less at the time of their response. There were 570 female MZ pairs in this young cohort, with mean age 23.77 years (SD = 3.65); and 349 DZ pairs, with mean age 23.66 years (SD = 3.93).

Using responses to the marital status item, pairs were subdivided into those who were concordant for being married (or living in a marriage type relationship);

those who were concordant for being unmarried; and those who were discordant
for marital status. In the discordant pairs, the data were reordered so that the first
twin was always unmarried. Depression scores were derived by summing the 7 DSSI
item scores, and then taking a log-transformation of the data $[x' = log_{10}(x + 1)]$ to
reduce heteroscedasticity. Covariance matrices of depression scores were computed
for the six zygosity groups after linear and quadratic effects of age were removed.
The matrices are provided in the LISREL 7 scripts in Appendices G.3 and G.4,
while the correlations and sample sizes are shown in Table 11.3. We note (i) that in
all cases, MZ correlations are greater than the corresponding DZ correlations; and
(ii) that for concordant married and discordant pairs, the MZ:DZ ratio is greater
than 2:1, suggesting the presence of genetic dominance.

Table 11.3: Sample sizes and correlations for Australian female twin depression
data.

Zygosity Group	N	r
MZ - Concordant single	254	0.409
DZ - Concordant single	155	0.221
MZ - Concordant married	177	0.382
DZ - Concordant married	107	0.098
MZ - Discordant	139	0.324
DZ - Discordant	87	0.059

Before proceeding with the G × E interaction analyses, we tested whether there
was a G – E correlation involving marital status and depression. To do so, cross-
correlations between twins' marital status and cotwins' depression score were computed. In all but one case (DZ twin 1's depression with cotwin's marital status;
$r = -0.156$, $p < 0.01$), the correlations were not significant. This near absence of
significant correlations implies that a genetic predisposition to depression does not
lead to an increased probability of remaining single, and indicates that a G – E
correlation need not be modeled.

Model-fitting Results

Table 11.4 shows the results of fitting several models: general G × E (I); full
common-effects G × E (II); three common-effects sub-models (III-V); scalar G x E
(VI); and no G × E interaction (VII). Parameter estimates subscripted s and m refer respectively to single (unexposed) and married twins. Models including genetic
dominance parameters, rather than common environmental effects, were fitted to
the data. The reader may wish to show that the overall conclusions concerning
G × E interaction do not differ if shared environment parameters are substituted

for genetic dominance.

Table 11.4: Parameter estimates obtained by fitting genotype × marriage interaction models to depression scores in Australian female twins.

Parameter	MODEL						
	I	II	III	IV	V	VI	VII
a_s	0.187	0.187	0.207	0.209	0.186	0.206	0.188
d_s	0.106	0.105	–	–	–	–	–
e_s	0.240	0.240	0.246	0.245	0.257	0.247	0.246
a_m	0.048	0.048	0.163	0.162	0.186	0.206	0.188
d_m	0.171	0.173	–	–	–	–	–
e_m	0.232	0.232	0.243	0.245	0.232	0.247	0.246
a'_m	0.008	–	–	–	–	–	–
k	–	–	–	–	–	0.916	–
χ^2	15.44	15.48	18.88	18.91	22.32	20.08	27.19
$d.f.$	11	12	14	15	15	15	16
p	0.16	0.22	0.17	0.22	0.10	0.17	0.04
AIC	-6.56	-9.52	-9.12	-11.09	-7.68	-9.92	-4.81

Model I is a general G × E model with environment-specific additive genetic
effects. It provides a reasonable fit to the data ($p = 0.16$), with all parameters of
moderate size, except a'_m. Under model II, the parameter a'_m is set to zero, and
the fit is not significantly worse than model I ($\chi^2_1 = 0.04$, $p = 0.84$). Thus, there
is no evidence for environment-specific additive genetic effects. As an exercise, the
reader may verify that the same conclusion can be made for environment-specific
dominant genetic effects.

Under model III, we test whether the dominance effects on single and married
individuals are significant. A χ^2 difference of 3.40 ($p = 0.183$, 2 df.) between
models III and II indicates that they are not. Consequently, model III, which
excludes common dominance effects while retaining common additive genetic and
specific environmental effects, is favored.

Models IV - VII are all sub-models of III: the first specifies no differences in
environmental variance components across exposure groups; the second specifies
no differences in genetic variance components across groups; the third constrains
the genetic and environmental variance components of single twins to be scalar
multiples of those of married twins; and the fourth specifies no genetic or environmental differences between the groups. When each of these is compared to model
III using a χ^2 difference test, only model VII (specifying complete homogeneity
across groups) is significantly worse than the fuller model ($\chi^2_2 = 8.28$, p = 0.004).
In order to select the best sub-models from IV, V and VI, Akaike's Information

Criteria were used. These criteria indicate that model IV — which allows for group differences in genetic, but not environmental, effects — gives the most parsimonious explanation for the data. Under model IV, the heritability of depression is 42% for single, and 30% for married twins. This finding supports our hypothesis that marriage or marriage type relationships act as a buffer against the expression of inherited liability to depression.

Chapter 12

Multivariate Analysis

12.1   Introduction

Until this point we have been concerned primarily with methods for analyzing single variables obtained from twin pairs; that is, with estimation of the relevant sources of genetic and environmental *variation* in each variable separately. Most studies, however, are not designed to consider single variables, but are trying to understand what factors make sets of variables correlate, or *co-vary*, to a greater or lesser extent. Just as we can partition variation into its genetic and environmental components, so too we can try to determine how far the covariation between multiple measures is due to genetic and environmental factors. This partitioning of covariation is one of the first tasks of multivariate genetic analysis, and it is one for which the classical twin study, with its simple and regular structure, is especially well-suited.

In Chapter 1 we described three of the main issues in the genetic analysis of multiple variables. These issues include

1. The contribution of genes and the environment to the correlation between variables

2. The direction of causation between observed variables

3. Genetic and environmental contributions to developmental change.

Each of these questions presumes either a different data collection strategy or a different model or both; for example, analysis of measurements of correlated traits taken at the same time (question 1) requires somewhat different methods than assessments of the same trait taken longitudinally (question 3). However, all of the multivariate issues share the requirement of multiple measurements from the same subjects. In this chapter we direct our attention to the first issue: genetic and environmental contributions to observed correlations among variables. We describe twin methods for the other two questions in Chapters 13 – 15.

231

The treatment of multivariate models presented here is intended to be introductory. There are many specific topics within the broad domain of multivariate genetic analysis, some of which we address in subsequent chapters. Here we exclude treatment of observed and latent variable means, analysis of singleton twins, and approaches using the constrained variable options in LISREL 8.

12.2   Phenotypic Factor Analysis

Factor analysis is one of the most widely used multivariate methods. The general idea is to explain variation within and covariation between a large number of observed variables with a smaller number of latent factors. Here we give a brief outline of the method — those seeking more thorough treatments are referred to e.g., Gorsuch (1983), Harman (1976), Lawley and Maxwell (1971). Typically the free parameters of primary interest in factor models are the *factor loadings* and *factor correlations*. Factor loadings indicate the degree of relationship between a latent factor and an observed variable, while factor correlations represent the relationships between the hypothesized latent factors. An observed variable that is a good indicator of a latent factor is said to "load highly" on that factor. For example, in intelligence research, where factor theory has its origins (Spearman, 1904), it may be noted that a vocabulary test loads highly on a hypothesized (latent) verbal ability factor, but loads to a much lesser extent on a latent spatial ability factor; i.e., the vocabulary test relates strongly to verbal ability, but less so to spatial ability. Normally a factor loading is identical to a path coefficient of the type described in Chapter 5.

In this section we describe factor analytic models and present some illustrative applications to observed measurements without reference to genetic and environmental causality. We turn to genetic factor models in Section 12.3.

12.2.1   Exploratory and Confirmatory Factor Models

There are two general classes of factor models: exploratory and confirmatory. In exploratory factor analysis one does not postulate an *a priori* factor structure; that is, the number of latent factors, correlations among them, and the *factor loading pattern* (the pattern of relative weights of the observed variables on the latent factors) is calculated from the data in some manner which maximizes the amount of variance/covariance explained by the latent factors. More formally, in exploratory factor analysis:

1. There are no hypotheses about factor loadings (all variables load on all factors, and factor loadings cannot be constrained to be equal to other loadings)

2. There are no hypotheses about interfactor correlations (either all correlations are zero — orthogonal factors, or all may correlate — oblique factors)

3. Only one group is analyzed

4. Unique factors (those that relate only to one variable) are uncorrelated,

5. All observed variables need to have specific variances.

These models often are fitted using a statistical package such as SPSS or SAS, in which one may *explore* the relationships among observed variables in a latent variable framework.

In contrast, confirmatory factor analysis requires one to formulate a hypothesis about the number of latent factors, the relationships between the observed and latent factors (the factor pattern), and the correlations among the factors. Thus, a possible model of the data is formulated in advance as a *factor structure,* and the factor loadings and correlations are estimated from the data[1]. As usual, this model-fitting process allows one to *test* the ability of the hypothesized factor structure to account for the observed covariances by examining the overall fit of the model. Typically the model involves certain constraints, such as equalities among certain factor loadings or equalities of some of the factor correlations. If the model fails then we may relax certain constraints or add more factors, test for significant improvement in fit using the chi-squared difference test, and examine the overall goodness of fit to see if the new model adequately accounts for the observed covariation. Likewise, some or all of the correlations between latent factors may be set to zero or estimated. Then we can test if these constraints are consistent with the data. Confirmatory factor models are the type we are concerned with using LISREL.

12.2.2 Building a Phenotypic Factor Model LISREL Script

Although it is possible to set up models in LISREL as described in the earlier chapters, using both x and y variables and their respective latent factors, in the present factor analysis examples it is more efficient to use only the Λ_y, Θ_ϵ, and Ψ matrices with observed y and latent η variables, or alternatively, the Λ_x, Θ_δ, and Φ matrices with observed x and latent ξ variables. Using the former, the factor model may be written as

$$y_{ij} = \lambda_i \eta_j + \epsilon_{ij}$$

with

$$i \;=\; 1, \cdots, p \;\text{(variables)}$$
$$j \;=\; 1, \cdots, n \;\text{(subjects)}$$

and where the measured variables y are a function of a subject's value on the underlying factor (η) (henceforth the j subscript indicating subjects in y will be

---

[1] In exploratory factor analysis the term "factor structure" is used to describe the correlations between variables and factors, but in confirmatory analysis, as described here, the term often describes the characteristics of a hypothesized factor model.

omitted). These subject values are called *factor scores*. Although the use of factor scores is always implicit in the application of factor analysis, they cannot be determined precisely but must be estimated, since the number of common and unique factors always exceeds the number of observed variables. In addition, there is a specific part (ϵ) to each variable. The λ's are the p–variate factor loadings of measured variables on the latent factors. To estimate these loadings we do not need to know the individual factor scores, as the expectation for the $p \times p$ covariance matrix ($\Sigma_{y,y}$) consists only of Λ_y, Ψ, and Θ_ϵ, where Λ_y is a $p \times m$ matrix of factor loadings (m equals the number of latent factors), Ψ is the $m \times m$ correlation matrix of factor scores, and Θ_ϵ is a $p \times p$ diagonal matrix of specific variances:

$$\Sigma_{y,y} = \Lambda_y \Psi \Lambda_y' + \Theta_\epsilon . \tag{12.1}$$

In problems with uncorrelated latent factors, $\Psi = I$, so equation 12.1 reduces to

$$\Sigma_{y,y} = \Lambda_y \Lambda_y' + \Theta_\epsilon . \tag{12.2}$$

Thus, the parameters in the model consist of factor loadings and specific variances (sometimes also referred to as error variances).

12.2.3   Fitting a Phenotypic Factor Model

Martin *et al.* (1985) obtained data on arithmetic computation from male and female twins who were measured once before and three times after drinking a standard dose of alcohol. To illustrate the use of a confirmatory factor analysis model in LISREL, we analyze data from MZ females (first born twin only). The observed variances and correlations are shown in Table 12.1. The confirmatory model is one in which a single latent factor is hypothesized to account for all the covariances among the four variables. The LISREL script below shows the model specifications and the 4×4 input matrix.

Table 12.1: Observed correlations (with variances on the diagonal) for arithmetic computation variables from female MZ twins before (time 0) and after (times 1 – 3) standard doses of alcohol.

	Time 0	Time 1	Time 2	Time3
Time 0	259.66			
Time 1	.81	259.94		
Time 2	.83	.87	245.24	
Time 3	.87	.87	.90	249.30

LISREL Script for Phenotypic Factor Analysis of Four Variables

```
SINGLE FACTOR PHENOTYPIC MODEL: 4 ARITH. COMP. VARIABLES
DA NG=1 NI=4 NO=42 MA=CM
CM
259.664
209.325 259.939
209.532 220.755 245.235
221.610 221.491 221.317 249.298
LA
Time1 Time2 Time3 Time4
MO NY=4 NE=1 LY=FU,FR PS=DI,FI TE=DI,FR
VA 1 PS 1
ST 9 ALL
OU NS RS
```

On the DAta line we have only NG=1 group (consisting of NO=42 subjects) and there are NI=4 input variables. The MOdel command is specified so that all of the NY=4 y variables load on the single common factor (NE=1) and their specific variances are estimated on the diagonal of TE (=DI,FR). In this phenotypic factor model, we have sufficient information to estimate factor loadings and specific variances for the four y variables, but we cannot simultaneously estimate the variance of the common factor because the model would then be underidentified. We therefore fix the variance of the latent factor to an arbitrary non-zero constant, which we choose to be unity in order to keep the factor loadings and specific variances in the original scale of measurement of y (VA 1 PS 1).

The LISREL output (after editing) from this common factor model is shown below. The PARAMETER SPECIFICATIONS section of the output depicts the single common factor structure of the model: there are free factor loadings for each of the four y variables on the common factor η, and specific variance parameters for each of the observed variables. Thus, the model has a total of 8 parameters to explain the $4(4+1)/2 = 10$ free statistics. The chi-squared goodness-of-fit value of 1.46 for 2 degrees of freedom suggests that this single factor model adequately explains the observed covariances ($p = .483$). This also may be seen by comparing the elements of the fitted covariance matrix and the observed covariance matrix, which are seen to be very similar. The fitted covariance matrix is printed by LISREL when the OUtput line includes (as in this case) the RS (residuals) keyword. The fitted covariance matrix is calculated by LISREL using expression 12.2 with the final estimated parameter values.

LISREL Output from Phenotypic Factor Model

PARAMETER SPECIFICATIONS
        LAMBDA Y
            ETA 1

TIME1   1
TIME2   2
TIME3   3
TIME4   4

THETA EPS
          TIME1   TIME2   TIME3   TIME4

        --------   --------   --------   --------
            5   6   7   8

LISREL ESTIMATES (MAXIMUM LIKELIHOOD)
        LAMBDA Y
            ETA 1

TIME1   14.431
TIME2   14.745
TIME3   14.699
TIME4   15.119

        PSI
            ETA 1

            1.000

        THETA EPS
          TIME1   TIME2   TIME3   TIME4

        --------   --------   --------   --------
         51.422   42.509   29.174   20.709

    CHI-SQUARE WITH   2 DEGREES OF FREEDOM =   1.46 (P = .483)

        FITTED COVARIANCE MATRIX
          TIME1   TIME2   TIME3   TIME4

        --------   --------   --------   --------
TIME1   259.670
TIME2   212.784   259.927
TIME3   212.115   216.736   245.229
TIME4   218.181   222.933   222.233   249.297

12.3 Simple Genetic Factor Models

The factor analytic approach outlined above can be readily applied to multivariate genetic problems. This was first suggested by Martin and Eaves (1977) for the analysis of twin data (although in their original publication they use matrices of mean squares and cross-products between and within twin pairs). As in the phenotypic example above, a single common factor is proposed to account for correlations among the variables, but now one such factor is hypothesized for each of the components of variation, genetic, shared environmental, and non-shared environmental. Data from genetically related individuals are used to estimate loadings of variables on common genetic and environmental factors, so that variances and covariances may be explained in terms of these factors.

12.3.1 Multivariate Genetic Factor Model

Using genetic notation, the genetic factor model can be represented as

$$P_{ij} = a_i A_j + c_i C_j + e_i E_j + U_{ij}$$

with

$$
\begin{aligned}
i &= 1, \cdots, p \text{ (variables)} \\
j &= 1, \cdots, n \text{ (subjects)}
\end{aligned}
$$

The measured phenotype (P) (again, omitting the j subscript) consists of multiple variables that are a function of a subject's underlying additive genetic deviate (A), common (between-families) environment (C), and non-shared (within-families) environment (E). In addition, each variable P_j has a specific component U_j that itself may consist of a genetic and a non-genetic part. In this initial application, we assume that U_j is entirely random environmental in origin, an assumption we relax later. Parameters a, c, and e are the p–variate factor loadings of measured variables on the latent factors.

In LISREL, we can model the genetic and environmental factors as η variables, so that η might, for example, consist of one genetic, one shared environment and one random environment factor for each twin ($A_1, A_2, C_1, C_2, E_1, E_2$). In this case there would be $m = 6$ factors and if there were four observed variables for each twin, Λ_y would be a $p \times m$ (8×6) matrix of the factor loadings, Ψ the $m \times m$ correlation matrix of factor scores, and Θ_ϵ a $p \times p$ diagonal matrix of unique variances. The expected covariance may then be calculated as in equation 12.1:

$$\Sigma_{y,y} = \Lambda_y \Psi \Lambda_y' + \Theta_\epsilon . \tag{12.3}$$

In a multivariate analysis of twin data according to this factor model, Σ is a $2p \times 2p$ predicted covariance matrix of observations on twin 1 and twin 2 and Λ_y is a $2p \times 2m$ matrix of loadings of these observations on latent genotypes and non-shared and common environments of twin 1 and twin 2. The factor loadings between A_1 and A_2, E_1 and E_2, and C_1 and C_2 are constrained to be equal for twin 1 and twin 2, similar to the path coefficients of the univariate models discussed in previous chapters. The unique variances also are equal for both members of a twin pair. These may be estimated on the diagonal of the $2p \times 2p$ Θ_ϵ matrix (e.g., Heath *et al.*, 1989c). To fit this model, Λ_y and Θ_ϵ are estimated from the data and Ψ ($2m \times 2m$) must be fixed *a priori* (for example, the correlation between A_1 for twin 1 and A_2 for twin 2 is 1.0 for MZ and 0.5 for DZ twins; the correlation between the C variables of twin 1 and twin 2 is 1.0).

12.3.2   Fitting the Multivariate Genetic Model

Table 12.2: Observed female MZ (above diagonal) and DZ (below diagonal) correlations for arithmetic computation variables.

	Twin 1			Twin 2			
T0	T1	T2	T3	T0	T1	T2	T3
DZ Twins							
297.92							
.89	229.41						
.85	.90	247.42					
.83	.86	.86	274.94				
.23	.31	.36	.34	281.96			
.22	.32	.34	.38	.81	359.70		
.16	.23	.27	.35	.79	.86	326.93	
.23	.31	.34	.37	.81	.86	.87	281.09
MZ Twins							
259.66							
.81	259.94						
.83	.87	245.24					
.87	.87	.90	249.30				
.78	.74	.73	.74	283.80			
.65	.74	.66	.71	.73	249.49		
.71	.74	.72	.74	.78	.86	262.09	
.68	.71	.70	.75	.79	.87	.87	270.93

Arithmetic assessments are shown as T0 — T3 to represent administration times 0—3 before and after standard doses of alcohol. Variances are shown on the diagonals of the matrices.

To illustrate the genetic common factor model we fit it to the arithmetic computation data, but now using both members of the female twin pairs and specifying two groups for the MZ and DZ twins. The observed variances and correlations examined in this analysis are presented in Table 12.2. Appendix E.1 shows the full LISREL script for this model. The DAta command of the script now defines the model for NG=2 groups and NI=8 variables, comprised of the four variables each for both members of twin pairs. The MOdel command appears as

MO NY=8 NE=6 LY=FU,FI PS=FI TE=DI,FR

which shows that we are treating all observed measures as y variables (NY=8) and the NE=6 latent factors as η variables. The (fixed) correlations between genetic factors and between shared environmental factors for twins are specified in the Ψ matrix, and the diagonal of this matrix contains the variances of the latent genetic and environmental factors, which we fix at unity as in the phenotypic model (VA 1 PS 1,1 ... PS 6,6). Also similar to the phenotypic model are the unique variances in the diagonal of Θ_ϵ. It is important to note that there are several EQuality statements to equate the factor loadings and unique variances for both twins in a pair, and that the LY and TE matrix are specified as INvariant in the second group. The INvariant statement equates all factor loadings and unique variances between MZ and DZ twins. The most notable difference between this genetic factor model and the phenotypic formulation is in the Λ_y matrix. For this we use the PAttern statement to express the confirmatory factor model specification. The PA LY usage forces the twin 1 and twin 2 variables to load only on their respective latent factors:

	A_1	C_1	E_1	A_2	C_2	E_2
Twin1-Time0	1	1	1	0	0	0
Twin1-Time1	1	1	1	0	0	0
Twin1-Time2	1	1	1	0	0	0
Twin1-Time3	1	1	1	0	0	0
Twin2-Time0	0	0	0	1	1	1
Twin2-Time1	0	0	0	1	1	1
Twin2-Time2	0	0	0	1	1	1
Twin2-Time3	0	0	0	1	1	1

The row and column headings are added here for clarity but must be omitted from the LISREL script. We equate the loadings between A_1 and A_2, C_1 and C_2, and E_1 and E_2 for the two twins using EQuality commands. We then fix the correlation between twins' additive genetic values at 1.0 (PS 4,1) in the first group (MZ twins) and at 0.5 in the second (DZ twins). The shared environment correlations are fixed at 1.0 for both groups (VA 1 PS 5,2). Note that this part of the model is simply an extension of the univariate model but with more rows of Λ_y for the additional phenotypes.

The LISREL output from this multivariate common factor model is shown below (after editing). The PARAMETER SPECIFICATIONS section illustrates the effects of the EQuality statements in the input script — the A1 and A2 factor loadings are equated, as are the C1 and C2 and the E1 and E2 loadings, and the TE variances for the twin 1 and twin 2 variables. The parameter estimates indicate a substantial genetic basis for the observed arithmetic covariances, as the genetic loadings are much higher than either the shared and non-shared environmental effects. The unique variances in THETA EPS also appear substantial but these do not contribute to covariances among the measures, only to the variance of each observed variable. The χ^2_{56} value of 46.77 suggests that this single factor model provides a reasonable explanation of the data. (Note that the 56 degrees of freedom are obtained from $2 \times 8(8+1)/2$ free statistics minus 16 estimated parameters).

LISREL Output from Full Genetic Common Factor Model

```
----------------------------------------------------------------------
```

PARAMETER SPECIFICATIONS
  LAMBDA Y

	A1	C1	E1	A2	C2	E2
Tw1-T0	1	2	3	0	0	0
Tw1-T1	4	5	6	0	0	0
Tw1-T2	7	8	9	0	0	0
Tw1-T3	10	11	12	0	0	0
Tw2-T0	0	0	0	1	2	3
Tw2-T1	0	0	0	4	5	6
Tw2-T2	0	0	0	7	8	9
Tw2-T3	0	0	0	10	11	12

THETA EPS

Tw1-T0	Tw1-T1	Tw1-T2	Tw1-T3	Tw2-T0	Tw2-T1
13	14	15	16	13	14

THETA EPS

Tw2-T2	Tw2-T3
15	16

LISREL ESTIMATES (MAXIMUM LIKELIHOOD)
  LAMBDA Y

	A1	C1	E1	A2	C2	E2
Tw1-T0	15.088	1.189	4.142	.000	.000	.000
Tw1-T1	13.416	5.119	6.250	.000	.000	.000
Tw1-T2	13.293	4.546	7.146	.000	.000	.000
Tw1-T3	13.553	5.230	5.765	.000	.000	.000

Tw2-T0	.000	.000	.000	15.088	1.189	4.142
Tw2-T1	.000	.000	.000	13.416	5.119	6.250
Tw2-T2	.000	.000	.000	13.293	4.546	7.146
Tw2-T3	.000	.000	.000	13.553	5.230	5.765

```
      THETA EPS
         Tw1-T0      Tw1-T1      Tw1-T2      Tw1-T3      Tw2-T0      Tw2-T1

        --------    --------    --------    --------    --------    --------
         46.208      39.171      31.522      34.684      46.208      39.171
      THETA EPS
         Tw2-T2      Tw2-T3

        --------    --------
         31.522      34.684
```

CHI-SQUARE WITH 56 DEGREES OF FREEDOM = 46.77 (P = .806)

Earlier in this chapter we alluded to the fact that confirmatory factor models allow one to statistically test the significance of model parameters. We can perform such a test on the present multivariate genetic model. The LISREL output above shows that the shared environment factor loadings are much smaller than either the genetic or non-shared environment loadings. We can test whether these loadings are significantly different from zero by modifying slightly the LISREL script to fix these parameters and then re-estimating the other model parameters. There are several possible ways in which one might modify the script to accomplish this task, but one of the easiest methods is simply to change the PA LY matrix to fix all of the C factor loadings to zero:

	A_1	C_1	E_1	A_2	C_2	E_2
Twin1-Time0	1	0	1	0	0	0
Twin1-Time1	1	0	1	0	0	0
Twin1-Time2	1	0	1	0	0	0
Twin1-Time3	1	0	1	0	0	0
Twin2-Time0	0	0	0	1	0	1
Twin2-Time1	0	0	0	1	0	1
Twin2-Time2	0	0	0	1	0	1
Twin2-Time3	0	0	0	1	0	1

Performing this modification in the first group effectively drops all C loadings from both groups because the LY=IN statement in the second group equates its loadings to those in the first. Thus, the modified script represents a model in which common factors are hypothesized for genetic and non-shared environment effects to account for covariances among the observed variables, and unique effects are allowed to contribute to measurement variances. All shared environment effects are omitted from the model.

Since the modified multivariate model is a sub- or nested model of the full common factor specification, comparison of the goodness-of-fit chi-squared values provides a test of the significance of the deleted C factor loadings (see Chapter 6). The full model has 56 degrees of freedom and the reduced one: $2 \times 8(8 + 1)/2 - 12 = 60$ d.f. Thus, the difference chi-squared statistic for the test of C loadings has $60 - 56 = 4$ degrees of freedom. As may be seen in the output fragment below, the χ^2_{60} of the reduced model is 51.08, and, therefore, the difference χ^2_4 is $51.08 - 46.77 = 4.31$, which is non-significant at the .05 level. This non-significant chi-squared indicates that the shared environment loadings can be dropped from the multivariate genetic model without significant loss of fit; that is, the arithmetic data are not influenced by environmental effects shared by twins.

Parameter estimates from this reduced model are given below.

LISREL Output from Reduced Common Factor Model (Omitting C)

```
-------------------------------------------------------------------
LISREL ESTIMATES (MAXIMUM LIKELIHOOD)
     LAMBDA Y
```

	A1	C1	E1	A2	C2	E2
Tw1-T0	14.756	.000	3.559	.000	.000	.000
Tw1-T1	14.274	.000	6.331	.000	.000	.000
Tw1-T2	14.081	.000	7.047	.000	.000	.000
Tw1-T3	14.405	.000	5.845	.000	.000	.000
Tw2-T0	.000	.000	.000	14.756	.000	3.559
Tw2-T1	.000	.000	.000	14.274	.000	6.331
Tw2-T2	.000	.000	.000	14.081	.000	7.047
Tw2-T3	.000	.000	.000	14.405	.000	5.845

```
     THETA EPS
         Tw1-T0    Tw1-T1    Tw1-T2    Tw1-T3    Tw2-T0    Tw2-T1
```

Tw1-T0	Tw1-T1	Tw1-T2	Tw1-T3	Tw2-T0	Tw2-T1
59.502	39.433	30.843	36.057	59.502	39.433

```
     THETA EPS
         Tw2-T2    Tw2-T3
```

Tw2-T2	Tw2-T3
30.843	36.057

```
CHI-SQUARE WITH  60 DEGREES OF FREEDOM =    51.08 (P = .787)
```

The estimates for the genetic and non-shared environment parameters differ somewhat between the reduced model and those estimated in the full common factor model. Such differences often appear when fitting nested models, and are not necessarily indicative of misspecification (of course, one would not expect the estimates to change in the case where parameters to be omitted are estimated as 0.0 in the full model). The fitting functions used in LISREL (see Chapter 7) are designed to produce parameter estimates that yield the closest match between the observed and estimated covariance matrices. Omission of selected parameters, for example, the C loadings in the present model, generates a different model Σ and thus may be expected to yield slightly different parameter estimates in order to best approximate the observed matrix.

12.3.3 Alternate Representation of the Multivariate Genetic Factor Model

One of the features of LISREL is its flexibility for specifying the same or very similar models in different ways. In this text we often make use of this flexibility, sometimes writing a model using the "y-side" of LISREL (i.e., using y, η, Λ_y, Θ_ϵ, and Ψ), other times using the "x-side" of the structural equations (x, ξ, Λ_x, Θ_δ, and Φ), and still other times using a combination of x and y variables. Frequently the choice of model specification is simply a matter of individual preference, convenience, or familiarity with LISREL variables and notation, particularly when a model can be written in several different ways with no change in the substantive or numerical outcome. However, at other times very subtle changes in the LISREL formulation of a model translate to a completely different substantive question. While it may be true that flexibility imparts confusion, it is important to recognize and distinguish alternative representations of genetic models in LISREL.

We present a different representation of the reduced multivariate genetic model of Section 12.2.3 in Appendix E.2. In this example, we use the x variables in LIS-REL, model the latent genetic and non-shared environmental factors as ξ variables, and estimate *all* parameters in the Λ_x matrix. Appropriate matrix representation allows us to fix all elements of the residual Θ_δ matrix to zero and estimate the unique variances in Λ_x. The MOdel line for this formulation is

```
MO NX=8 NK=12 LX=FU,FI PH=FI TD=ZE
```

which shows that all NX=8 observed variables are modeled in the x vector and that we now have NK=12 latent factors. These 12 factors comprise the ξ vector (A_1, A_2, E_1, T_1U_1, T_1U_2, T_1U_3, T_1U_4, E_2, T_2U_1, T_2U_2, T_2U_3, T_2U_4). The Φ matrix is similar to that of the preceding example, having fixed variances of unity and an off-diagonal element representing the genetic correlation between MZ or DZ twins, except it is now extended to include the unique variance factors. Also as in the preceding example, the factor loadings are equated for twin 1 and twin 2 and across the MZ and DZ groups.

Aside from the switch from x to y variables in LISREL, the biggest alteration of this model is in the factor pattern matrix PA LX. The pattern for Λ_x now appears as

	A_1	A_2	E_1	T_1U_1	T_1U_2	T_1U_3	T_1U_4
Twin1-Time0	1	0	1	1	0	0	0
Twin1-Time1	1	0	1	0	1	0	0
Twin1-Time2	1	0	1	0	0	1	0
Twin1-Time3	1	0	1	0	0	0	1
Twin2-Time0	0	1	0	0	0	0	0
Twin2-Time1	0	1	0	0	0	0	0
Twin2-Time2	0	1	0	0	0	0	0
Twin2-Time3	0	1	0	0	0	0	0

	E_2	T_2U_1	T_2U_2	T_2U_3	T_2U_4
Twin1-Time0	0	0	0	0	0
Twin1-Time1	0	0	0	0	0
Twin1-Time2	0	0	0	0	0
Twin1-Time3	0	0	0	0	0
Twin2-Time0	1	1	0	0	0
Twin2-Time1	1	0	1	0	0
Twin2-Time2	1	0	0	1	0
Twin2-Time3	1	0	0	0	1

where again the factor loadings are equated across twins. Close inspection of this matrix reveals that the factor patterns for A and E of twin 1 and twin 2 are identical to that in Section 12.2.3. The main difference lies in the treatment of the unique variances. In the earlier example these were estimated as variances on the diagonal of Θ_ϵ, but now they are modeled as the *square roots of the variances*, using Λ_x. These quantities are now square roots because the unique variances are calculated as the product $\Lambda_x \Phi \Lambda_x'$ in the expected covariance expression

$$\Sigma_{x,x} = \Lambda_x \Phi \Lambda_x' , \qquad (12.4)$$

whereas in the previous example the quantities were estimated as the unproducted quantity Θ_ϵ. In other words, the relationship between residual parameters in Λ_x in this example and the unique variances of Θ_ϵ in the last example is $\Lambda_{x_{i,j}}^2 = \Theta_{\epsilon_{i,i}}$ ($i = 1, ..., 8$; $j = 4, ..., 7, 9, ..., 12$). One might expect that this subtle change would have no effect on the model (as indeed it does not in this example), but on occasion these alternative residual specifications may produce different outcomes. The problem arises when LISREL estimates $\theta_{\epsilon_{i,i}} < 0.0$. This occurrence cannot be replicated in the present formulation because λ_x^2 can never be less than zero[2]. The situation of $\theta_\epsilon < 0.0$ makes little sense in genetic analyses because it implies an impossible negative variance component. Consequently, although it may be possible to make alternative representations like this in LISREL, we recommend the model of equation 12.4, as it constrains unique variances to be ≥ 0.0. Nevertheless, both methods give identical solutions when fitted to the arithmetic computation data used in these examples.

---

[2] We make use of this fact to specify non-negativity constraints in Chapter 11.

12.3.4 Fitting a Second Genetic Factor

The genetic common factor model we introduced in Sections 12.3.2 and 12.3.3 may be extended to address more specific questions about the data. In the arithmetic computation measures, for example, it is reasonable to hypothesize two genetic factors: one general factor contributing to all measurements of arithmetic computation, and a second "alcohol" factor which influences the measures taken after the challenge dose of alcohol. The most parsimonious extension of our common factor model may involve the addition of only 1 free parameter which represents each of the factor loadings on the alcohol factor (that is, the alcohol loadings may be equated for all alcohol measurements). We present a LISREL script for this model in Appendix E.3.

The LISREL script in Appendix E.3 corresponds very closely to that used in section 12.3.3, using x variables and placing all common factors and unique variances in the ξ vector. The biggest change in this example is in the Λ_x matrix. We add the latent alcohol factors for twins 1 and 2 as ξ variables, and, thus, must modify the Λ_x matrix accordingly. The PA LX statement now shows the pattern

	A_1	$Aalc_1$	A_2	$Aalc_2$	E_1	T_1U_1	T_1U_2	T_1U_3	T_1U_4
Tw1-T0	1	0	0	0	1	1	0	0	0
Tw1-T1	1	1	0	0	1	0	1	0	0
Tw1-T2	1	1	0	0	1	0	0	1	0
Tw1-T3	1	1	0	0	1	0	0	0	1
Tw2-T0	0	0	1	0	0	0	0	0	0
Tw2-T1	0	0	1	1	0	0	0	0	0
Tw2-T2	0	0	1	1	0	0	0	0	0
Tw2-T3	0	0	1	1	0	0	0	0	0

	E_2	T_2U_1	T_2U_2	T_2U_3	T_2U_4
Tw1-T0	0	0	0	0	0
Tw1-T1	0	0	0	0	0
Tw1-T2	0	0	0	0	0
Tw1-T3	0	0	0	0	0
Tw2-T0	1	1	0	0	0
Tw2-T1	1	0	1	0	0
Tw2-T2	1	0	0	1	0
Tw2-T3	1	0	0	0	1

with all loadings within and between $Aalc_1$ and $Aalc_2$ equated using EQuality statements. The addition of the single parameter for all alcohol loadings reflects a model having 13 parameters and $2 \times 8(8 + 1)/2 - 13 = 59$ degrees of freedom. We can, therefore, test the significance of the alcohol factor by comparing the goodness-of-fit chi-squared value for this model with that obtained from the model of Section 12.3.3 for a $60 - 59 = 1$ d.f. test.

The edited LISREL output from the two-factor multivariate genetic model is as follows:

LISREL Output from Two Factor Genetic Model

PARAMETER SPECIFICATIONS
    LAMBDA X

	A1	Aalc1	A2	Aalc2	E1	T1U1
Tw1-T0	1	0	0	0	2	3
Tw1-T1	4	11	0	0	5	0
Tw1-T2	7	11	0	0	8	0
Tw1-T3	10	11	0	0	12	0
Tw2-T0	0	0	1	0	0	0
Tw2-T1	0	0	4	11	0	0
Tw2-T2	0	0	7	11	0	0
Tw2-T3	0	0	10	11	0	0

    LAMBDA X

	T1U2	T1U3	T1U4	E2	T2U1	T2U2
Tw1-T0	0	0	0	0	0	0
Tw1-T1	6	0	0	0	0	0
Tw1-T2	0	9	0	0	0	0
Tw1-T3	0	0	13	0	0	0
Tw2-T0	0	0	0	2	3	0
Tw2-T1	0	0	0	5	0	6
Tw2-T2	0	0	0	8	0	0
Tw2-T3	0	0	0	12	0	0

    LAMBDA X

	T2U3	T2U4
Tw1-T0	0	0
Tw1-T1	0	0
Tw1-T2	0	0
Tw1-T3	0	0
Tw2-T0	0	0
Tw2-T1	0	0
Tw2-T2	9	0
Tw2-T3	0	13

LISREL ESTIMATES (MAXIMUM LIKELIHOOD)
    LAMBDA X

	A1	Aalc1	A2	Aalc2	E1	T1U1
Tw1-T0	15.067	.000	.000	.000	4.408	6.674
Tw1-T1	13.701	4.270	.000	.000	6.091	.000

Tw1-T2	13.518	4.270	.000	.000	6.800	.000
Tw1-T3	13.832	4.270	.000	.000	5.695	.000
Tw2-T0	.000	.000	15.067	.000	.000	.000
Tw2-T1	.000	.000	13.701	4.270	.000	.000
Tw2-T2	.000	.000	13.518	4.270	.000	.000
Tw2-T3	.000	.000	13.832	4.270	.000	.000

LAMBDA X

	T1U2	T1U3	T1U4	E2	T2U1	T2U2
Tw1-T0	.000	.000	.000	.000	.000	.000
Tw1-T1	6.277	.000	.000	.000	.000	.000
Tw1-T2	.000	5.644	.000	.000	.000	.000
Tw1-T3	.000	.000	5.928	.000	.000	.000
Tw2-T0	.000	.000	.000	4.408	6.674	.000
Tw2-T1	.000	.000	.000	6.091	.000	6.277
Tw2-T2	.000	.000	.000	6.800	.000	.000
Tw2-T3	.000	.000	.000	5.695	.000	.000

LAMBDA X

	T2U3	T2U4
Tw1-T0	.000	.000
Tw1-T1	.000	.000
Tw1-T2	.000	.000
Tw1-T3	.000	.000
Tw2-T0	.000	.000
Tw2-T1	.000	.000
Tw2-T2	5.644	.000
Tw2-T3	.000	5.928

CHI-SQUARE WITH 59 DEGREES OF FREEDOM = 47.52 (P = .858)

The estimated genetic factor loading for the alcohol variables ($\lambda_x = 4.27$) is reasonably large, but much smaller than the loadings on the general genetic factor. This difference is more apparent when we consider proportions of genetic variance accounted for by these two factors, being $4.27^2/(13.70^2 + 4.27)$ or 9% for the alcohol factor, and $100 - 9 = 91\%$ for the general genetic factor. The model yields a $\chi^2_{59} = 47.52$ ($p = .86$), indicating a good fit to the data. The chi-squared test for the significance of the alcohol factor loadings is $51.08 - 47.52 = 3.56$, which is not quite significant at the .05 level. Thus, while the hypothesis of there being genetic effects on the alcohol measures additional to those influencing arithmetic skills fits the observed data better, the increase in fit obtained by adding the alcohol factor does not reach statistical significance.

12.4   Multiple Genetic Factor Models

12.4.1   Genetic and Environmental Correlations

We now turn from the one- and two-factor multivariate genetic models described above and consider more general multivariate formulations which may encompass many genetic and environmental factors. These more general approaches subsume the simpler techniques described above.

Consider a simple extension of the one- and two-factor AE models for multiple variables (sections 12.3.3–12.3.4). The total phenotypic covariance matrix in a population, C_p, can be decomposed into an additive genetic component, A, and a random environmental component, E:

$$C_p = A + E , \tag{12.5}$$

We are leaving out the shared environment in this example just for simplicity. More complex expectations for 12.5 may be written without affecting the basic idea. "A" is called the *additive genetic covariance matrix* and "E" the *random environmental covariance matrix*. If A is diagonal, then the traits comprising A are genetically independent; that is, there is no "additive genetic covariance" between them. One interpretation of this is that different genes affect each of the traits. Similarly, if the environmental covariance matrix, E, is diagonal, we would conclude that each trait is affected by quite different environmental factors.

On the other hand, suppose A were to have significant off-diagonal elements. What would that mean? Although there are many reasons why this might happen, one possibility is that at least some genes are having effects on more than one variable. This is known as *pleiotropy* in the classical genetic literature (see Chapter 3). Similarly, significant off-diagonal elements in E (or C, if it were included in the model) would indicate that some environmental factors influence more than one trait at a time.

The extent to which the same genes or environmental factors contribute to the observed phenotypic correlation between two variables is often measured by the *genetic* or *environmental correlation* between the variables. If we have estimates of the genetic and environmental covariance matrices, A and E, the genetic correlation (r_g) between variables i and j is

$$r_{g_{ij}} = \frac{a_{ij}}{\sqrt{(a_{ii} \times a_{jj})}} \tag{12.6}$$

and the environmental correlation, similarly, is

$$r_{e_{ij}} = \frac{e_{ij}}{\sqrt{(e_{ii} \times e_{jj})}} . \tag{12.7}$$

The analogy with the familiar formula for the correlation coefficient is clear. The genetic covariance between two phenotypes is quite distinct from the genetic correlation. It is possible for two traits to have a very high genetic correlation yet have little genetic covariance. Low genetic covariance could arise if either trait had low genetic variance. Vogler (1982) and Carey (1988) discuss these issues in greater depth.

12.4.2 Cholesky Decomposition

Clearly, we cannot resolve the genetic and environmental components of covariance without genetically informative data such as those from twins. Under our simple AE model we can write, for MZ and DZ pairs, the expected covariances between the multiple measures of first and second members very simply:

$$c_{MZ} = A$$
$$c_{DZ} = \alpha A$$

with the total phenotypic covariance matrix being defined as in expression 12.5. The coefficient α in DZ twins is the familiar additive genetic correlation between siblings in randomly mating populations (i.e., 0.5).

The method of maximum likelihood, implemented in LISREL, can be used to estimate A and E. However, there is an important restriction on the form of these matrices which follows from the fact that they are covariance matrices: they *must* be positive definite. It turns out that if we try to estimate A and E without imposing this constraint they will very often not be positive definite and thus give nonsense values (greater than or less than unity) for the genetic and environmental correlations. It is very simple to impose this constraint in LISREL by recognizing that any positive definite matrix, F, can be decomposed into the product of a *triangular matrix* and its transpose:

$$F = TT' , \tag{12.8}$$

where T is a triangular matrix (i.e., one having fixed zeros in all elements above the diagonal). This is sometimes known as a *triangular decomposition* or a *Cholesky factorization* of F. Figure 12.1 shows this type of model as a path diagram for three variables. In our case, we represent the genetic and environmental covariance matrices in LISREL by their respective Cholesky factorizations:

$$A = HH' \tag{12.9}$$

and

$$E = WW' , \tag{12.10}$$

where H and W are triangular matrices of additive genetic and within-family environment factor loadings.

A triangular matrix such as T, H, or W is square, having the same number of rows and columns as there are variables. The first column has non-zero entries in

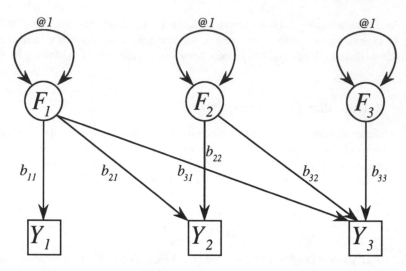

Figure 12.1: Phenotypic Cholesky decomposition model for three variables. The symbol denotes a fixed parameter

every element; the second has a zero in the first element and free, non-zero elements everywhere else, and so on. Thus, the Cholesky factors of $\mathbf{F}$, when $\mathbf{F}$ is a 3×3 matrix of the product $\mathbf{TT}'$, will have the form:

$$\mathbf{T} = \begin{pmatrix} b_{11} & 0 & 0 \\ b_{21} & b_{22} & 0 \\ b_{31} & b_{32} & b_{33} \end{pmatrix} .$$

It is important to recognize that common factor models such as the one described in Section 12.3 are simply reduced Cholesky models with the first column of parameters estimated and all others fixed at zero.

12.4.3   Analyzing Genetic and Environmental Correlations

We illustrate the estimation of the genetic and environmental covariance matrices for a simple case of skinfold measures made on 11.5 year-old male twins from the Medical College of Virginia Twin Study (Schieken *et al.*, 1989)[3]. Our skinfold assessments include four different measures which were obtained using standard anthropometric techniques. The measures were obtained for biceps, subscapular, suprailiac, and triceps skinfolds. The raw data were averaged for the left and right sides and subjected to a logarithmic transformation prior to analysis in order to remove the correlation between error variance and skinfold measure. The 8×8 covariance matrices for the male MZ and DZ twins are given in Table 12.3.

---

[3] We are grateful to Dr. Richard Schieken for making these data available prior to publication.

Table 12.3: Covariance matrices for skinfold measures in MZ and DZ male twins.

	BIC1	SSC1	SUP1	TRI1	BIC2	SSC2	SUP2	TRI2
				Dizygotic Male Pairs (N=33)*				
BIC1	.1538							
SSC1	.1999	.3007						
SUP1	.2266	.3298	.3795					
TRI1	.1285	.1739	.2007	.1271				
BIC2	.0435	.0336	.0354	.0376	.1782			
SSC2	.0646	.0817	.0741	.0543	.2095	.3081		
SUP2	.0812	.0901	.0972	.0666	.2334	.3241	.3899	
TRI2	.0431	.0388	.0376	.0373	.1437	.1842	.2108	.1415
				Monozygotic Male Pairs (N=84)*				
	BIC1	SSC1	SUP1	TRI1	BIC2	SSC2	SUP2	TRI2
BIC1	.1285							
SSC1	.1270	.1759						
SUP1	.1704	.2156	.3031					
TRI1	.1035	.1101	.1469	.1041				
BIC2	.0982	.1069	.1491	.0824	.1233			
SSC2	.0999	.1411	.1848	.0880	.1295	.1894		
SUP2	.1256	.1654	.2417	.1095	.1616	.2185	.2842	
TRI2	.0836	.0907	.1341	.0836	.1010	.1134	.1436	.1068

Variable Labels: BIC=Biceps; SSC=Subscapular; SUP=Suprailiac;
TRI=Triceps. "1" and "2" refer to measures made on first and
second twins.
* Data kindly supplied by R.M. Schieken, gathered as part of a
project supported by NHLBI award HL-31010.

An example LISREL program for estimating the Cholesky factors of the additive genetic and within-family environmental covariance matrices is given in Appendix E.4. We specify NI=8 observed variables (4 measures each from twin 1 and twin 2) and use the x and ξ variables for the LISREL model. We have NK=16 latent variables, comprised of four genetic and four environmental factors for each twin. Λ_x contains both of the triangular matrices, **H** and **W**, and the factor pattern is established using PA LX. As in the multivariate models described earlier, the additive genetic and within-family environment factor loadings are EQuated across twins. We use off-diagonal elements of the Φ matrix to set the genetic correlations 1.0 and 0.5 for the MZ and DZ twins, respectively.

When this program is run with the data from male twins, we obtain a goodness-of-fit chi-squared of 68.92 for 52 d.f. ($p = .058$) suggesting that the AE model gives a reasonable fit to these data. Setting the off-diagonal elements of the genetic factors to zero yields a chi-squared that may be compared using the difference test to see whether the measures can be regarded as genetically independent. This chi-squared turns out to be 110.96 for 6 d.f. which is highly significant. Therefore, the genetic correlations between these skinfold measures cannot be ignored. Similarly, setting the environmental covariances to zero yields a significant increase in chi-squared of 356.98, also for 6 d.f. Clearly, there are also highly significant environmental covariances among the four variables.

Table 12.4 gives the estimates of the Cholesky factors of the genetic and environmental covariance matrices produced by LISREL. Carrying out the pre- and

Table 12.4: LISREL estimates of the cholesky factors in the genetic and environmental covariance matrices.

| | Factor | | | | | | | |
| | Genetic | | | | Environmental | | | |
Variable	1	2	3	4	1	2	3	4
Biceps	0.340	0.000	0.000	0.000	0.170	0.000	0.000	0.000
Subscapular	0.396	0.182	0.000	0.000	0.160	0.138	0.000	0.000
Suprailiac	0.487	0.159	0.148	0.000	0.180	0.117	0.093	0.000
Triceps	0.288	0.016	0.036	0.110	0.117	0.039	-0.004	0.085

post-multiplication of the Cholesky factors (see equations 12.9 and 12.10) gives the maximum-likelihood estimates of the genetic and environmental covariance matrices, which we present in the upper part of Table 12.5. The lower part of Table 12.5 gives the matrices of genetic and environmental correlations derived from these covariances (see 12.6 and 12.7).

We see that the genetic correlations between the four skin-fold measures are

Table 12.5: Maximum-likelihood estimates of genetic and environmental covariance and correlation matrices for skinfold measures.

Variable	Genetic				Environmental			
	Bicep	Subsc	Supra	Tricep	Bicep	Subsc	Supra	Tricep
Biceps	0.116	0.135	0.166	0.098	0.029	0.027	0.030	0.020
Subsc	0.909	0.190	0.222	0.117	0.759	0.044	0.045	0.024
Supra	0.914	0.955	0.284	0.148	0.769	0.908	0.054	0.025
Triceps	0.927	0.863	0.894	0.097	0.778	0.757	0.716	0.023

Note: The variances are given on the diagonals of the two matrices; covariances are the elements above the diagonals; correlations are given below the diagonals.

indeed very large, suggesting that the amount of fat at different sites of the body is almost entirely under the control of the same genetic factors. However, in this example, the environmental correlations also are quite large, suggesting that environmental factors which affect the amount of fat at one site also have a generalized effect over all sites.

12.5 Common vs. Independent Pathway Genetic Models

As another example of multivariate analysis we consider four atopic symptoms reported by female twins in a mailed questionnaire study (Duffy *et al.*, 1990; 1992). Twins reported whether they had ever (versus never) suffered from asthma, hayfever, dust allergy and eczema. Tetrachoric correlation matrices were calculated with PRELIS and are shown in the LISREL script in Appendix E.5 and in Table 12.6. Analysis of tetrachoric matrices such as these requires the statement MA=PM on the DAta line. The script shows that asymptotic covariance matrices are stored in files named ahdemzf.acv and ahdedzf.acv respectively for MZ and DZ twins. This is indicated to LISREL by the lines beginning with AC, which is also the flag indicating that weighted least squares minimization (WLS) is required, rather than the default of maximum likelihood. Maximum-likelihood estimation is not appropriate when there are glaring departures from normality; the dichotomous items used in this example are inevitably non-normal.

Table 12.6: Tetrachoric correlations for female MZ (above diagonal) and DZ (below diagonal) twins for asthma (A), hayfever (H), dust allergy (D), and eczema (E).

			Twin 1				Twin 2		
		A	H	D	E	A	H	D	E
Twin 1	Asthma		.56	.57	.27	.59	.41	.43	.09
	Hayfever	.52		.76	.26	.37	.59	.42	.20
	Dust Allergy	.59	.75		.31	.40	.45	.52	.19
	Eczema	.29	.31	.28		.23	.15	.19	.59
Twin 2	Asthma	.26	.17	.04	.14		.55	.64	.15
	Hayfever	.13	.32	.26	.09	.40		.77	.12
	Dust Allergy	.08	.17	.21	.02	.68	.72		.22
	Eczema	.22	.11	.09	.31	.25	.22	.28	

12.5.1   Independent Pathway Model for Atopy

Inspection of the correlation matrices in Table 12.6 reveals that the presence of any one of the symptoms is associated with an increased risk of the others within an individual (hence the concept of "atopy"). All four symptoms show higher MZ correlations (0.592, 0.593, 0.518, 0.589) than DZ correlations in liability (0.262, 0.318, 0.214, 0.313) and there is a hint of genetic dominance (or epistasis) for asthma and dust allergy (DZ correlations less than half their MZ counterparts). Preliminary multivariate analysis suggests that dominance is acting at the level of a common factor influencing all symptoms, rather than as specific dominance contributions to individual symptoms. Our first model for covariation of these symptoms is shown in the path diagram of Figure 12.2

Because each of the three common factors (A, D, E) has its own paths to each of the four variables, this has been called the *independent pathway model* (Kendler *et al.*, 1987) or the *biometric factors model* (McArdle and Goldsmith, 1990). This is translated into LISREL in the Appendix E.5 script. For this example, we model the observed variables in the y vector and equate the y variables to latent η variables using an identity matrix in Λ_y. The latent genetic and environmental factors are specified in the ξ vector. For each twin there are three general factors (A, D, E) and eight specific factors (four A_i's and four E_i's), hence NK=22. The order in which the common and specific factors appear in the columns of the GAmma matrix is listed on the line providing labels for the ξ variables (LK line). The PHi matrices are used to set the values 1.0 and 0.5 for the genetic resemblance between MZ and DZ twins, respectively. The elements of Φ may be specified more economically using

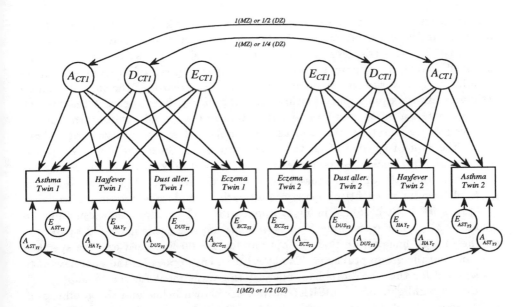

Figure 12.2: Independent pathway model for asthma, hayfever, dust allergy, and eczema. All labels for path-coefficients have been omitted. All four correlations at the bottom of the figure are fixed at 1 for MZ and .5 for DZ twins.

the VA line, but the MAtrix specification has the advantage of being easily checked.

One important new feature of the model shown in Figure 12.2 is the treatment of variance specific to each variable. Such residual variance does not generally receive much attention in regular non-genetic factor analysis, for at least two reasons. First, the primary goal of factor analysis (and of many multivariate methods) is to understand the covariance between variables in terms of reduced number of factors. Thus the residual, variable specific, components are not the focus. A second reason is that with phenotypic factor analysis, there is simply no information to further decompose the variable specific variance. However, in the case of data on groups of relatives, we have two parallel goals of understanding not only the within-person covariance for different variables, but also the across-relatives covariance structure both within and across variables. The genetic and environmental factor structure at the top of Figure 12.1 addresses the genetic and environmental components of variance common to the different variables. However, there remains information to discriminate between genetic and environmental components of the residuals, which in essence answers the question of whether family members correlate for the variable specific portions of variance.

A second important difference in this example — using correlation matrices in which diagonal variance elements are standardized to one — is that the degrees of freedom available for model testing are different from the case of fitting to covariance matrices in which all NI(NI+1)/2 elements are available. We encountered this difference in the univariate case in Section 8.10.1, but it is slightly more complex in multivariate analysis. For correlation matrices, since the NI diagonal elements are fixed to one, we apparently have NG×NI fewer degrees of freedom than if we were fitting to covariances. However, since for a given variable the sum of squared estimates always equals unity (within rounding error), it is apparent that not all the parameters are free, and we may conceptualize the unique environment specific standard deviations (i.e., the e_i's) as being obtained as the square roots of one minus the sum of squares of all the other estimates. Since there are N_V (number of variables) such constrained estimates, we actually have N_V more degrees of freedom than the above discussion indicates, the correct adjustment to the degrees of freedom when fitting genetic multivariate models to correlation matrices is $-(\text{NG} \times \text{NI} - N_V)$. Since in most applications $\text{NI} = 2N_V$, the adjustment is usually $-3N_V$. In our example $N_V = 4$ and the adjustment is indicated by DF=-12 on the first OU line. (Note that the options for the OU line need only be specified once in multiple group problems. The DF adjustment applies for the goodness-of-fit chi-squared for the whole problem, not just the adjustment for that group).

Edited highlights of the LISREL output are shown below and the goodness-of-fit chi-squared indicates an acceptable fit to the data. Note that the adjustment of −12 to the degrees of freedom which would be available were we working with covariance matrices (72) leaves 60 statistics. We have to estimate 3×4 factor loadings and 2×4 specific loadings (20 parameters in all), so there are $60 - 20 = 40$ d.f. It is a wise precaution always to go through this calculation of degrees of freedom — not because LISREL is likely to get them wrong, but as a further check that the model has been specified correctly.

LISREL Output from Independent Pathway Model

```
-----------------------------------------------------------------------
LISREL ESTIMATES (WEIGHTED LEAST SQUARES)
        GAMMA
```

	EATOPY1	HATOPY1	DATOPY1	H (spec)	E (spec)
ASTHMA1	.320	.431	.466	.441	.548
HAYFVR1	.494	.772	.095	.000 [4]	.388
DUSTAL1	.660	.516	.431	.297	−.159 [5]
ECZEMA1	.092	.221	.260	.712	.606

---

[4] A parameter on the lower bound generates the diagnostic that GA(2,8) may not be identified. Fixing this parameter to zero removes the diagnostic and does not affect the chi-squared.

[5] Note that the sign of this estimate is negative, but since factors (including specific factors) are independent of each other, the loadings within a factor may be multiplied by −1 without affecting the fit.

```
CHI-SQUARE WITH  40 DEGREES OF FREEDOM =    38.44 (P = .540)
```

We can test variations of the above model by dropping the common factors one at a time, or by setting additive genetic specifics to zero. This is easily done by fixing the appropriate elements in Γ. Note that fixing E specifics to zero usually results in model failure since it generates singular expected covariance matrices $(\Sigma)^6$. Neither does it make biological sense since it is tantamount to saying that a variable can be measured without error; it is hard to think of a single example of this in biology! We could also elaborate the model by specifying a third source of specific variance components, or by substituting shared environment for dominance, either as a general factor or as specific variance components.

12.5.2 Common Pathway Model for Atopy

In this section we focus on a much more stringent model which hypothesizes that the covariation between symptoms is determined by a single 'phenotypic' latent variable called "atopy." Atopy itself is determined by additive, dominance and individual environmental sources of variance. As in the independent pathway model, there are still specific genetic and environmental effects on each symptom. The path diagram for this model is shown in Figure 12.3. Because there is now a latent variable ATOPY which has direct phenotypic paths to each of the symptoms, this has been called the *common pathway model* (Kendler *et al.*, 1987) or the *psychometric factors model* (McArdle and Goldsmith, 1990).

The LISREL script corresponding to this path diagram, given in Appendix E.6, contains several new features. One useful feature of LISREL is its ability to reorder variables using the SE command; in this example the variables are reordered so that each symptom for the first twin is followed by that for the second. This reordering clearly has consequences for the pattern of the parameter specifications in the Γ and other matrices. In the Γ matrix we must now specify the contributions to the latent phenotype ATOPY from additive (AATOPY), dominant (DATOPY) and unique environmental (EATOPY) sources. The Γ matrix also allows space to test hypotheses concerning shared environmental influences on atopy (CATOPY), although this factor is fixed to zero in the example below.

The most important new feature, however, is the introduction of the BEta matrix to represent the phenotypic paths from the latent phenotypic variable ATOPY to the latent variables corresponding to each of the four measured symptoms. The number of η variables is now 10 (as opposed to 8 in the independent pathway model above) because we have added ATOPY1 and ATOPY2 as latent variables. The identity of the four latent variables (for each twin) corresponding to symptoms with their measured counterparts is specified in the Λ_y (LY) matrix, which has dimensions NY×NE (8×10). Note that this identity is specified by fixing the diagonal

---

[6] This problem is extreme when maximum likelihood is the fit function, because the inverse of Σ is required (see Chapter 7).

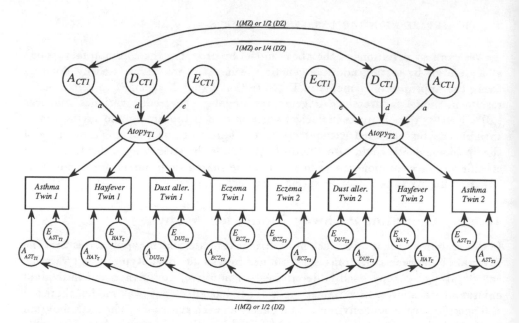

Figure 12.3: Common pathway model for asthma, hayfever, dust allergy, and eczema.

elements of the first 8 columns of the LY matrix to unity (using the VA command). These LY paths are seen as the paths with value 1 from the latent variables to measured symptoms in the path diagram.

One final feature of the model is that since ATOPY is a latent variable whose scale (and hence variance) is not indexed to any measured variable, we must fix its residual variance term (EATOPY) to unity (VA 1 GA 9 7) to make the model identified. This inevitably means that the estimates for the Γ loadings contributing to ATOPY are arbitrary and hence so are the β paths leading from ATOPY to the symptoms. It is thus particularly important to standardize the solution so that the total variance explained for each symptom is unity. This is done by placing SC (for Standardized Completely) on the OU line. The fixing of the loading on EATOPY clearly has implications for the calculation of degrees of freedom, as we shall see below.

The condensed output for this model is presented below, showing the completely standardized estimates which give unit variance for each variable.

LISREL Output from Common Pathway Model

WITHIN GROUPS COMPLETELY STANDARDIZED SOLUTION

	BETA	GAMMA				
	ATOPY	HATOPY1	DATOPY1	EATOPY2	H (spec)	E (spec)
A1	.671	–	–	–	.531	.517
H1	.814	–	–	–	.456	.358
D1	.941	–	–	–	-.059	.334
E1	.301	–	–	–	.735	.608
ATOPY1	–	.686	.397	.610	–	–

CHI-SQUARE WITH 46 DEGREES OF FREEDOM =   51.37 (P = .238)

Note that here NI=8 so there are 56 $(2 \times NI(NI-1)/2)$ unique correlations. From the above table it appears that 15 parameters have been estimated, but in fact EATOPY was fixed and the four E specifics are obtained by difference, so there are only 10 free parameters in the model, hence 46 degrees of freedom.

The latent variable ATOPY has a broad heritability of over 0.6 ($1 - .610^2 = .686^2 + .397^2$) of which approximately a quarter is due to dominance, and this factor has an important phenotypic influence (β paths) on all symptoms, particularly dust allergy (0.941) and hayfever (0.814). There are still sizeable specific genetic influences not accounted for by the ATOPY factor on all symptoms except dust allergy ($.059^2$). However, despite the appeal of this model, it does not fit as well as the independent pathway model and the imposition of constraints that covariation between symptoms arises purely from their phenotypic relation with the latent variable ATOPY has worsened fit by $\chi^2 = 12.93$ for 6 degrees of freedom, which is significant at the 5% level.

We conclude that while there are common environmental, additive, and non-additive genetic factors which influence all four symptoms of atopy, these have *differential* effects on the symptoms; the additive and non-additive factors, for example, having respectively greater and lesser proportional influence on hayfever than the other symptoms. While it is tempting to interpret this as evidence for at least two genes, or sets of genes, being responsible for the aggregation of symptoms we call atopy, this is simplistic as in fact such patterns could be consistent with the action of a single gene — or indeed with polygenic effects. For a full discussion of this important point see Mather and Jinks (1982) and Carey (1988).

Chapter 13

Direction of Causation

13.1 Introduction

The past 15 years have seen a broadening of the focus of studies in behavioral genetics and genetic epidemiology. Rather than concentrating exclusively on a single behavioral domain (e.g., IQ or personality or psychiatric disorder or a behavioral risk-factor for major chronic disease), researchers have attempted to assess numerous behavioral domains and environmental risk-factors in a single study. There has been a corresponding growth of interest in identifying 'intervening' or 'mediating' variables in the causal pathway pathway from genotype and environment to outcome. In alcoholism research, for example, the hypothesis has been advanced (e.g., Tartar *et al.*, 1985; Cloninger, 1987) that the genetic influence on risk of alcoholism (Heath *et al.*, 1990) is in part explained by the inheritance of temperamental or personality factors which in turn influence an individual's risk of becoming alcoholic. The growing interest in genotype-environment correlation, particularly the extent to which an individual's genotype shapes the environment to which she or he is exposed (Eaves *et al.*, 1977; Plomin *et al.*, 1977; Scarr and McCartney, 1983; Plomin and Bergeman, 1991), has led to the formulation of competing hypotheses about *how* inherited differences in personality, temperament, or other behavioral variables might influence the environment to which an individual exposes herself (e.g., adverse life-events). These environmental agents in turn may increase the risk of psychiatric disorder (e.g., depression: Kendler *et al.*, 1992d). In such cases we need to go beyond merely demonstrating that an outcome variable is influenced by genetic factors, in tests of univariate genetic models (Chapter 8), or merely demonstrating that this variable loads on the same genetic factor(s) as measures of temperament and personality or measures of environmental exposure, in a multivariate genetic analysis (Chapter 12). Instead, we need to consider more precise hypotheses, that the association between, say, alcoholism and temperament arises from the *causal* influence of temperament on alcoholism (temperament ⟶

261

Table 13.1: Causes of the association between two variables.

$A \longrightarrow B$	Unidirectional causation	A is the cause of B
$B \longrightarrow A$	Unidirectional causation	B is the cause of A
$A \Longleftrightarrow B$	Reciprocal causation	A is the cause of B and B is the cause of A
$A \longleftarrow C \longrightarrow B$	Indirect association	A and B are correlated because C causes both A and B

alcoholism) rather than because of the influence of alcohol abuse on personality (alcoholism $\longrightarrow$ temperament). Another good example is the association between life-events and depression, in which life-events could be a cause of depression (events $\longrightarrow$ depression) or depressed individuals may be less successful at avoiding stressful events (depression $\longrightarrow$ events). Some ways in which we may test such hypotheses will be the principal concern of this chapter.

Table 13 1 summarizes four plausible alternatives that we should think about when testing hypotheses about the causes of the association between a pair of variables, A and B. We shall consider the two unidirectional hypotheses only in the strong form where $A \longrightarrow B$ implies that the association between A and B arises *solely* because of the causal influence of A on B. Likewise we regard the hypothesis of reciprocal causation only in the strong form, that $A \Longleftrightarrow B$ implies that the association between A and B arises *solely* because of the reciprocal causal influences of A on B and B on A (a 'feedback loop' between A and B). Thus, the case of indirect association ($A \longleftarrow C \longrightarrow B$) subsumes the cases where the association between A and B arises partly through the causal influence of a third, unmeasured variable C on both A and B, and partly through the unidirectional or reciprocal causal influences of A on B or B on A. (Of course, if C were also a measured variable, we would be able to include it in our causal model, and test the hypothesis that there is no residual association between A and B after allowing for the effects of C on A and B). We may view the process of testing hypotheses about direction of causation as one of attempting to falsify (Popper, 1961) the strong unidirectional or reciprocal causal hypotheses and demonstrate that an association between two variables is in part 'spurious' (Kenny, 1975; Kessler *et al.*, 1992; Heath *et al.*, 1992), i.e., determined by other unmeasured variables.

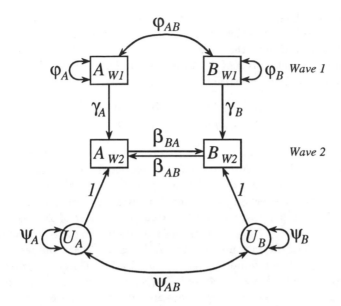

Figure 13.1: Instrumental variable model for two-panel data on unrelated individuals (after Kessler, 1983). The two variables A and B are measured on two waves $W1$ and $W2$.

13.2   Models for Data from Unrelated Individuals: Instrumental Variables Method

By and large, it is not possible to make experimental interventions to provide a direct test of our causal hypotheses. For example, we cannot impose adverse life-events on subjects in order to determine whether such events, occurring independently of any preexisting risk-factors, increase risk of depression. Even if such an intervention were feasible, we would still be uncertain about generalizing our findings to naturally occurring events arising in non-experimental settings. Most attempts to derive inferences about causation in the behavioral sciences are therefore based on observational studies. In studies of samples of unrelated individuals, a widely used strategy has been to employ longitudinal data, most commonly two-wave panel ('cross-lagged correlation') data on the two variables whose possible reciprocal causal influence is under investigation (Campbell, 1963; Duncan, 1969; Kenny, 1975; Biddle *et al.*, 1985, Friedrich *et al.*, 1989; however see Rogosa, 1980). In cases where the reciprocal causal influences of A on B and B on A are essentially instantaneous, we can consider this approach as but one special case of the the *instrumental variables* method (Kessler, 1983; Heath *et al.*, 1992), which has been broadly used in econometrics (Johnston, 1972).

Given two variables A and B (e.g., measures of temperament and alcoholism) with reciprocal causal influences on each other, we seek to identify 'instruments' for A and B, i.e., variables that are direct causes of A but not of B (IA), and variables that are direct causes of B but not of A (IB). Thus, when we have single instruments for A and B, the structural equations are

$$A = \gamma_A IA + \beta_{AB} B + UA \qquad (13.1)$$
$$B = \gamma_B IB + \beta_{BA} A + UB \qquad (13.2)$$

where UA and UB represent residual effects on A and B respectively. A path diagram of this model for two waves of measurement is shown in Figure 13.1. As applied to two-wave panel data the instrumental variable model thus assumes that there is no direct effect of A measured in wave one of data-collection (A_{W1}, equivalent to IA) on B measured in wave two (B_{W2}), nor of B measured in wave one (B_{W1}, equivalent to IB) on A measured in wave two (A_{W2}). Violation of the assumptions (i) that the instruments for A have no direct influence on B, and (ii) those for B no direct influence on A, can lead to seriously biased estimates of the reciprocal paths between A and B (Kessler, 1983). Also critical in the application of the instrumental variable approach are the assumptions (iii) that UA is uncorrelated with IA; and (iv) that UB is independent of IB. However, in practice these premises are often violated in panel data (Kessler and Greenberg, 1981).

The full model as specified in Figure 13.1 has 10 parameters, and would perfectly fit any 4×4 covariance matrix for A, B, IA, and IB. Thus, given that assumptions (i) and (ii) are valid, we have one degree of freedom to test the hypothesis that the covariance between the residuals UA and UB, ψ_{AB}, is zero. A second interpretation of the goodness-of-fit of the model with ψ_{AB} fixed at zero is that the covariance between A and B at wave 2 is due entirely to their reciprocal causation (via β_{BA} and β_{AB}), and their initial correlation at wave 1 (via $\gamma_A \psi_{AB} \gamma_B$). Two further hypotheses may also be considered: that there is no causal effect of B on A ($\beta_{AB} = 0$); and no causal effect of A on B ($\beta_{BA} = 0$).

To understand why the instrumental variable model can be used to estimate the effects of reciprocal causation, it is helpful to consider simpler submodels. In the absence of any direct causal influence of A on B or vice versa, given the model of Figure 13.1, by the rules of path analysis for non-standardized variables, the cross-temporal cross-trait ('cross-lagged') covariances will be $\psi_{AB} \gamma_A$ for B_{W1} with A_{W2} and $\psi_{AB} \gamma_B$ for A_{W1} with B_{W2}. If there is a causal influence of A on B but not of B on A (i.e., $\beta_{AB} = 0$), then the expected covariance of B_{W1} with A_{W2} would still be $\psi_{AB} \gamma_A$, but the expected covariance of A_{W1} with B_{W2} would become $(\psi_{AB} \gamma_B + \beta_{BA} \gamma_A \psi_A)$. Comparable predictions would apply if the causal influence is of B on A only ($\beta_{BA} = 0$). Thus, we see that in the instrumental variable approach information about causality depends critically upon the *cross-covariances* between each of the reciprocally interacting variables and the instrument for the other variable.

13.3   Modeling Causation with Data from Twins

Recent work has suggested that, even in the absence of panel data or other measured instruments, cross-sectional data on genetically informative constellations of relatives (e.g., MZ and DZ twin pairs, or adoptees and their adoptive and biological relatives) may, at least under certain circumstances, permit the resolution of competing hypotheses about direction of causation (Heath *et al.*, 1989; Neale *et al.*, 1989c; Duffy and Martin, 1992; Neale *et al.*, 1992; Heath *et al.*, 1991a,b). In this Section we illustrate how the method works, and develop a LISREL script for bivariate data from twins.

13.3.1   The Principle of the Method

At first glance, it may be difficult to understand how cross-sectional data from twins provide information about direction of causation. To illustrate how the method might work at all, we shall begin with the simplified example shown in Figure 13.2.

Here we assume for illustrative purposes that, in the absence of any effects mediated through causal influences between A and B, twin pair resemblance for variable A is determined by shared environmental factors, and that twin pair resemblance for variable B is determined by additive and dominance genetic effects. For both traits we also allow for within-family environmental effects, that is, we do not assume that MZ twin pairs correlate unity! In Figure 13.2a we represent the case $A \longrightarrow B$, i.e., the only causal influence is of A on B. In Figure 13.2b, we represent the alternative case $B \longrightarrow A$[1]. In parallel to what we noted for the instrumental variable case, where the cross-covariances between each trait and the instrument for the other trait were critical, in the present example cross-trait twin pair covariances, i.e., the covariances between trait A measured in one twin and trait B measured in the cotwin, are particularly informative. From Figure 13.2a, the expected cross-trait covariance between twin pairs is given by $c_{AS}^2 i_B$, and will therefore be predicted to be the same for DZ as for MZ twin pairs. Under the alternative hypothesis that $B \longrightarrow A$ (Figure 13.2b), however, the expected cross-trait covariance will be $(a_{AS}^2 + d_{AS}^2) i_A^2$ in MZ pairs, but only $(0.5 a_{AS}^2 + 0.25 d_{AS}^2) i_A^2$ in DZ pairs, i.e., the cross-trait covariance will be higher in MZ than in DZ pairs. Although this simplified example is an extreme one, the same rationale applies when the relative magnitude of genetic and shared environmental influences is different for the two traits. If A was more strongly influenced by shared environmental influences than by genetic influences, but B was more strongly influenced by genetic influences than by shared environmental factors, then $A \longrightarrow B$ would predict predominantly shared environmental influences on the twin pair cross-trait covariances, whereas $B \longrightarrow A$ would predict predominantly genetic influence.

---

[1]Note that we use subscripts e_{AS}, e_{BS} in Figure 13.2, rather than merely e_A and e_B etc. used in previous chapters, because some of the genetic or environmental variance in B is mediated through the causal influence of A on B. Hence the estimates e_{BS} (in Figure 13.2a) and e_{AS} (in Figure 13.2b) will not be equal to their counterparts e_B and e_A estimated in a univariate analysis.

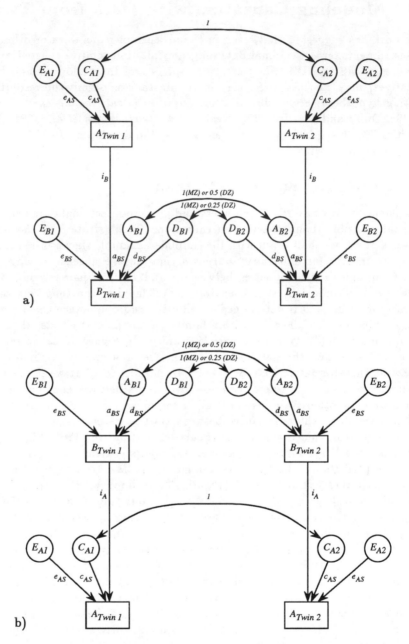

Figure 13.2: Simplified model of causes of resemblance among two variables, A and B, measured on a pair of twins. a) Trait A causes Trait B and b) Trait B causes Trait A.

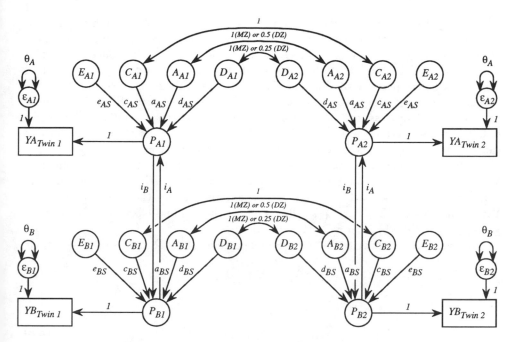

Figure 13.3: Basic direction of causation model.

13.3.2 LISREL Script for the Direction of Causation Model

We shall illustrate the testing of direction of causation models using the example of data on MZ and DZ twin pairs reared together; examining other relationships involves no new principles. Figure 13.3 summarizes our basic model in the form of a path diagram. In terms of structural equations, we have for first twins

$$P_{A1} = i_A P_{B1} + e_{AS} E_{A1} + c_{AS} C_{A1} + a_{AS} A_{A1} + d_{AS} D_{A1} \quad (13.3)$$
$$P_{B1} = i_B P_{A1} + e_{BS} E_{B1} + c_{BS} C_{B1} + a_{BS} A_{B1} + d_{BS} D_{B1} \quad (13.4)$$
$$YA_{Twin1} = P_{A1} + \varepsilon_{A1} \quad (13.5)$$
$$YB_{Twin1} = P_{B1} + \varepsilon_{B1} \quad (13.6)$$

with corresponding equations for second twins relating P_{A2} and P_{B2} to E_{A2} etc., and E_{B2} etc., and relating YA_{Twin2} and YB_{Twin2} to P_{A2} and P_{B2} and error terms ε_{A2} and ε_{B2}. The explicit inclusion of residual error terms is a new feature that we have not encountered in previous chapters: when we are testing direction of causation models, we can no longer assume that measurement error will be confounded with within-family environmental effects, leaving estimates of other parameters unbiased (Heath *et al.*, 1992). We assume that the covariances of the genetic and environmental determinants of P_A with those of P_B are all zero.

That is to say, the association between trait B (P_B) and the within-family and shared environmental and additive and dominance genetic factors which determine trait A $(E_A, C_A, A_A,$ and $D_A)$ arises *solely* because of the influence of trait A on trait B, and likewise that the association between P_A and $E_B, C_B, A_B,$ and D_B arises *solely* because of the causal influence of trait B on trait A. Thus we are interested in testing strong hypotheses of the form $A \Longleftrightarrow B$ or $A \longrightarrow B$ or $B \longrightarrow A$. We also assume that there is no genotype-environment correlation for either variable, because any such effects will be confounded with our estimates of shared environmental effects when we have data only on twins reared together (see Chapter 8). Further, all variables are assumed to be scaled as deviations from zero. We also have assumed, in Figure 13.3, that all latent genetic and environmental variables are standardized to unit variance, except that for the residual effects on YA we have $\text{var}(\varepsilon_{A1}) = \text{var}(\varepsilon_{A2}) = \theta_{\varepsilon A}$, and for the residual effects on YB we have $\text{var}(\varepsilon_{B1}) = \text{var}(\varepsilon_{B2}) = \theta_{\varepsilon B}.$[2]

As usual, we can rewrite the structural equations 13.3– 13.6 as matrix equations

$$\eta = \mathbf{B}\eta + \mathbf{\Gamma}\xi \tag{13.7}$$

and

$$y = \mathbf{\Lambda}_y\eta + \epsilon, \tag{13.8}$$

with $\mathbf{\Lambda}_y = \mathbf{I}$. In the present application we will have

$$\xi' = (E_{A1}, C_{A1}, A_{A1}, D_{A1}, E_{B1}, C_{B1}, A_{B1}, D_{B1}, E_{A2}, \ldots D_{B2})$$

i.e., for the number of independent variables we will have NK=16. For the latent dependent variables we will have $\eta' = (P_{A1}, P_{B1}, P_{A2}, P_{B2})$, thus NE=4. The (4×16) matrix of paths from the independent to dependent variables is

$$\mathbf{\Gamma} = \begin{pmatrix} e_{AS} & c_{AS} & a_{AS} & d_{AS} & 0 & 0 & 0 & 0 & 0 & 0 & 0 & 0 \\ 0 & 0 & 0 & 0 & e_{BS} & c_{BS} & a_{BS} & d_{BS} & 0 & 0 & 0 & 0 \\ 0 & 0 & 0 & 0 & 0 & 0 & 0 & 0 & e_{AS} & c_{AS} & a_{AS} & d_{AS} \\ 0 & 0 & 0 & 0 & 0 & 0 & 0 & 0 & 0 & 0 & 0 & 0 \end{pmatrix}$$

$$\begin{pmatrix} 0 & 0 & 0 & 0 \\ 0 & 0 & 0 & 0 \\ 0 & 0 & 0 & 0 \\ e_{BS} & c_{BS} & a_{BS} & d_{BS} \end{pmatrix}$$

---

[2] We note, however, that the model could be equally reparameterized as a variance components problem, estimating variance components $VE_A, VE_B, VC_A, VC_B, VA_A, VA_B, VD_A,$ and VD_B as well as reciprocal causal paths i_A and i_B and error variances $\theta_{\varepsilon A}$ and $\theta_{\varepsilon B}$, and fixing $e_{AS} = e_{BS} = c_{AS} = c_{BS} = a_{AS} = a_{BS} = d_{AS} = d_{BS} = 1$, for use with LISREL 8.

and the matrix of paths from the dependent variables to other dependent variables is

$$\mathbf{B} = \begin{pmatrix} 0 & i_A & 0 & 0 \\ i_B & 0 & 0 & 0 \\ 0 & 0 & 0 & i_A \\ 0 & 0 & i_B & 0 \end{pmatrix}$$

We still set the $\mathbf{\Lambda}_y$ matrix equal to the identity matrix, but also have

$$\mathbf{\Theta}_\epsilon{}' = (\theta_A, \theta_B, \theta_A, \theta_B).$$

The matrices $\mathbf{\Gamma}$, $\mathbf{B}$, and $\mathbf{\Theta}_\epsilon$ will be invariant across zygosity groups (assuming there are no gender differences in these parameters). The only matrix that differs across groups is (as usual) the fixed matrix $\mathbf{\Phi}$, giving the covariances of the latent genetic and environmental variables. For the parameterization in terms of path coefficients, all groups will have the diagonal elements of the $\mathbf{\Phi}$ matrix fixed to unity. For MZ pairs, we have $\phi(2, 10) = \phi(3, 11) = \phi(4, 12) = \phi(6, 14) = \phi(7, 15) = \phi(8, 16) = 1$; and, for DZ pairs, we have $\phi(2, 10) = \phi(6, 14) = 1$ (the covariances of C_A in twin pairs, and of C_B in twin pairs), $\phi(3, 11) = \phi(7, 15) = 0.5$ (the covariances of the additive genetic deviations), and $\phi(4, 12) = \phi(8, 16) = 0.25$ (the covariances of the dominance genetic deviations). Appendix I.1 gives an example LISREL 7 script for fitting a reciprocal causation model.

13.4   General Bivariate Models

For indirect causation ($A \longleftarrow C \longrightarrow B$), with C an unmeasured variable or set of variables, we can use a general bivariate genetic model. Figure 13.4 represents two equivalent parameterizations of the general bivariate model, each drawn as a path diagram for the causes of individual variation for two traits. (Note that we represent only individuals, not twin pairs, in Figure 13.4). The parameterization of Figure 13.4a estimates latent genetic and environmental effects for each variable, and covariances of these effects across traits, a traditional parameterization used by Eaves and Eysenck (1975), Heath *et al.* (1989), and others. The parameterization of Figure 13.4b uses a bivariate cholesky decomposition, with common factor effects on both traits A and B (E_A, C_A, A_A, and D_A), and specific-factor effects for one variable, chosen arbitrarily to be trait B in this example (e.g., E_B, C_B, A_B, and D_B). The parameterization of Figure 13.4a is awkward to implement in LISREL 7, since it requires the use of dummy variables (Heath *et al.*, 1989), but is more easily specified in LISREL 8 or Mx. The cholesky parameterization of Figure 13.4b is easily implemented in LISREL 7, and has the advantage of generalizing more readily to other types of problems.

Under the parameterization of the model in Figure 13.4a, in terms of structural equations, we have for first twins,

$$P_{A1} = e_A E_{A1} + c_A C_{A1} + a_A A_{A1} + d_A D_{A1} \tag{13.9}$$

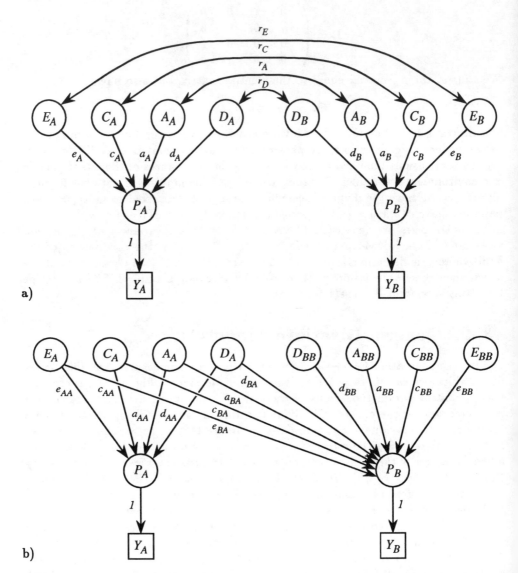

Figure 13.4: Two equivalent bivariate models for covariation between traits due to latent genetic and environmental factors: a) correlated factors, and b) Cholesky or triangular decomposition.

and

$$P_{B1} = e_B E_{B1} + c_B C_{B1} + a_B A_{B1} + d_B D_{B1} \qquad (13.10)$$

with corresponding expressions for the second twins, substituting PA_2 and PB_2 for PA_1 and PB_1, EA_2 and EB_2 for EA_1 and EB_1, and so on. Thus, there are sixteen elements of the vector ξ of independent variables (NK=16), and four elements of the vector η of dependent variables (NE=4). The matrix Γ, representing paths from the independent to the dependent variables, will be of the same form as under the reciprocal causation model. Since there are no paths from dependent variables in the general bivariate model, the **B** matrix is zero. Measurement error effects on the two traits are confounded with within-family environmental effects, and cannot be estimated separately without retest data, so we set the Λ_y matrix to be an identity matrix, and the Θ_ϵ matrix to zero. The Φ matrix differs from that used with the direction of causation model, because we must specify additional non-zero elements. First, for the across-trait covariances of each individual's genetic and environmental determinants of the two traits, we have:

- $\phi(1,5) = \phi(9,13) = r_E$ (the covariance of E_A and E_B)

- $\phi(2,6) = \phi(10,14) = r_C$ (the covariance of C_A and C_B)

- $\phi(3,7) = \phi(11,15) = r_A$ (the covariance of A_A and A_B)

- $\phi(4,8) = \phi(12,16) = r_D$ (the covariance of D_A and D_B)

These elements are the same for MZ as for DZ twin pairs. The cross-trait cross-twin covariances for the genetic and environmental variables depend upon zygosity. For MZ pairs, we have:

- $\phi(2,14) = \phi(6,10) = r_C$ (covariances of C_{A1} with C_{B2} and of C_{B1} with C_{A2})

- $\phi(3,15) = \phi(7,11) = r_A$ (covariances of A_{A1} with A_{B2} and A_{B1} with A_{A2})

- $\phi(4,16) = \phi(8,12) = r_D$ (covariances of D_{A1} with D_{B2} and D_{B1} with D_{A2})

Corresponding elements of the Φ matrix for DZ pairs are:

- $\phi(2,14) = \phi(6,10) = r_C$

- $\phi(3,15) = \phi(7,11) = 0.5r_A$

- $\phi(4,16) = \phi(8,12) = 0.25r_D$

In LISREL 8, we can use constraints to specify the two latter equalities for the DZ groups, i.e.,

```
CO PH(3,15)= 0.5*PH(1,3,15)
CO PH(7,11)= 0.5*PH(1,3,15)
CO PH(4,16)=0.25*PH(1,4,16)
CO PH(8,12)= 0.25*PH(1,4,16)
```

where PH(1,3,15) and PH(1,4,16) refer back to the corresponding elements in the first group of MZ pairs. All other elements of the Φ matrix are the same as for the direction of causation model. An example LISREL 8 script for fitting a bivariate genetic model using this parameterization is included in Appendix I.2. Using this parameterization with LISREL 7, which does not handle constraints, requires the use of dummy variables (Heath *et al.*, 1989) and is difficult to implement. In addition, this specification allows nonsensical estimates of correlations between latent variables (e.g., $r_A > 1$ or $r_C < -1$). While interval constraints are planned for LISREL 8, they are not working properly at the time of writing and are not available in LISREL 7. For these reasons, an alternative parameterization is to be preferred.

The parameterization of the model in Figure 13.4b is simply the cholesky model discussed in Section 12.4.2 applied to the two-variable case, and so will not be detailed here. This latter parameterization generalizes more readily to tests of genotype × environment or genotype × sex interaction in bivariate or multivariate data, giving us another reason to prefer this approach. An example script for LISREL 7 for this parameterization is included in Appendix I.3.

We can easily convert from the parameter estimates of 13.4b to the parameters of 13.4a. For the variable with no specific-factor parameters in the cholesky decomposition (A in our example), estimates of genetic and environmental parameters will be the same as under the model of 13.4a; i.e., $e_{AA} = e_A$, $c_{AA} = c_A$, $a_{AA} = a_A$, and $d_A = d_{AA}$. Genetic and environmental effects on the second variable are split into two components in Figure 13.4b — those due to the latent variables of A and those specific to B. We must combine these to obtain the total genetic and environmental variances for B (e.g., $e_B = e_{BB}^2 + e_{BA}^2$, $c_B = c_{BB}^2 + c_{BA}^2$). The correlation of two variables is defined as their covariance divided by the square root of the product of their variances (see Chapter 2) so we have

$$r_E = \frac{e_{AA}e_{BA}}{e_{AA}\sqrt{e_{BA}^2 + e_{BB}^2}} \qquad (13.11)$$

$$r_C = \frac{c_{AA}c_{BA}}{c_{AA}\sqrt{c_{BA}^2 + c_{BB}^2}} \qquad (13.12)$$

$$r_A = \frac{a_{AA}a_{BA}}{a_{AA}\sqrt{a_{BA}^2 + a_{BB}^2}} \qquad (13.13)$$

$$r_E = \frac{d_{AA}d_{BA}}{d_{AA}\sqrt{d_{BA}^2 + d_{BB}^2}} \qquad (13.14)$$

It also can be shown (Heath *et al.*, 1992) that the reciprocal causation model of the previous section is a submodel of the general bivariate genetic model. In particular, if there is reciprocal causation between two variables ($A \Longleftrightarrow B$) but we fit a bivariate genetic model, we can interpret the estimates using the equalities:

$$a_A^2 = \frac{a_{AS}^2 + i_A^2 a_{BS}^2}{(1 - i_A i_B)^2} \tag{13.15}$$

$$a_B^2 = \frac{a_{BS}^2 + i_B^2 a_{AS}^2}{(1 - i_A i_B)^2} \tag{13.16}$$

$$r_G = \frac{i_B a_{AS}^2 + i_A a_{BS}^2}{\sqrt{(a_{AS}^2 + i_A^2 h_{BS}^2)(a_{BS}^2 + i_B^2 a_{AS}^2)}} \tag{13.17}$$

together with expressions for dominance genetic and shared and within-family environmental components obtained by making the appropriate substitutions[3]. Thus, the unidirectional causation and reciprocal causation models are nested submodels of the general bivariate model, and their fit can be compared to that of the latter by likelihood-ratio chi-squared test.

13.5 Considerations in Causal Models

Many of the issues that arise when testing reciprocal causation models using twin data have been explored by Heath *et al.* (1992), and we will review these only briefly here, illustrating them with concrete examples.

The treatment of measurement error is of primary concern in reciprocal causation models. If we do not consider measurement error in our model, when measurement error exists, we are at risk of reaching false inferences about causality. To demonstrate this, we shall use LISREL to simulate expected covariance matrices for a variety of sets of parameter values of the direction of causation model, by fixing all parameters of the model at values assigned with VAlue statements. If we specify RS on the output line, LISREL will report the expected or 'fitted' covariance matrices for the specified parameter values. We can then use these as observed covariance matrices, assume some arbitrary sample size for MZ and for DZ twin pairs (e.g., N=5000 pairs for each group), and explore the consequences of fitting alternative false models, by maximum-likelihood, as we would do when performing power calculations (see Chapter 9).

13.5.1 Data Simulation under the Causal Model

Tables 13.2 and 13.3 give six sets of covariance matrices, generated under either a reciprocal ($A \Longleftrightarrow B$) or a unidirectional causation model ($A \longrightarrow B$). For all six data-sets, we have used the same values for the genetic and environmental

---

[3]Heath *et al.* (1992) use h instead of A_{AS} and h' instead of a_{BS}, c instead of c_{BS} and so on. The notation used here is intended to assist the reader and to facilitate future multivariate generalization of the model.

Table 13.2: Covariance matrices generated under a reciprocal causation model, allowing for measurement error. The data simulate twins ($T1$ and $T2$) measured on two traits (A and B). We assume $e_{AS} = 0.5, c_{AS} = 0.868, e_{BS} = 0.5, a_{BS} = 0.866, i_B = 0.2$, and $i_A = 0.4$. (Note: only the lower triangle of each matrix is given).

	\multicolumn{8}{c}{Reciprocal Causation $A \Longleftrightarrow B$}

Reciprocal Causation $A \Longleftrightarrow B$

Example 1: 20% of variance in each trait is due to measurement error ($\theta_A = 0.343, \theta_B = 0.307$)

	\multicolumn{4}{c}{MZ Pairs}	\multicolumn{4}{c}{DZ Pairs}
	$T1_A$	$T1_B$	$T2_A$	$T2_B$	$T1_A$	$T1_B$	$T2_A$	$T2_B$
Twin 1 A	1.713				1.713			
Twin 1 B	0.709	1.536			0.709	1.536		
Twin 2 A	1.028	0.532	1.713		0.957	0.354	1.713	
Twin 2 B	0.532	0.922	0.709	1.536	0.354	0.478	0.709	1.536

Example 2: 33.4% of variance in trait A, 0% of trait B is due to measurement error ($\theta_A = 0.685; \theta_B = 0$)

	\multicolumn{4}{c}{MZ Pairs}	\multicolumn{4}{c}{DZ Pairs}
	$T1_A$	$T1_B$	$T2_A$	$T2_B$	$T1_A$	$T1_B$	$T2_A$	$T2_B$
Twin 1 A	2.056				2.056			
Twin 1 B	0.709	1.229			0.709	1.229		
Twin 2 A	1.028	0.532	2.056		0.957	0.354	2.056	
Twin 2 B	0.532	0.922	0.709	1.229	0.354	0.478	0.709	1.229

Example 3: 0% of variance of trait A, 33.4% of trait B is due to measurement error ($\theta_B = 0.614; \theta_A = 0$)

	\multicolumn{4}{c}{MZ Pairs}	\multicolumn{4}{c}{DZ Pairs}
	$T1_A$	$T1_B$	$T2_A$	$T2_B$	$T1_A$	$T1_B$	$T2_A$	$T2_B$
Twin 1 A	1.370				1.370			
Twin 1 B	0.709	1.843			0.709	1.843		
Twin 2 A	1.028	0.532	1.370		0.957	0.354	1.370	
Twin 2 B	0.532	0.922	0.709	1.843	0.354	0.478	0.709	1.843

Table 13.3: Covariance matrices generated under a unidirectional causal model, allowing for measurement error. The data simulate twins ($T1$ and $T2$) measured on two traits (A and B). We assume $e_{AS} = 0.5, c_{AS} = 0.868, e_{BS} = 0.5, a_{BS} = 0.866, i_B = 0.4$ and $i_A = 0$. (Note: only the lower triangle of each matrix is given).

	\multicolumn{8}{c}{Unidirectional Causation $A \longrightarrow B$}

Unidirectional Causation $A \longrightarrow B$

Example 4: 20% of variance in each trait is due to measurement error ($\theta_A = 0.25, \theta_B = 0.29$)

| | \multicolumn{4}{c}{MZ Pairs} | \multicolumn{4}{c}{DZ Pairs} |

	$T1_A$	$T1_B$	$T2_A$	$T2_B$	$T1_A$	$T1_B$	$T2_A$	$T2_B$
Twin 1 A	1.250				1.250			
Twin 1 B	0.400	1.450			0.400	1.450		
Twin 2 A	0.750	0.300	1.250		0.750	0.300	1.250	
Twin 2 B	0.300	0.870	0.400	1.450	0.300	0.500	0.400	1.450

Example 5: 33.4% of variance of trait A, 0% of trait B is due to measurement error ($\theta_A = 0.5, \theta_B = 0$)

| | \multicolumn{4}{c}{MZ Pairs} | \multicolumn{4}{c}{DZ Pairs} |

	$T1_A$	$T1_B$	$T2_A$	$T2_B$	$T1_A$	$T1_B$	$T2_A$	$T2_B$
Twin 1 A	1.500				1.500			
Twin 1 B	0.400	1.160			0.400	1.160		
Twin 2 A	0.750	0.300	1.500		0.750	0.300	1.500	
Twin 2 B	0.300	0.870	0.400	1.160	0.300	0.495	0.400	1.160

Example 6: 0% of variance of trait A, 33.4% of trait B is due to measurement error ($\theta_A = 0; \theta_B = 0.58$)

| | \multicolumn{4}{c}{MZ Pairs} | \multicolumn{4}{c}{DZ Pairs} |

	$T1_A$	$T1_B$	$T2_A$	$T2_B$	$T1_A$	$T1_B$	$T2_A$	$T2_B$
Twin 1 A	1.000				1.000			
Twin 1 B	0.400	1.740			0.400	1.740		
Twin 2 A	0.750	0.300	1.000		0.750	0.300	1.000	
Twin 2 B	0.300	0.870	0.400	1.740	0.300	0.870	0.400	1.740

parameters of the direction of causation model: $e_{AS} = 0.5, c_{AS} = 0.868, a_{AS} = d_{AS} = 0, e_{BS} = 0.5, a_{BS} = 0.868, c_{BS} = d_{BS} = 0$. For the reciprocal examples, we use values of $i_B = 0.2, i_A = 0.4$; and for the unidirectional case, we set $i_B = 0.4, i_A = 0$. By considering an example where A and B have very different modes of inheritance, we have chosen an example where the power of resolving direction of causation models in twin data is greatest. To make life more difficult, however, we have assumed that there is measurement error, but no test-retest data. For both the reciprocal and the unidirectional causation examples, we explore three cases: (i) 20% of the observed variation in each of the traits is attributable to measurement error; (ii) one-third of the observed variation in trait A is due to measurement error, which is negligible in trait B; and (iii) the same as (ii) but B has error and A does not. Values of θ_A and θ_B for these examples are given in Tables 13.2 and 13.3. We can now review the effects of fitting direction of causation models which ignore error, and examine the estimates of model parameters which are recovered.

13.5.2   Fitting False Models to Simulated Data

For the reciprocal causation examples, when the true values are $i_B = 0.2$ ($A \longrightarrow B$) and $i_A = 0.4$ ($B \longrightarrow A$), but 20% of the variance in each trait is due to error, we recover estimates of $i_B = 0.3$ and $i_A = 0.1$; i.e., the variable that has the stronger impact under the true model (trait B) appears to have the weaker impact. When error for trait B is negligible, but accounts for one-third of the variation in trait A, the causal influence of B on A is overestimated ($i_A = 0.53$), and no reciprocal influence of A on B is found ($i_B = 0.02$). In the third example, where we assume that there is no measurement error in trait B but one-third of the variance in A is due to measurement error, parameter estimates for the reciprocal paths are $i_B = 0.357$ and $i_A = 0.13$; thus, again we overestimate the influence $A \longrightarrow B$ and underestimate the reciprocal effect $B \longrightarrow A$.

For the unidirectional examples, with true values for the causal paths of $i_B = 0.4$ and $i_A = 0$ (i.e., $A \longrightarrow B$), when we assume that 20% of the variance in each trait is attributable to error, but fit models that ignore error, we recover estimates of $i_B = 0.47$ and $i_A = -0.17$. Thus we overestimate the effect of $A \longrightarrow B$, and incorrectly infer a negative feedback effect $B \longrightarrow A$. For the true model of no error in B, and one-third error variance in A, parameter estimates are $i_B = 0.06$ and $i_A = 0.225$ — underestimating the effect of $A \longrightarrow B$, overestimating $B \longrightarrow A$, and leading to entirely the wrong conclusion about the direction of causation. For the final example, with measurement error in B only, estimates of i_B and i_A are unbiased, i.e., maximum-likelihood estimates are $i_B = 0.4, i_A = 0$. This last result is to be expected: the prediction for the within-person covariance in traits A and B under unidirectional causation, for the case $A \longrightarrow B$, will be $i_B(a_{AS}^2 + d_{AS}^2 + c_{AS}^2 + e_{AS}^2)$. Provided that errors of measurement are uncorrelated between family members (the standard assumption used in family studies, which we attempt to ensure by scheduling independent testing of family members by different testers), measurement error inflates the estimate of within-family environmental effects. However, in this example since A is assumed to be measured without error, e^2_{AS} is unbiased, and is not inflated by error variance. Thus, in the case of unidirectional causation, if the variable which is a postulated cause of the other variable is measured with negligible error, we should be able to obtain an unbiased estimate of the causal parameter i_B or i_A.

13.5.3 Discussion of Simulation Exercise

Unidirectional causation

Given the sensitivity of the direction of causation model to measurement error effects on the two traits with reciprocal causal influence, it is clearly desirable that causal hypotheses be tested using test-retest or other multiple-indicator data on family members. In the absence of such data, a critical consideration is the number of 'sources of variation' (Jinks and Fulker, 1970) for the two traits under study, counting additive genetic, dominance genetic, shared environmental, and random environmental effects each as a separate source of variation. For example, in the simulated data sets of Tables 13.2 and 13.3 there are three sources of variation: additive genetic effects, shared environmental effects and within-family environmental effects. If there are really only two sources of variation, (e.g., additive genetic effects and within-family environmental effects), then unless we know that measurement error effects for both traits are negligible, or have retest or other data about the magnitude of error variances, we cannot draw any trustworthy inferences from fitting direction of causation models. On the other hand, if there are three sources of variation, it still is possible to test unidirectional causation models which allow for measurement error in the postulated causal variable. As we discuss elsewhere, this is possible because when fitting direction of causation models we are in essence testing constraints on the general bivariate model implied by equation 13.17 and the equivalent expressions for r_E and r_C or r_D. Provided that there are at least three sources of variation in the two traits, when we fit unidirectional causal models, by estimating an error variance for one trait, we are in effect relaxing the constraint on r_E, but retaining one degree of freedom to test the remaining constraints on r_A and r_D. Thus, we can still test 'unidirectional causation with error' models against the general bivariate genetic models. When we reanalyze data sets for examples 4 and 5 from Table 13.3, but include a parameter θ_A to allow for error variance in trait A (still fixing $\theta_B = 0$), then we indeed recover an unbiased estimate of $i_B = 0.4$ (and $i_A = 0$). In example 5, since these data were generated assuming no measurement error in B, all recovered parameter estimates are unbiased. In example 4, all estimates are unbiased except that of the within-family environmental variance for B, e^2_{BS}, which is inflated by the error variance for trait B. However, though it is possible to test the two unidirectional causal models $A \longrightarrow B$ and $B \longrightarrow A$ even if there is no information about measurement error, the power of our data for rejecting false causal models increases considerably when test-retest or other multiple-indicator data are used (Heath *et al.*, 1992). If there are only two sources of variability, we can test the unidirectional causal models only if we use multiple-indicator data to provide estimates of measurement error effects. Otherwise the fit of the unidirectional causal model allowing for measurement error should be the same as that of the general bivariate genetic one estimating r_E and either r_A or r_C.

Reciprocal Causation with Negligible Error

Under the reciprocal causation model, the expected within-person covariance of traits A and B involves both e_{AS}^2 and e_{BS}^2, so error variances of the variables are important. If one of the two traits can be assumed to be measured with negligible error, we can still estimate an error variance for the second, provided that there are at least three sources of variation[4]. When we did this for example data sets 2 and 3 in Table 13.2, we recovered unbiased estimates of $i_B = 0.2$ and $i_A = 0.4$. However, by estimating an additional parameter we lose a degree of freedom, and so can no longer compare the fit of the reciprocal causation model against that of the general bivariate, to see whether the indirect hypothesis gives a significant improvement in fit. This problem disappears if there are at least four sources of variation for the two traits — for example if we are looking at the causes of the association between a personality trait which is influenced by additive plus dominance genetic effects and within-family environment (Eaves *et al.*, 1989; 1992), and a measure of perceived family background influenced by shared and within-family environmental factors (Parker, 1983; 1990; Neale *et al.*, 1992). The effects of dominance and shared environment are confounded if we have data only on twin pairs reared together (Eaves, 1969, 1970; Martin *et al.*, 1978); but with additional data on separated twins (Jinks and Fulker, 1970) or parents and other relatives (Fulker, 1982; Heath, 1983), these effects may be resolved. Thus a one degree of freedom likelihood-ratio test of the reciprocal causation against the general bivariate model would still be possible. However, cases where we can safely assume that a variable is measured with negligible error are likely to be rare. Smoking status, defined as whether or not an individual has ever smoked, approximates this ideal, at least as assessed by self-report in general population surveys.

Reciprocal Causation with Equal Errors

Under the reciprocal causation model, we do not have sufficient information to estimate two separate error variances, since all our information about error is derived from relaxing the single constraint on r_E. However, if two traits have nearly identical error variances, we can assume that they are equal and estimate one error

---

[4]If there are only two sources of variation, even if both traits are measured without error, the reciprocal causation model will in any case give the same fit as the general bivariate, so no test of the model is available.

parameter. When we used this approach with example data set 1, we were able to recover almost unbiased estimates of the reciprocal paths: $i_B = 0.199, i_A = 0.401$. In many instances, however, the assumption of equal error variances will not be valid. For such cases, it will be possible to provide a convincing test of the reciprocal causation model only if test-retest data or other multiple indicators are used to provide information about measurement error. To illustrate, we applied the simulation procedure with marked differences in error variance in example 1. When measurement error accounts for 50% of the variance in trait B, but only 20% of the variance in trait A, our estimates of i_A and i_B are quite seriously biased $(i_A = 0.247, i_B = 0.301)$, compared to the true values of $i_A = 0.4$ and $i_B = 0.2$. This is also true, albeit to a lesser degree, if measurement error accounts for 50% of the variance in trait A, and only 20% of trait B: we recover estimates of $i_A = 0.441$ and $i_B = 0.157$. For the example data sets of Table 13.2, inferences about reciprocal causation are surprisingly robust to modest differences in error variance. If we assume that measurement error accounts for 20% of the variance in A, and one-third of B, or vice versa, and estimate a single error variance for both traits, our maximum-likelihood estimates are $i_A = 0.401$ and $i_B = 0.199$. However, we must emphasize that we have used as an illustration an example where traits A and B have very different modes of inheritance. In other cases the impact of modest differences in error variance on inferences about direction of causation is likely to be more pronounced.

13.6 Application to Alcohol Data

To illustrate the issues surrounding unidirectional and reciprocal causation models, we reanalyze data from an Australian alcohol challenge study of volunteer twin pairs aged 18-34 years, conducted by Martin and colleagues (Martin et al., 1985; Heath and Martin, 1991a,b). In this study, after baseline assessments, 206 twin pairs were given a standard body-weight adjusted dose of ethanol, followed by measures of psychomotor performance and subjective ratings of intoxication taken over a three-hour period. Sample sizes in this study are small, so that only tentative conclusions can be drawn. Nonetheless, these data will suffice to illustrate many of the practical problems which arise when testing causal models.

A substantial literature, including studies of adoptees (Cadoret et al., 1980; Cloninger et al., 1981; Goodwin et al., 1974), half-siblings (Schuckit et al., 1972), and twins (Kaij, 1960; Hrubec and Omenn, 1981; Kaprio et al., 1987; Pickens et al., 1991) supports a genetic contribution to vulnerability to alcoholism. One hypothesis to explain this genetic predisposition is that there are genetically determined differences in reactivity to alcohol, and individuals who are less reactive are at greater risk of developing alcohol-related problems (Schuckit, 1984a,b). A practical problem which arises when attempting to falsify this hypothesis is that ethical considerations make it impossible to study the reactions to alcohol of previously alcohol-naive subjects — particularly those with a family history of alcoholism!

Thus, observed differences in alcohol reactivity between offspring of alcoholics and controls[5] might also be a consequence of differences in drinking history between these two groups. Results of univariate genetic analyses of data from the alcohol challenge study support a genetic contribution to differences in post-alcohol deterioration in psychomotor performance (Martin *et al.*, 1985; Heath and Martin, 1991b), and to differences in subjective ratings of intoxication (Neale and Martin, 1989; Martin and Boomsma, 1989). However, there is considerable evidence for a genetic influence on alcohol consumption patterns, including measures of average frequency of alcohol use, quantity consumed per drinking occasion, and average weekly consumption[6], raising the possibility that genetic differences in alcohol reactivity are a secondary consequence of genetically influenced differences in drinking history. In other words, this is a case where two alternative strong causal hypotheses may be advanced (Reactivity $\longrightarrow$ Consumption, versus Consumption $\longrightarrow$ Reactivity), as well as the more general hypothesis of reciprocal causation.

Data Summary

Table 13.4 summarizes 4×4 covariance matrices for twin pairs' history of alcohol consumption (reported average number of drinks per week, assessed at baseline) and subjective ratings of intoxication. Average weekly consumption was transformed by taking $\log(x + 1)$ where x was the number of 'standard drinks' of beer, wine, spirits, sherry, or other alcoholic beverages taken per week. For the measure of intoxication, subjects were asked to rate on a 10-point scale their response to the question "How drunk do you feel now", with 1="quite sober", and 10="the most drunk I have ever been." We have treated this measure as a continuous variable, and also have reversed the ordering of the categories, so that high scores indicate low reactivity to alcohol. We have correspondingly reversed the sign of estimates of genetic and environmental correlations, or causal paths, to correct for this in the parameter estimates reported in Table 13.5. Both variables were standardized to unit variance, separately for males and females, so that we could equate error variances for the Consumption and Intoxication measures when testing the reciprocal causation model.

Results of Fitting Causal Models to Data from Males

We discuss only the results of separate analyses of data from the male like-sex and female like-sex pairs, without testing for genotype $\times$ sex interaction. Table 13.5 summarizes the results of model-fitting, and reports standardized parameter estimates under the best-fitting models. All models were fitted by maximum-likelihood. First we address the results for male like-sex pairs, in whom the association between

---

[5](e.g., Schuckit, 1984a,b; Schuckit and Gold, 1988; Pollock *et al.*, 1986; O'Malley and Maisto, 1989; Moss *et al.*, 1989)

[6](Cederloff, 1977; Clifford *et al.*, 1981; Heath *et al.*, 1989; Heath *et al.*, 1991a,b; Kaprio *et al.*, 1981;1987)

Table 13.4: Covariance matrices for self-reported history of alcohol consumption (drinks/week) and intoxication after a challenge dose of alcohol. Data are from the Australian alcohol challenge twin study (Martin *et al*, 1985; Heath and Martin, 1991b)

		$T1_C$	$T1_I$	$T2_C$	$T2_I$
	MZ Female Pairs (N=43 pairs)				
Twin 1	Consumption	0.9927			
	Intoxication	0.5329	0.9829		
Twin 2	Consumption	0.5332	0.4859	0.9134	
	Intoxication	0.2731	0.5214	0.4285	1.2121
	MZ Male Pairs (N=42 pairs)				
Twin 1	Consumption	1.0727			
	Intoxication	0.6686	0.9773		
Twin 2	Consumption	0.6970	0.5751	0.9093	
	Intoxication	0.6167	0.5238	0.6794	1.2041
	DZ Female Pairs (N=42 pairs)				
Twin 1	Consumption	0.8390			
	Intoxication	0.2731	0.7283		
Twin 2	Consumption	0.3578	0.0584	1.2359	
	Intoxication	0.0698	-0.0208	0.2157	1.1453
	DZ Male Pairs (N=37 pairs)				
Twin 1	Consumption	1.0766			
	Intoxication	0.5710	1.0918		
Twin 2	Consumption	0.2606	0.2732	1.0561	
	Intoxication	0.0509	0.1410	0.3836	1.8570
	Opposite-Sex Pairs (N=39 pairs)				
Twin 1	Consumption	0.9970			
	Intoxication	0.0993	0.7778		
Twin 2	Consumption	0.2457	0.0668	0.9718	
	Intoxication	0.1012	0.0652	0.3646	0.8887

Table 13.5:

Results of fitting direction of causation models to alcohol challenge data on history of alcohol consumption ('Drinks') and self-report intoxication after a challenge dose of alcohol ('Intox')

	Goodness of Fit			Standardised Parameter Estimates															
				Drinks					Intoxication					Covariance (Intox, Drinks)					
Model	d.f.	χ^2	p	e_{AS}	c_{AS}	a_{AS}	d_{AS}	θ_C	e_{HS}	c_{HS}	a_{HS}	d_{HS}	θ_I	i_D	i_I	e_{HH}	c_{HH}	a_{HH}	d_{HH}
									Male Like-Sex Pairs										
1. Drinks $\longrightarrow$ Intox, no error	13	11.31	0.58	0.54	—	0.49	0.69	—	0.77	—	0.21	0.21	—	-0.56	—	—	—	—	—
2. Drinks $\longrightarrow$ Intox, error in Drinks	12	7.33	0.83	0.28	—	0.63	0.72	0.25	0.74	—	0.20	0.00	—	-0.65	—	—	—	—	—
3. Intox $\longrightarrow$ Drinks, no error	13	23.27	0.04	0.63	—	0.29	0.54	—	0.73	—	0.39	0.56	—	—	-0.49	—	—	—	—
4. Intox $\longrightarrow$ Drinks, error in Intox[a]	12	8.00	0.78	0.51	—	0.23	0.35	—	0.32	—	0.64	0.70	0.46	—	-0.75	—	—	—	—
5. Reciprocal causation, no error	12	7.34	0.83	0.64	—	0.69	0.79	—	0.83	—	0.20	—	—	-0.76	0.35	—	—	—	—
6. Reciprocal causation, equal error	11	7.33	0.77	0.00	—	0.58	0.66	0.30	0.56	—	0.23	0.00	0.29	-0.73	-0.16	—	—	—	—
7. General bivariate genetic model[b]	11	7.33	0.77	0.55	—	0.55	0.63	—	-0.08	—	-0.42	-0.46	—	—	—	0.75	—	0.20	0.00
									Female Like-Sex Pairs										
1. Drinks $\longrightarrow$ Intox, no error	13	16.33	0.23	0.65	0.31	0.69	—	—	0.75	0.00	0.56	—	—	-0.34	—	—	—	—	—
2. Drinks $\longrightarrow$ Intox, error in Drinks	12	15.81	0.20	0.53	0.28	0.80	—	0.20	0.74	0.00	0.55	—	—	-0.39	—	—	—	—	—
3. Intox $\longrightarrow$ Drinks, no error	13	17.62	0.17	0.67	0.38	0.56	—	—	0.75	0.00	0.66	—	—	—	-0.31	—	—	—	—
4. Intox $\longrightarrow$ Drinks, error in Intox[a]	12	14.75	0.25	0.63	0.44	0.42	—	—	0.44	0.00	0.90	—	0.48	—	-0.49	—	—	—	—
5. Reciprocal causation, no error	12	16.18	0.18	0.68	0.24	0.77	—	—	0.77	0.00	0.55	—	—	-0.46	0.13	—	—	—	—
6. Reciprocal causation, equal error	11	14.83	0.19	0.00	0.53	0.61	—	0.40	0.49	0.00	0.80	—	0.41	-0.11	-0.52	—	—	—	—
7. General bivariate genetic model[b]	11	14.75	0.19	0.09	—	0.45	0.41	—	-0.76	-0.04	-0.65	—	—	—	—	0.66	0.43	0.00	—

[a] Constrained solution with unstandardised $i_I < 1$; i_I fixed on its upper bound (unconstrained solution gives $\theta_I = .54$, $i_I = .83$ and $\chi^2 = 7.34$).

[b] Specific components estimated for consumption.

drinking history and post-alcohol challenge intoxication ratings is stronger (see Table 13.4), and, therefore, in whom our statistical power for resolving alternative models is likely to be greater. We fitted the bivariate genetic cholesky model (model 7) using LISREL 7. The general bivariate genetic model gives an excellent fit to the male like-sex data $(\chi^2_{11} = 7.33, p = 0.77)$, and yields estimates for the genetic and environmental correlations $r_E = -0.19, r_G = -0.77$ and $r_D = -1.00$. This suggests that substantially the same genetic factors are determining differences in consumption patterns and differences in alcohol reactivity, but that within-family environmental influences are more highly variable-specific. (Note that we expect these correlations to be negative, since high consumption levels are associated with low alcohol reactivity, and high alcohol reactivity with low consumption.) From the maximum-likelihood parameter estimates, we also computed the proportion of the total variation in Consumption and Reactivity explained by within-family environmental, additive genetic, and dominance effects. Our estimates for Consumption are: 30% within-family environment, 30% additive genetic, and 40% dominance genetic effects; for Intoxication: 57% within-family environment, 22% additive genetic, and 21% dominance genetic effects.

Turning to the results of fitting direction of causation models to the male data, if we consider only the results of fitting models which ignore measurement error (as did Heath and Martin, 1991b), a rather perplexing finding emerges. The hypothesis that differences in alcohol reactivity lead to differences in drinking history (Model 3) is rejected by chi-squared test of goodness-of-fit. The alternative unidirectional causal hypothesis, that differences in drinking history cause differences in alcohol reactivity (Model 1) gives an excellent fit to the data $(\chi^2_{13} = 11.31, p = 0.58)$, and a fit which is not significantly worse that that of the general bivariate model $(\chi^2_2 = 3.98, p = 0.26)$. Thus, on the basis of this likelihood-ratio comparison, we would prefer the unidirectional causal hypothesis DRINKS $\longrightarrow$ INTOX on the principle of parsimony. However, reciprocal causation (Model 5) gives a significant improvement in fit over Model 1: the difference between the goodness-of-fit chi-squared of these two models yields a likelihood-ratio χ^2, of 3.97 with one degree of freedom, $(p < 0.05)$. Thus, we must infer that reciprocal causation is the most parsimonious model considered so far. Unexpectedly, however, while our estimate of the causal path from drinking history to intoxication rating is strong and negative (-0.76), the reciprocal effect of intoxication rating on drinking history is positive (0.35). This implies that, once we allow for the effects of drinking history on alcohol reactivity, those with high reactivity to alcohol exhibit increased consumption, rather than the predicted decrease (Schuckit, 1984a). Estimates of genetic and environmental parameters under Model 5 indicate that most of the genetic variance in intoxication may be explained by the causal influence of consumption on intoxication; only 4% of the variance is explained by additive genetic effects specific to the intoxication measure, and this effect is non-significant with these sample sizes.

Including Measurement Error

We have to qualify our interpretations once we include the effects of measurement error. Neither of the two unidirectional causal models allowing for measurement error (Models 2 and 4) gives a significantly worse fit than the general bivariate model, implying that we have little power to resolve what is causing what. Under the model DRINKS ⟶ INTOX (Model 2), we obtain a plausible estimate for the error variance for consumption (25%), and a sensible estimate for the causal effect of drinking history on intoxication rating (−0.65). When we fit the alternative unidirectional model with error, however, we get an implausibly high estimate for the effects of alcohol reactivity on consumption pattern. The unstandardized value is $i_A = 1.78$. If we constrain this parameter to be less than or equal to unity, using the interval restriction option in LISREL 8,

```
IR B(1,2) < 1.0
```

the (unstandardized) maximum-likelihood estimate is unity; and the estimate of the proportion of the observed variance in intoxication ratings explained by measurement error is 45%. Since it was not possible to reject either unidirectional model by likelihood-ratio test against the full model, once we allowed for measurement error, we examined the parameter estimates obtained under a reciprocal causation model assuming equal error variances for each trait (Model 6). The fit then appears slightly worse than that of the general bivariate genetic model, because one of its parameters (the estimate of within-family environmental effects, excluding measurement error, for consumption) has gone to its lower bound of zero. The reciprocal causal paths are now both of the same sign, with the predominant causal influence being that of drinking history on post-alcohol challenge intoxication rating (−0.73), with a much more modest effect of intoxication (i.e., alcohol reactivity) on drinking history (−0.16). Measurement error is estimated to account for 30% of the variance in the two variables. Once again, under Model 6, we find that almost all of the genetic variance in self-ratings of intoxication is mediated through the effects of drinking history on intoxication, with the direction effects of additive gene action on post-alcohol challenge intoxication accounting for a modest 5.3% of the variance. Such a conclusion, though tantalizing, is based on very small sample sizes, and would be more convincing if replicated in the female data.

Results of Fitting Causal Models to Data from Females

To the female twin data we fit a genetic cholesky model incorporating additive and dominance genetic and within-family environmental effects on both consumption and intoxication measures, together with additive genetic and shared and within-family environmental effects specific to consumption. This general bivariate model gives a moderately good fit to the data ($\chi^2_{11} = 14.75, p = 0.19$). The specific-factor additive genetic parameter is estimated as zero, indicating that all genetic effects on the two traits are common-factor effects, but substantial specific-factor shared and within-family environmental effects are apparent. However, we find marked dominance but no additive genetic effects on intoxication, a result which makes little biological sense (e.g., Mather and Jinks, 1971), but may simply reflect the poor resolution of additive versus non-additive genetic effects in twin data (Martin *et al.*, 1978). The association between drinking history and intoxication rating is much weaker for female respondents, perhaps because in the female twins the challenge dose of alcohol exceeded the maximum amount previously experienced in many cases. Our statistical power of resolving alternative models is correspondingly weak. Even if we ignore measurement error, neither of the unidirectional causal models (1 and 3) gives a significantly worse fit than the general bivariate one (Model 7). The hypothesis DRINKS $\longrightarrow$ INTOX yields a lower χ^2, if measurement error is ignored, but comparing the fit of Models 2 and 4 we see that this ordering is reversed once we allow for measurement error. Under reciprocal interaction, the relative magnitude of the causal paths is consistent with what we observed in males ($i_B = -0.46, i_A = 0.13$). Once measurement error is included in the model, however, this finding is reversed; the major effect appears to be that alcohol reactivity causes consumption pattern ($i_A = -0.52$), with a relatively modest effect of drinking history on reactivity ($i_B = -0.11$). We are forced to conclude that the female data do not replicate the pattern observed in males.

13.7 Multivariate Direction of Causation Models

Measurement error greatly reduces the statistical power for resolving alternative causal hypotheses in family data, but the use of multiple measures of the underlying constructs A and B ('multiple indicator variables', in the terminology of structural equation modeling) lessens this problem (Heath *et al.*, 1992). Figure 13.5a illustrates a reciprocal causation model, and Figure 13.5b shows the more general bivariate genetic model against which it may be compared (the 'correlated factors' psychometric model of McArdle and Goldsmith, 1990), for the case where there are three indicator variables for each of variables A and B. Once again, Figure 13.5 shows the causes of variation within-individuals: the path diagrams for twin pairs are rather more complex, but introduce no new principles. Figures 13.5a and 13.5b differ from the single-variable indicator models of Figures 13.3 and 13.4a principally through the use of three indicators of trait A (Y_{A1}, Y_{A2}, and Y_{A3}) of trait B (Y_{B1}, Y_{B2}, and Y_{B3}) each Y variable having its own residual or specific-factor term ε_{Ai} or ε_{Bj}. The structural equations for P_A and P_B remain the same as in the single-indicator case (equations 13.3 and 13.4 for the reciprocal causation model, or 13.9 and 13.10 for the general bivariate genetic model); but equations relating the observed indicator variables to the underlying latent constructs P_A and P_B are now of the form

$$YA_{i(T1)} = \lambda_{iA} P_{AT1} + \varepsilon_{Ai(T1)} \quad (i = 1, 3) \tag{13.18}$$

$$YB_{j(T1)} = \lambda_{jB} P_{BT1} + \varepsilon_{Bj(T1)} \quad (j = 1, 3). \tag{13.19}$$

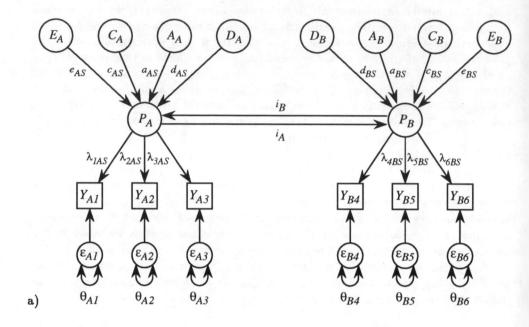

a)

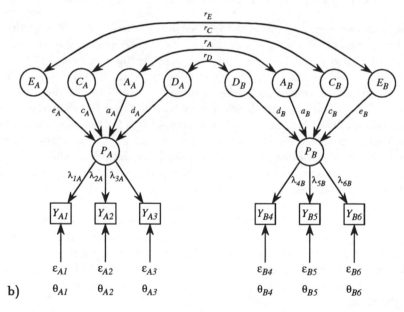

b)

Figure 13.5: Path diagrams of (a) reciprocal interaction model and (b) correlated factors model for three indicators of each of the latent variables A and B.

Here the λ's are factor loadings of the indicator variables on the underlying traits A and B. As in the more general 'psychometric' or 'latent phenotype' model, the ϵ terms represent specific-factor effects, i.e., within-family and shared environmental and additive and dominance genetic effects which are specific to a particular indicator variable, rather than merely measurement error (which forms part of within-family environmental specific-factor effects). The modeling of specific-factor effects has already been described in the context of multivariate genetic analysis (Chapter 12), so we shall not elaborate here. As in the psychometric model, we must fix the scale of traits P_A and P_B, either by giving a loading on each factor equal to unity, or by setting the within-family environmental parameters $e_A = e_B = 1$, as we have done in the present applications.

Provided that measurement error effects occur at the level of the indicator variable and are uncorrelated across such variables, use of the multiple-indicator direction of causation model allows us to include error effects explicitly; it is no longer necessary to test the unidirectional-with-error and reciprocal causation-with-error models. At least three sources of variability will still be needed to test reciprocal-causation against general bivariate genetic models; but tests of unidirectional causal models will be possible even if only two sources of variability in traits A and B are present.

13.8 Concluding Remarks

Heath *et al.* (1992) review the power of the classical twin study for resolving direction of causation models and conclude that it is greatest when traits A and B have very dissimilar modes of inheritance, as in the extreme case illustrated in Figure 13.2. In practice, this implies that methods for resolving causal hypotheses are likely to be most useful for such examples as investigating relationships between (i) measures of perceived early environment (Parker, 1990; Neale *et al.*, 1992), (ii) measures of attitudes (Eaves *et al.*, 1989; Truett *et al.*, 1991), or (iii) habits (e.g., alcohol use: Heath *et al.*, 1991a,b), which exhibit possible effects of shared family environment, and inherited personality or temperamental traits (Eaves *et al.*, 1989; Eaves *et al.*, 1992) for which family resemblance appears to be largely determined by additive and non-additive genetic factors. Although most attention has been given to the application of these methods using data on twin pairs, in practice they are likely to be more powerful using adoption data. It is our hope that their application will lead to increasing precision of the causal hypotheses which behavioral geneticists and genetic epidemiologists are able to test.

Chapter 14

Repeated Measures

14.1 Introduction

This chapter deals with the genetic analysis of repeated measures. Examples of data that are collected in repeated measures designs include: dietary intake measured over several days or weeks; blood pressure taken under different conditions of rest and stress; psychophysiological data such as EEG that may be sampled with frequencies of 100 Hz or more (i.e., 100 times per second); performance measured during learning experiments; IQ measures taken at several different ages; or behavioral indices of development collected over several years of childhood. Two fundamental questions are important for analysis of these data:

1. Are there changes in the magnitude of the genetic and environmental effects over time? For example, are there changes in heritability?

2. Do the same genetic and environmental influences operate throughout time? For example, are the genes that influence behavior early in life different from the genes that influence the same trait later in life?

If there are no cohort effects, the first question can be addressed in a cross-sectional study that measures subjects of different ages, but the second question can only be answered in a longitudinal setting. Data collected in this way are essentially multivariate, if we consider the 'multi' to refer to the multiple occasions of measurement. However, the direct application of the multivariate methods described in Chapters 12 and 13 would not take full advantage of our *a priori* knowledge of the data structure. By definition, causation is unidirectional through time; earlier causes can have only later effects. This constraint gives added power to the study of genetic and environmental variability — we may assess whether "new" genes or new environmental factors start to operate at specific points in time. Given sufficient occasions of measurement, we may be able to discriminate between: (i)

Table 14.1: Within-person correlations for weight measured at six-month intervals on 66 females (Fischbein, 1977).

	Weight 1	Weight 2	Weight 3	Weight 4	Weight 5	Weight 6
Weight 1	1.000					
Weight 2	0.985	1.000				
Weight 3	0.968	0.981	1.000			
Weight 4	0.957	0.970	0.985	1.000		
Weight 5	0.932	0.940	0.964	0.975	1.000	
Weight 6	0.890	0.897	0.927	0.949	0.973	1.000

completely transient factors including, but not restricted to, measurement error; (ii) the long-term consequences of experience at one point in time; and (iii) the continuous presence and influence of a causal factor.

We shall start our treatment of longitudinal genetic analysis with a simplex model for phenotypic correlations. Phenotypic simplex models are relatively easy to implement in LISREL and elucidate some important features of longitudinal measurements. Given this basic understanding of the potential of time series data, the reader should have no difficulty understanding the extension to genetically informative data.

14.2   Phenotypic Simplex Model

Data that are measured repeatedly in time on the same subjects are often characterized by a specific correlation structure among the measures at the different time points. More specifically, it can be seen quite often that correlations are highest among adjoining occasions and that they fall away systematically as the distance between time points increases. Such a pattern is called a *simplex structure* after Guttman (1954; see also Wohlwill, 1973). The simplex structure of repeated observations is illustrated in Table 14.2 with correlations for repeated assessments of weight (in kilograms) in 66 females from a sample of opposite sex DZ twins in a longitudinal study by Fischbein (1977). In this example, the data were taken at 6 month intervals starting when subjects were on average 11.5 years of age. Although all correlations are high, it is clear that they decrease systematically as the time between measurements increases (i.e., as one moves further down the columns away from the principal diagonal). This correlation pattern can be explained well by a simplex model, such as that illustrated graphically in the path diagram in Figure 14.1 (see also Jöreskog, 1970). In this figure, following the general LISREL model, the observed measurements (i.e., weight) are shown as y variables which serve as indicators of the latent η variables, weighted by the factor loadings λ_i. Measurement errors are shown as ϵ variables, and factor residuals as ζ's. The

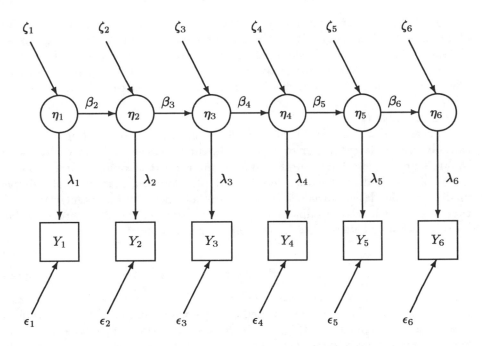

Figure 14.1: Simplex model for a phenotypic time series.

regression coefficients of η_i on η_{i-1}, the β weights, are solely responsible for the covariation of measurements over time.

We will first illustrate the use of the simplex model in LISREL for a phenotypic analysis with the weight data in Table 14.2.

14.2.1 Formulation of the Phenotypic Simplex Model in LIS-REL

As described in Chapter 6, the general LISREL model consists of two parts: the measurement model and the structural equation model. The measurement model describes how latent variables are related to observed variables and can be thought of as a confirmatory factor analysis model. For an observed variable y with latent variable η and measurement error ϵ, we can write the measurement model at time each point as follows:

$$y = \lambda\eta + \epsilon \tag{14.1}$$

$$\text{var}(y) = \lambda^2\text{var}(\eta) + \text{var}(\epsilon) \tag{14.2}$$

To define the units of measurement in the latent η variables, the factor loadings (λ_i) can be fixed at unity so that the measurement scale of the latent variables is the same as in the observed variables. This implies that the variance of the latent factors is to be estimated. Alternatively, the latent factors can be standardized to have unit variance and the factor loadings can be estimated. As we have noted elsewhere, it is not possible to estimate both the variance of and the regression on a latent variable (see Chapter 13).

The second part of the LISREL model is the structural equation model that causally relates latent variables to other latent variables. We have already encountered examples of structural models in the context of sibling interactions and direction of causation (see Chapters 10 and 13). Another example is the simplex model, in which latent variables at time i are influenced by the latent variables at time $i - 1$. Such relationships amongst latent variables are often termed *autoregressive* and may be described by the following equation:

$$\eta_i = \beta_i\eta_{i-1} + \zeta_i \tag{14.3}$$

$$\text{var}(\eta_i) = \beta_i^2\text{var}(\eta_{i-1}) + \text{var}(\zeta_i) \tag{14.4}$$

where η_i is the latent variable at time i ($i > 0$), β_i is the regression of the latent factor on the previous latent factor, and ζ represents a random input term (innovation) that is uncorrelated with η_{i-1}. There is an important conceptual distinction between innovations of latent factors and measurement errorsof observed variables. The innovations are that part of the latent factor at time i that is not caused by the latent factor at time $i - 1$, but are part of every subsequent time point $i + 1$. On the other hand, the ϵ terms are random errors of measurement that do not influence subsequent observed variables.

The parameters of this model are:

1. λ_i: the factor loadings of the observed on the latent factors;

2. $\psi_0 = \text{var}(\eta_0)$: the variance of the latent factor at time $t = 0$;

3. $\psi_i = \text{var}(\eta_i)$: the variances of the innovations at times $t > 0$;

4. β_i: the regression of the latent factor at time i on time $i - 1$;

5. θ_i: the variances of the measurement errors.

The weight data that were introduced above can be analyzed according to a simplex model using the following two LISREL scripts [the covariance matrix for these data (FISCHBEIN.COV) is given in Appendix J.1] In both scripts for the phenotypic simplex we specify only NY and NE which automatically selects submodel 3B in the LISREL program (see Jöreskog & Sörbom, 1989, p. 11).

LISREL Script 1 for Phenotypic Simplex Model

Our first script looks like this:

```
Phenotypic Simplex: PSI is free diagonal matrix and LAMBDA is fixed
DA NI=6 NO=66 MA=CM
CM FI=FISCHBEIN.COV
MO NY=6 NE=6 LY=DI,FI BE=FU,FI PS=DI,FR TE=DI,FR
ST 9 PS 1 PS 2 PS 3 PS 4 PS 5 PS 6
ST 1 LY 1 LY 2 LY 3 LY 4 LY 5 LY 6
FR BE 2 1 BE 3 2 BE 4 3 BE 5 4 BE 6 5
EQ TE 1 TE 2 TE 3 TE 4 TE 5 TE 6
OU SE SS NS AD=OFF IT=200
```

In this script the factor loadings in Λ_y are fixed at 1 so that the latent variables have the same measurement scale as the observed data (kilograms in this case). At each time point we estimate the variances of the innovations on the diagonal of the Ψ matrix. Of course, at the first measurement occasion the first latent factor cannot be explained by factors associated with an earlier point in time and, therefore, this first factor is itself regarded as an innovation (i.e., $\eta_1 = \zeta_1$). In **B** we estimate the autoregression coefficients that tell us how much of the variance in the latent factors at each occasion is accounted for by the previous factor. Parameters on the diagonal of the Θ_ϵ matrix estimate the residual, non-transmissible, variances that include measurement error. To identify the error variances at the first and the last measurement occasions additional constraints are needed, because error variances at these occasions cannot be distinguished from innovation variance. In the examples below we have constrained all error variances to be equal.

LISREL Script 2 for Phenotypic Simplex Model

In this second script the innovations are standardized to have unit variance and at each time point the factor loadings are estimated in the Λ_y matrix.

```
Phenotypic Simplex: LAMBDA is a free matrix and PSI is fixed
DA NI=6 NO=66 MA=CM
CM FI=FISCHBEIN.COV
MO NY=6 NE=6 LY=DI,FR BE=FU,FI PS=DI,FI TE=DI,FR
ST 1 PS 1 PS 2 PS 3 PS 4 PS 5 PS 6
ST 3 LY 1 LY 2 LY 3 LY 4 LY 5 LY 6
FR BE 2 1 BE 3 2 BE 4 3 BE 5 4 BE 6 5
EQ TE 1 TE 2 TE 3 TE 4 TE 5 TE 6
OU NS SE SS AD=OFF IT=200
```

The first latent factor in this specification may be thought of as an innovation because it cannot be explained by factors associated with an earlier point in time.

Again we use the **B** matrix to specify the occasion to occasion transmission but here the transmission is of the standardized η variables.

In the edited LISREL output for the first setup it can be seen that the β's are relatively high and the variances of the innovations small. Variances associated with measurement error also are small and — as judged against their standard errors — not significant.

LISREL Output from Script 1

```
-------------------------------------------------------------------------------
LAMBDA Y
          ETA 1       ETA 2       ETA 3       ETA 4       ETA 5       ETA 6
        --------    --------    --------    --------    --------    --------
          1.000       1.000       1.000       1.000       1.000       1.000

  BETA
        --------    --------    --------    --------    --------    --------
Est.      .000       1.049       1.029       1.056        .969        .942
SE        .000        .023        .025        .023        .027        .028

  PSI
        --------    --------    --------    --------    --------    --------
Est.   51.336       1.499       2.072       1.856       3.272       3.272
SE      9.030        .435        .491        .476        .674        .678

  THETA EPS
          VAR 1       VAR 2       VAR 3       VAR 4       VAR 5       VAR 6
        --------    --------    --------    --------    --------    --------
Est.      .134        .134        .134        .134        .134        .134
SE        .154        .154        .154        .154        .154        .154

        CHI-SQUARE WITH    9 DEGREES OF FREEDOM =       13.02 (P = .162)
```

From the output the total variances at each measurement occasion can be obtained according to equations 14.2 and 14.4:

Time	$\text{var}(\eta_t)$		$\text{var}(\epsilon_t)$	total variance
$t = 1$		51.336	0.134	51.470
$t = 2$	$1.049^2 \times 51.336 + 1.499 =$	57.968	0.134	58.102
$t = 3$	$1.029^2 \times 57.968 + 2.072 =$	63.402	0.134	63.536
$t = 4$	$1.056^2 \times 63.402 + 1.856 =$	72.549	0.134	72.683
$t = 5$	$0.969^2 \times 72.549 + 3.272 =$	71.322	0.134	71.456
$t = 6$	$0.942^2 \times 71.322 + 3.272 =$	66.534	0.134	66.668

At the second time point the total variance of the latent factor is 57.968. This is (within rounding error) equal to the second diagonal element of the covariance matrix of η that is given in the LISREL output. Only a small proportion of this variance is due to innovation: $1.499/57.968 = 0.026$, the vast majority comes from amplification of existing variance at the first time point. At $t = 6$ we see that the variance of the latent factor is decreasing and that the contribution of new influences becomes somewhat larger.

LISREL Output from Script 2

```
---------------------------------------------------------------------

LAMBDA Y
         ETA 1      ETA 2      ETA 3      ETA 4      ETA 5      ETA 6

       --------   --------   --------   --------   --------   --------
Est.   7.165      1.224      1.440      1.362      1.809      1.809
SE      .630       .178       .170       .175       .186       .187


BETA

       --------   --------   --------   --------   --------   --------
Est.    .000      6.140       .875      1.116       .730       .942
SE      .000      1.056       .131       .160       .106       .129


PSI

       --------   --------   --------   --------   --------   --------
       1.000      1.000      1.000      1.000      1.000      1.000


THETA EPS
         VAR 1      VAR 2      VAR 3      VAR 4      VAR 5      VAR 6

       --------   --------   --------   --------   --------   --------
Est.    .134       .134       .134       .134       .134       .134
SE      .154       .154       .154       .154       .154       .154


       CHI-SQUARE WITH   9 DEGREES OF FREEDOM =      13.02 (P = .162)
```

The output for the second LISREL setup gives the estimates of the factor loadings of the observed variables on latent variables in LAMBDA Y. As may be seen, these loadings correspond to the square roots of the variances that were estimated in PSI (first setup). The estimates in BETA, however are quite different. In this case they can be conceived of as "scaled" regression coefficients and their absolute values have to be interpreted with care. As the χ^2 and degrees of freedom for both LISREL specifications are the same, it is clear that these differences in parameter estimates do not affect the goodness-of-fit of the model. As is easily verified (by specifying SS on the OUtput statement) the standardized solutions for both LISREL setups are identical. The standardized solution also gives the correlation matrix among latent factors:

```
CORRELATION MATRIX OF ETA
         ETA 1    ETA 2    ETA 3    ETA 4    ETA 5    ETA 6

         --------  -------  -------  -------  -------  --------
ETA 1    1.000
ETA 2     .987    1.000
ETA 3     .971     .984    1.000
ETA 4     .958     .971     .987    1.000
ETA 5     .936     .948     .964     .977    1.000
ETA 6     .913     .925     .940     .953     .975    1.000
```

The correlations on the first subdiagonal are the standardized β's. This correlation matrix of the latent factors clearly reflects the simplex structure we observe in the data.

14.3   Genetic Simplex Model

In a behavior genetics context we usually want to analyze more than one latent construct, for example, genetic and environmental components of variance. To estimate such effects we can divide each of the η factors into a genetic and a non-genetic part. In the context of simplex models we want to fit a genetic and an environmental time series[1], and we can specify both of these time series using the η variables in LISREL.

14.3.1   LISREL Formulation of the Genetic Simplex Model

Letting A_i and E_i represent the additive genetic and within-family environmental factors at each occasion (the η variables), the measurement model at each occasion becomes:

$$y = \lambda_{ai} A_i + \lambda_{ei} E_i + \epsilon_i.$$

And for the structural part of the model we can write:

$$A_i = \beta_{ai} A_{i-1} + \zeta_{ai} \tag{14.5}$$

$$E_i = \beta_{ei} E_{i-1} + \zeta_{ei} \tag{14.6}$$

---

[1] Here we fit the simplex only to additive genetic and *within-family* environmental effects. See Section 14.5 for a discussion of extended simplex formulations involving other variance components.

For $t = 3$ the covariance matrix of these latent processes then equals:

$$
\begin{pmatrix}
\text{var}(A_1) + \text{var}(E_1) & & \\
\beta_{a2}\text{var}(A_1) + \beta_{e2}\text{var}(E_1) & \text{var}(A_2) + \text{var}(E_2) & \\
\beta_{a2}\beta_{a3}\text{var}(A_1) + & \beta_{a3}\text{var}(A_2) + \beta_{e3}\text{var}(E_2) & \text{var}(A_3) + \text{var}(E_3) \\
\beta_{e2}\beta_{e3}\text{var}(E_1) & &
\end{pmatrix}
$$

where

$$
\begin{aligned}
\text{var}(A_i) &= \beta_{ai}^2\,\text{var}(A_{i-1}) + \text{var}(\zeta_{ai}) \\
\text{var}(E_i) &= \beta_{ei}^2\,\text{var}(E_{i-1}) + \text{var}(\zeta_{ei}) .
\end{aligned}
$$

This genetic simplex model is shown diagrammatically in Figure 14.2 for the more complete case of 6 variables, as in the Fischbein weight data.

When covariance matrices of Twin 1 and Twin 2 are used as input we cannot estimate the variances of the genetic and environmental innovations in $\boldsymbol{\Psi}$, because $\boldsymbol{\Psi}$ has to be used to specify the correlations between latent genetic and environmental factors for Twin 1 and Twin 2. More specifically, it is not possible in LISREL 7 to specify the 0.5 correlation between the genotypes of DZ twins if the diagonal of $\boldsymbol{\Psi}$ contains the variances of ζ instead of 1's. Thus, the scale of measurement of the latent factors has to be defined by standardizing their innovations at unit variance (similar to our second formulation of the phenotypic simplex model). The free parameters of this model are:

1. λ_{ai} and λ_{ei}: the factor loadings of the observations on the genetic and environmental factors;

2. β_{ai} and β_{ei}: the regression of the latent factors at $t = i$ on $t = i - 1$;

3. Θ_i, the variances of the measurement errors[2].

14.3.2 Application to Longitudinal Data on Weight

From the same study by Fischbein (1977) we have weight data for 32 MZ and 51 DZ female twin pairs. Appendix J.2 gives the LISREL setup for the genetic analysis of these data. The MOdel statement for the first group (DZ twins) of this script appears as:

```
MO NY=12 NE=24 PS=FI LY=FU,FI TE=ZE BE=FU,FI
```

---

[2] Although we only estimate environmental residuals in this example, it is possible to estimate both genetic and environmental residuals. Figure 14.2 is drawn for the more complete model.

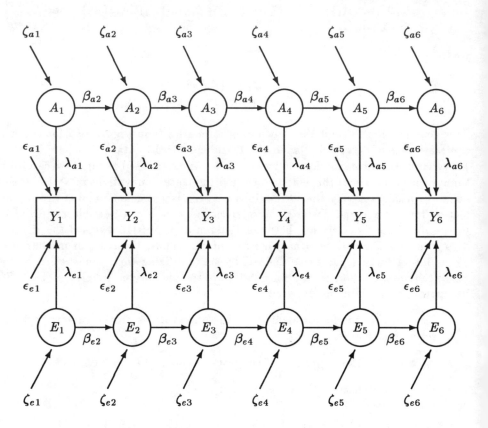

Figure 14.2: Simplex model of genetic and within-family environmental time series. Latent variables A_i and E_i ($i = 1, ..., 6$) correspond to η variables in LISREL. The figure is drawn for one twin.

This line shows that we are specifying all 12 weight measurements (6 measurements each from Twin 1 and Twin 2) as y variables (NY=12) and that we model 24 η variables (NE=24). The η vector comprises additive genetic and non-shared environmental factors for each twin at each occasion of measurement: $(A_1T_1, ..., A_6T_1, A_1T_2, ..., A_6T_2, E_1T_1, ..., E_6T_1, E_1T_2, ..., E_6T_2)$. The Ψ matrix is set as a symmetric correlation matrix with no free elements (PS=FI). Subsequently, we fix all of the diagonal elements of this matrix at 1.0, and some of the off-diagonal elements at 0.5 for the genetic resemblance between DZ twins. Specifically, we fix at 0.5: $\psi_{7,1}$ $(r_{A1T1,A1T2})$, $\psi_{8,2}$ $(r_{A2T1,A2T2})$, $\psi_{9,3}$ $(r_{A3T1,A3T2})$, $\psi_{10,4}$ $(r_{A4T1,A4T2})$, $\psi_{11,5}$ $(r_{A5T1,A5T2})$, and $\psi_{12,6}$ $(r_{A6T1,A6T2})$. The Λ_y matrix is set as FUll and FIxed on the MOdel statement; subsequently we free elements of this matrix corresponding to the factor loadings of each of the weight measurements on the respective genetic and environmental factors. For example, the first weight measurement of Twin 1, y_1, loads on η_1 (A_1T_1) and η_{13} (E_1T_1) by writing FR LY 1,1 LY 1,13. These loadings are equated for Twin 1 and Twin 2 (y_7, η_7, η_{19}):

```
EQ LY 1,1 LY 7,7
EQ LY 1,13 LY 7,19
```

Similar procedures are carried out for the other measurement occasions. Note that we do not specify any measurement errors on the MOdel statement (TE=ZE), since these were found to be non-significant in the previous analysis. Finally, the **B** matrix containing the genetic and environmental regression coefficients is set at full and fixed for this example. Later in the script we free the subdiagonal elements of this matrix that correspond to the regression of each A_i on A_{i-1} and E_i on E_{i-1}, and equate these regression coefficients across twins.

The model specification for the second (MZ) group is identical to that described for the first group, except the off-diagonal elements of Ψ that were fixed at 0.5 for DZ twins are now set to 1.0 for the MZ pairs. The MZ and DZ covariance matrices for weight in Twin 1 and weight in Twin 2 at six occasions each (i.e., 12 × 12 input matrices) are given in Appendix J.3. Note that this model has 22 free parameters $(6\lambda_a + 6\lambda_e + 5\beta_a + 5\beta_e)$ and, thus, $2[12(12+1)]/2 - 22 = 156 - 22 = 134$ degrees of freedom.

Results

Parameter estimates from this model are shown in Table 14.2; Appendix J.4 gives the edited LISREL output. With the parameter estimates from the output we can calculate the genetic and environmental variances at each time point and then compute the heritabilities.

The total genetic variance at time point i, $i > 0$, is computed as:

$$\text{var}(A_i) = \lambda_{ai}^2 \left(\beta_{ai}^2 \text{var}(A_{i-1}) + \text{var}(\zeta_i)\right)$$

This reduces to

$$\text{var}(A_i) = \lambda_{ai}^2 \left(\beta_{ai}^2 \text{var}(A_{i-1}) + 1\right)$$

Table 14.2: Parameter estimates from genetic simplex model applied to Fischbein's (1977) weight measures.

Time	Genetic Parameters λ_{at}	β_{at}	ψ^*_{at}	Environmental Parameters λ_{et}	β_{et}	ψ^*_{et}
$t = 1$	4.79	–	1.0	1.82	–	1.0
$t = 2$	1.12	4.50	1.0	0.56	2.96	1.0
$t = 3$	1.50	0.78	1.0	0.98	0.61	1.0
$t = 4$	1.23	1.24	1.0	0.96	0.87	1.0
$t = 5$	1.39	0.92	1.0	0.82	0.99	1.0
$t = 6$	1.39	0.97	1.0	0.99	0.82	1.0

*Parameters fixed for all occasions.

since the variance of the innovations is standardized at 1. The term in brackets $(\beta^2_{ai}\text{var}(A_{i-1}) + 1)$ represents the variance of the latent genetic factor at time i; to obtain the total genetic variance this term is multiplied by the genetic factor loading at $t = i$. The environmental variances are computed in the same way. To obtain the genetic and environmental variances at the first time point, we simply square the factor loadings because the variance of the first latent genetic and environmental factors is fixed at 1. The genetic, environmental, and total (phenotypic) variances estimated from this model are shown in Table 14.3.

As in the phenotypic analysis, we see that there is an increase in total variance over time (26.25 to 41.92), and here we see that this is caused by an increase in the genetic part of the variance, whereas the environmental variances do not change very much. We can now address the questions that were raised in the introduction to this chapter, i.e., are there changes in heritabilities over time?, and do the same genetic and environmental influences operate throughout time? For the first question we can calculate the heritabilities by dividing the genetic variance at each time point by the total variance, which yields the heritability estimates 0.89, 0.89, 0.87, 0.89, 0.91 and 0.89. Clearly there is little change in the magnitude of genetic influence on weight over time. For the second question, we can partition the heritable variation at each time into (i) genetic influences novel to the occasion, and (ii) genetic effects persisting from the previous occasion. That is, a portion of each heritability is due to new genetic influences impacting weight assessments at each point in time, and a portion is due to the genetic effects which were already operating at the previous measurement point. The former can be calculated from the parameter estimates as $\lambda^2_{ai}\psi_{ai}/\text{var}(\text{total}) = \lambda^2_{ai}/\text{var}(\text{total})$, since all ψ_{ai} are fixed at 1.0, and the latter as $\lambda^2_{ai}\beta^2_{ai}\text{var}(A_{i-1})/\text{var}(\text{total})$. For example, on the second occasion $1.25/29.61 = 4\%$ of the total variance consists of new genetic variance and $1.25 \times 20.25/29.61 = 85\%$ of the total variance consists of

Table 14.3: Genetic, environmental, and total phenotypic variances estimated from the genetic simplex model applied to Fishbein's (1977) data on weight

	Variance		
Time	Genetic	Environmental	Total
$t = 1$	$4.79^2 \times (1) = 22.94$	$1.82^2 \times (1) = 3.31$	26.25
$t = 2$	$1.12^2 \times \left(4.50^2 \times 1 + 1\right)$	$0.56^2 \times \left(2.96^2 \times 1 + 1\right)$	
	$= 1.12^2 \times (21.25) = 26.56$	$= 0.56^2 \times (9.76) = 3.05$	29.61
$t = 3$	$1.50^2 \times \left(0.78^2 \times 21.25 + 1\right)$	$0.98^2 \times \left(0.61^2 \times 9.76 + 1\right)$	
	$= 1.50^2 \times (13.75) = 30.93$	$= 0.98^2 \times (4.61) = 4.41$	34.34
$t = 4$	$1.23^2 \times \left(1.24^2 \times 13.75 + 1\right)$	$0.96^2 \times \left(0.87^2 \times 4.61 + 1\right)$	
	$= 1.23^2 \times (22.03) = 33.32$	$= 0.96^2 \times (4.45) = 4.10$	37.42
$t = 5$	$1.39^2 \times \left(0.92^2 \times 22.03 + 1\right)$	$0.82^2 \times \left(0.99^2 \times 4.45 + 1\right)$	
	$= 1.39^2 \times (19.50) = 37.66$	$= 0.82^2 \times (5.36) = 3.59$	41.25
$t = 6$	$1.39^2 \times \left(0.97^2 \times 19.50 + 1\right)$	$0.99^2 \times \left(0.82^2 \times 5.36 + 1\right)$	
	$= 1.39^2 \times (19.33) = 37.33$	$= 0.99^2 \times (4.59) = 4.59$	41.92

amplification of existing variance at the first time point. At the other time points also ($i = 3 \ldots 6$), only a small part of the total variance is due to genetic innovation terms (6%, 4%, 4%, and 4%). Thus, we see that the genetic effects do not change dramatically during this period of development; i.e., the same genetic influences are operating over time.

As in the phenotypic example, we can get the correlations among the latent factors by including the SS statement on the OUtput statement in LISREL. In this case, the latent variables are genetic and non-shared environmental factors; thus, the standardized solution gives the genetic and environmental correlations for the weight data. We present these correlations in Table 14.3.2. It may be seen that both of these matrices conform to a simplex structure and from these matrices it also is clear that both genetic and environmental stabilities are high. Evidence for genetic simplex patterns in morphological traits also has been found in studies of animal development (Arnold, 1990).

14.3.3 Application of Common Factor Model to Longitudinal Twin Data

Since the above analyses indicate that the genetic and environmental correlations are high, we may ask if a factor model also would give a good fit to the data [see, e.g., Boomsma and Molenaar (1987), Cardon and Fulker (1991) and Cardon et al., (1992) for empirical assessments of this question]. To address this question we fit a model that includes a common genetic and a common within-family environmental

Table 14.4: Estimated correlations among latent genetic and environmental factors in a genetic simplex model fitted to weight data.

| | Correlation matrix of genetic factors | | | | | |
	A_1T_1	A_2T_1	A_3T_1	A_4T_1	A_5T_1	A_6T_1
A1T1	1.000					
A2T1	.976	1.000				
A3T1	.941	.964	1.000			
A4T1	.919	.942	.977	1.000		
A5T1	.896	.917	.952	.974	1.000	
A6T1	.872	.893	.927	.949	.974	1.000

| | Correlation matrix of environmental factors | | | | | |
	E_1T_1	E_2T_1	E_3T_1	E_4T_1	E_5T_1	E_6T_1
E1T1	1.000					
E2T1	.947	1.000				
E3T1	.837	.884	1.000			
E4T1	.738	.779	.881	1.000		
E5T1	.665	.702	.794	.902	1.000	
E6T1	.589	.622	.704	.799	.886	1.000

factor and measurement-specific environmental factors to the weight covariances (genetic specific factors were either not identified or not different from zero). The LISREL specification for this model is described in detail in Section 12.3.3 of Chapter 12 and an example script is given in Appendix E.2 for the case of 4 measures. The extension to 6 variables in the present case is fairly trivial and is left to the reader. Appendix J.5 gives the output from the genetic common factor model. Although the factor model represents a more parsimonious account of the data (18 vs. 22 free parameters), the goodness-of-fit chi-squared for this model is much higher than for the one obtained from the simplex model (common factor $\chi^2_{138} = 359.11$, $p = .000$ vs. simplex $\chi^2_{134} = 161.00$, $p = .056$). Thus, the simplex model appears to provide a better explanation of the weight observations.

14.4 Problems with Repeated Measures Data

Analysis of repeatedly measured variables may create some specific numeric problems. Covariance matrices associated with highly intercorrelated repeated measures can become nearly singular. As a consequence, the chi-squared goodness-of-fit statistic may be positively biased (in contrast to parameter estimates, which are generally unbiased). Secondly, even if there are no singularity problems, the large number of variables in a covariance analysis of repeated measures may lead to indeterminacies during computation. This situation resembles the occurrence of collinearity in regression analysis, which usually can be counteracted by the invocation of ridge regression. A similar approach can be used in LISREL by

1. the addition of a small positive constant to the diagonal of the observed covariance matrix, and

2. correcting the model for this perturbation by fixing the diagonal of Θ_ϵ at the same positive constant (see Boomsma *et al.*, 1989a,b)

14.5 Discussion

The genetic analysis of development and age-related changes in human behavior involves more issues, such as modeling age of onset for example, than the questions that have been addressed here. An overview of some of these other issues is given by Eaves *et al.*, (1990a). The genetic analysis of repeated measures as outlined in this chapter is a very flexible approach to the analysis of change and continuity . The simplex model allows for both differential heritabilities and environmental variances at different time points, as well as different genetic and environmental correlations between time points. This model can be extended in several ways. An additional latent simplex structure may be specified to test the influence of common-environmental components (see, e.g., Eaves *et al.*, 1986; Hewitt *et al.*, 1988; Phillips and Fulker, 1989; Cardon *et al.*, 1992) The model also can be used for the analysis of multivariate time series. In this case, each single time series may conform to a simplex structure, while the relationship between different types of variables can be analyzed with a confirmatory factor analysis model (see e.g., Cardon, 1992). The simplex model used here in the analysis of the weight data specifies a so called *first-order autoregressive model*, where a measure is influenced only by the previous one. It is also possible to specify higher-order autoregressive models, where variables at $t = i$ are influenced for example by variables at time $i - 1$ as well as at time $i - 2$. All of these analyses can be carried out with LISREL.

Chapter 15

Longitudinal Mean Trends

15.1 Introduction

Our next task is to take the genetic simplex model as described in Chapter 14 and see whether the predicted change in variance over time is mirrored by a similar change in means. Although we said in the first chapter that inferences about means are not the primary focus of the study of individual differences, the longitudinal study is one in which changes in mean over time or *growth*, is of itself of considerable interest. This Chapter is not the first time that we have modeled information on means as well as covariances; in Chapter 8 we tested for the effects of sampling bias with the pairs concordant and discordant for study participation. Thus while at first glance the algebra and model formulation may seem a little intimidating, it covers what should by now be relatively familiar material.

15.2 Genetic Analysis of Longitudinal Trends in Mean

In the foregoing chapter it was shown how a behavior genetic analysis of longitudinal variances and covariances can be carried out. A univariate phenotypic variable P measured at consecutive occasions $t = 1, 2, ..., T$, was decomposed into genetic and environmental time-dependent components:

$$P(t) = A(t) + E(t)$$

where $A(t)$ and $E(t)$ denote latent additive genetic and within-family environmental time series, respectively, which are described by simplex models. Of course such elementary models can be generalized in several ways, to multivariate phenotypic covariances, for example, but for the moment we will turn to extensions of the simplex model involving *means* (Dolan *et al.*, 1991; Fischbein *et al.*, 1990).

305

Suppose that a genetic analysis of longitudinal covariances has yielded a sat-
isfactorily fitting model. For instance, assume that the elementary model $P(t) = A(t) + E(t)$ has been selected. In fact, this model (like all those considered in this
book so far) pertains to individual phenotypic differences or *deviations* (at each
occasion t); hence its complete specification should read:

$$P(t) - \mathcal{E}[P(t)] = A(t) + E(t), \quad t = 1, 2, \ldots, T, \tag{15.1}$$

where $\mathcal{E}[P(t)]$ denotes the expected value (average or mean) of $P(t)$. That is, the
genetic model pertains to centered phenotypic scores obtained by subtracting (an
efficient estimate of) the longitudinal mean trend from the observations[1]. This
implies that $\mathcal{E}[A(t)] = 0$ and $\mathcal{E}[E(t)] = 0$. Given the satisfactory fit of this model,
however, we would now like to consider the question of whether the same model
also applies to the original, uncentered, phenotypic scores. In other words, we wish
to test the hypothesis that the genetic model explaining longitudinal phenotypic
variation and covariation can also account for the time-dependent *mean* phenotypic variation making up the longitudinal mean trend. This chapter describes the
LISREL implementation of a model in which variances and means are proportional.

Developmental psychologists in particular have long been interested in the genetic and environmental processes underlying observed human growth curves. Yet,
any analysis along these lines is attended by special difficulties because phenotypic
mean trends obtained in a genetically heterogeneous population do not in themselves enable the identification of these underlying processes (Mather and Jinks,
1977). Hence, we shall consider a more indirect approach in which the genetic
model for longitudinal covariation serves as an anchor. To do so, we shall impose
sufficient additional constraints in order to arrive at an identifiable genetic model
of longitudinal means. The need for additional constraints is easily appreciated
when we attempt to extend model 15.1 to accommodate both longitudinal means
and covariances:

$$P(t) - \mathcal{E}[P(t)] = \{A(t) - \mathcal{E}[A(t)]\} + \{E(t) - \mathcal{E}[E(t)]\}, \tag{15.2}$$
$$\mathcal{E}[P(t)] = \mu + \mathcal{E}[A(t)] + \mathcal{E}[E(t)] \tag{15.3}$$

where either $\mathcal{E}[A(t)]$ or $\mathcal{E}[E(t)]$ or both may be non-zero. Notice that the longitudinal mean, $\mathcal{E}[P(t)]$, $t = 1, 2, \ldots, T$, is made up of T data points and thus involves
a total of T parameters. Likewise, $\mathcal{E}[A(t)]$, $t = 1, 2, \ldots, T$, involves a total of T
parameters, as does the $\mathcal{E}[E(t)]$. Hence, model 15.3 is severely over-parameterized:
$2T + 1$ parameters are used to model only T statistics.

15.2.1   Assumptions of the Model

In this chapter we shall develop one particular constrained means model. This
model is based on the assumptions that:

---

[1] The use of deviation phenotypes has been discussed in Chapters 8 and 10.

1. the same genetic and environmental processes underlying the longitudinal covariance structure of phenotypic individual differences also account for the time-dependent variation of the longitudinal mean,

2. the means and variances of these underlying processes are linearly related.

Assumption 1 is standard when we wish to relate mean and covariance structures, and assumption 2 describes the form of this relationship, which is specific to the current treatment and could be replaced by alternatives. In fact, assumption 2 gives rise to a considerable reduction of the number of parameters in the means model. For instance, it will be shown that T, the original number of parameters, of $\mathcal{E}[A(t)]$ now is reduced to one, which is the constant of proportionality in the assumed linear relationship between $\mathcal{E}[A(t)]$ and the genetic variances (the same remark applies to $\mathcal{E}[E(t)]$). Using the principles of the simplex model described in the preceding chapter, we will now fill in the details of the complete model 15.3 based on these assumptions:

$$A(t) - \mathcal{E}[A(t)] = \beta_{at}\left\{G(t-1) - \mathcal{E}[G(t-1)]\right\} + \left\{\zeta_{at} - \mathcal{E}[\zeta_{at}]\right\} \quad (15.4)$$

$$E(t) - \mathcal{E}[E(t)] = \beta_{et}\left\{E(t-1) - \mathcal{E}[E(t-1)]\right\} + \left\{\zeta_{et} - \mathcal{E}[\zeta_{et}]\right\} \quad (15.5)$$

$$\mathcal{E}[A(t)] = \beta_{at}\mathcal{E}[G(t-1)] + \mathcal{E}[\zeta_{at}] \quad (15.6)$$

$$\mathcal{E}[\zeta_{at}] = \alpha_a\sqrt{\psi_{at}} \quad (15.7)$$

$$\mathcal{E}[E(t)] = \beta_{et}\mathcal{E}[E(t-1)] + \mathcal{E}[\zeta_{et}] \quad (15.8)$$

$$\mathcal{E}[\zeta_{et}] = \alpha_e\sqrt{\psi_{et}} \quad (15.9)$$

First, notice that 15.2, 15.4, and 15.5 together constitute the model for longitudinal variance and covariance described in Chapter 14. As either or both of the genetic and environmental series may now be non-zero, they have to be centered in 15.2 by subtracting $\mathcal{E}[A(t)]$ and $\mathcal{E}[E(t)]$, respectively. Second, 15.3, 15.6, and 15.8 together constitute the means model. Since it is assumed that the same genetic and environmental processes underlie both the longitudinal means and covariances (assumption 1), the β_{at} transmission-coefficients in 15.4 and 15.6 are identical, as are the β_{et}'s in 15.5 and 15.8. Third, according to assumption 2, the time-dependent means and variances of $A(t)$ are linearly related, just like the means and variances of $E(t)$. The variance of $A(t)$ is a function of β_{at} and ψ_{at}. Since the transmission coefficient β_{at} in 15.6 is the same as in 15.4, it follows that the assumed linear relationship can be expressed by taking $\mathcal{E}[\zeta_{at}] = \alpha_a\sqrt{\psi_{at}}$, where α_a is the coefficient of proportionality in the linear relationship.

In this model the β and ψ parameters are identified solely by the longitudinal phenotypic variances and covariances. This implies that only three new parameters are introduced in the means model: α_a, α_e, and μ. Hence, if the number of repeated measurements, T, is greater than three, the genetic means model given by 15.3, 15.6, and 15.8 is identified. We will now turn to an application of the full mean/covariance model 15.2 to the same longitudinal weight data analyzed in Chapter 14.

15.2.2   Building a LISREL Script for Longitudinal Means

For the sake of conciseness, the details of fitting the genetic simplex to the longitudinal covariances will not be repeated here. We take it for granted that the LISREL script and outcomes of this analysis are available (see Appendices J.2 – J.4), and proceed by modifying it.

The selected genetic model for the data is 15.1 above, involving a latent genetic and within-families environmental series. To start with, we repeat the fit of this particular model to the data with one minor modification of the script: the following statement is added to the OU line.

```
OU ... LY=LYBE BE=LYBE
```

In this way, the parameter estimates in LY (involving $\sqrt{\psi_{at}}$ and $\sqrt{\psi_{et}}, t = 1, 2, ..., 6$) and BE (involving β_{at} and $\beta_{et}, t = 1, 2, ...6$) are saved in file LYBE in order to serve as starting values for the fit of model 15.2 (see pp. 72-73 of the LISREL 7 manual). Unfortunately, adding the means structure to the LISREL script takes a bit more work!

It turns out that the LISREL script for the means model 15.3, 15.6, and 15.8 can be appended quite easily to the given LISREL setup for the covariance structure model for repeated measures (Appendix J.2). Based on Section 10.1 of the LISREL 7 manual we can see that the μ parameter in 15.3 can be estimated in TY (τ_y) (see Table 10.1 in the LISREL 7 manual), while the α_a and α_e parameters can be estimated in AL (α). Using basic matrix algebra it can be shown that this surprisingly straightforward LISREL implementation is indeed the correct setup for the genetic means submodel of 15.2. Accordingly, the following additions to and modifications of the LISREL script for genetic and environmental time series should be made.

After the covariance matrix is read in each group (i.e., after CM...) we add the MEans card and list the observed means for the group (the means of the weight measures are given below). For example, in the first group, we add:

```
ME
35.906   38.116   40.794   42.941   45.476   47.890
35.208   37.435   40.155   42.659   45.073   47.159
```

In the first group we also add to the model lines:

```
MO ... AL=FU,FI TY=FU,FI
```

And in the second group:

```
MO ... AL=IN TY=IN
```

We insert the following lines after the model line in the first group:

```
FR AL(1) AL(13)
FR TY(1)
EQ AL(1) AL(2) AL(3) AL(4) AL(5) AL(6)
EQ AL(1) AL(7) AL(8) AL(9) AL(10) AL(11) AL(12)
EQ AL(13) AL(14) AL(15) AL(16) AL(17) AL(18)
EQ AL(13) AL(19) AL(20) AL(21) AL(22) AL(23) AL(24)
EQ TY(1) TY(2) TY(3) TY(4) TY(5) TY(6)
EQ TY(1) TY(7) TY(8) TY(9) TY(10) TY(11) TY(12)
```

and replace all starting values by:

```
MA LY FI=LYBE
MA BE FI=LYBE
ST 1 AL(1) AL(7)
ST 30 TY(1)
```

The `MA LY FI=LYBE` and `MA BE FI=LYBE` lines read in the parameter estimates of LY and BE, obtained in Chapter 14 as starting values to LY and BE in the present fit of model 15.2. If the hypothesis expressed by this model is not rejected, in particular if the genetic model explaining the longitudinal phenotypic covariances also accounts for the longitudinal mean trend, then the parameter estimates in LY and BE should not differ (significantly) from those saved in file LYBE. Hence, LYBE should provide excellent starting values for LY and BE. The level parameter μ in 15.3 corresponds to TY(1). Note that TY(1) is invariant at all 6 occasions and for both twins. The coefficient of proportionality between the variance and mean trend of the genetic series, α_a, is expressed by AL(1), while the corresponding coefficient for the environmental series is expressed by AL(13). TY(1), AL(1), and AL(13) constitute the complete set of free parameters associated with the means submodel 15.2.

15.2.3   Application to data on weight

The main output obtained by fitting our model 15.2 is as follows. First, the $\chi^2 = 173.38$ for df= 155 has probability level $p = .149$, indicating an adequate fit. Second, the new parameter estimates in LY and BE are almost equal to those already obtained for the longitudinal covariances. This is also the case with the standard errors. Third, the (STANDARDIZED) FITTED RESIDUALS for the phenotypic covariances as well as the associated ROOT MEAN SQUARE RESIDUALS are also almost identical to the corresponding values in the analysis of model 15.1. Finally, submodel 15.2 yields the following parameter estimates:

LISREL element	Model parameter	Estimate	Standard error
TY(1)	μ	28.098	.898
AL(1)	α_a	1.576	.253
AL(13)	α_e	0.122	.571

The observed means for twin 1 and twin 2 in the MZ and DZ groups are:

			Occasion			
Group	$t = 1$	$t = 2$	$t = 3$	$t = 4$	$t = 5$	$t = 6$
MZ1	36.763	39.059	41.759	43.850	45.997	48.119
MZ2	36.153	38.522	41.209	43.694	46.200	48.247
DZ1	35.906	38.116	40.794	42.941	45.476	47.890
DZ2	35.208	37.435	40.155	42.659	45.073	47.159

and the fitted longitudinal trends are:

			Occasion			
Estimate	$t = 1$	$t = 2$	$t = 3$	$t = 4$	$t = 5$	$t = 6$
$\mathcal{E}[P(t)]$	35.857	38.102	40.841	43.140	45.588	47.748
$\mathcal{E}[A(t)]$	7.536	9.731	12.330	14.580	16.997	19.041
$\mathcal{E}[E(t)]$	0.223	0.273	0.413	0.462	0.493	0.609

It turns out that model 15.2 yields (i) an acceptable fit to the data as assessed by the χ^2 statistic; (ii) close similarity of the results for the covariance submodel defined by equations 15.2, 15.4, 15.5 to those obtained for model 15.1; and (iii) the small discrepancies between observed and fitted longitudinal trends. Regarding the parameters of the means model, it appears that TY(1)$= \mu$ and AL(1)$= \alpha_a$ and that

$$\mathcal{E}[P(t)] = \mu + \mathcal{E}[A(t)] . \tag{15.10}$$

That is, the within-family environmental process does not seem to contribute to the phenotypic time-dependent variation in mean weight. This is confirmed by fitting a reduced model 15.2* in which AL(13) (and those entries of AL which are constrained to be equal to AL(13)) are fixed at zero. The fitted χ^2 is now virtually unchanged: 173.38; $df = 156$; $p = .162$, and all parameter estimates and standard errors associated with the covariance model remain almost identical. The estimates associated with the reduced means model are:

LISREL element	Model parameter	Estimate	Standard error
TY(1)	μ	28.094	.923
AL(1)	α_a	1.622	.120

and the fitted longitudinal trends are:

			Occasion			
Estimate	$t = 1$	$t = 2$	$t = 3$	$t = 4$	$t = 5$	$t = 6$
$\mathcal{E}[P(t)]$	35.855	38.101	40.817	43.134	45.571	47.749
$\mathcal{E}[A(t)]$	7.761	10.007	12.723	15.040	17.477	19.655

15.3 Discussion

The fit of model 15.2 to the body weight data appears to be satisfactory. Hence, it can be concluded that the hypothesis expressed by this model is supported: both the longitudinal covariances and mean trend of body weight can be explained by the same genetic and within-family environmental time series. Moreover, the time-dependent variation of mean body weight with respect to the constant level μ appears to be completely due to genetic influences. Note that this constant level by itself is of an unknown constitution and may, apart from an arbitrary origin of measurement scale, include genetic and environmental contributions in an unspecified manner.

A qualification should be made regarding the conceptual interpretation of the findings; such interpretation is conditional upon whether the longitudinal covariances and means obey the same genetic model. That is, the results are conditional on assumption 2, which stipulates a linear relationship between the time-dependent means and variances of the latent genetic and environmental series, respectively. Of course, the satisfactory fit of model 15.2 may have some bearings on the *a posteriori* plausibility of this particular assumption. Still, any conclusion regarding the genetic and/or environmental causes underlying the phenotypic time-dependent variation of mean body weight depends on assumption 2. Moreover, other assumptions than proportionality between latent means and variances in the genetic simplex could be made. It would then become apparent, however, that such alternative models are not at all easy to implement using LISREL.

Chapter 16

Observer Ratings

Rather than measuring an individual's phenotype directly, we often have to rely on ratings of the individual made by an observer. An important example is the assessment of children via ratings from parents and teachers. In this chapter we consider in some detail the assessment of children by their parents. Since the ratings obtained in this case are a function of both parent and child, disentangling the child's phenotype from that of the rater becomes an important methodological problem. For the analysis of genetic and environmental contributions to children's behavior, solutions to this are available when multiple raters, e.g., two parents, rate multiple children, e.g., twins. This chapter describes and illustrates simple LISREL models for the analysis of parental ratings of children's behavior. We show how the assumption that mothers and fathers are rating the same behavior in children can be contrasted with the weaker alternative that parents are rating correlated behaviors. Given the stronger assumption, which appears adequate for ratings of some children's behavior problems, the contribution of rater bias and unreliability may be separated from the shared and non-shared environmental components of variation of the true phenotype of the child.

16.1 Introduction

A primary source of information about a child's behavior is the description of that behavior by his or her parents. In the study of child and adolescent psychopathology for example, parental reports are fundamental to the widely used assessment system developed by Achenbach and Edelbrock (1981). However, different informants do not generally agree in detail about a given child's behavior (Achenbach *et al.*, 1987; Loeber *et al.*, 1989) and, of course, there are very good reasons why this should be so (Cox and Rutter, 1985). Different informants, such as the child, parents, teachers or peers, have different situational exposure, different degrees of insight, and different perceptions, evaluations and normative standards that may create rater differences of various kinds in reporting problem behaviors. How we analyze parental ratings of children's behavior, and the models we employ in the course of our analyses, will depend on the assumptions we make. In this chapter we discuss the application of three classes of models — biometric, psychometric, and bias models.

First, suppose we took an agnostic view of the relationship between the ratings by different informants by thinking of them as assessing different phenotypes of the child. The phenotypes may be correlated but for unspecified reasons. This view may be appropriate if mothers and fathers reported on behaviors observed in distinct situations, or if they did not share a common understanding of the behavioral descriptions. In such a case it would be appropriate to treat the analysis of mothers' and fathers' ratings as a standard bivariate genetic and environmental analysis where the two variables are the mothers' ratings and fathers' ratings. We shall refer to the class of standard bivariate factor model as *biometric models* (see Chapter 12 for examples).

Second, suppose we made the more restrictive assumption that there is (a) a common phenotype of the children which is assessed both by mothers and by fathers, and (b) a component of each parent's ratings which results from an assessment of an independent aspect of the child. Mothers' ratings and fathers' ratings would correlate because they are indeed making assessments based on shared observations and have a shared understanding of the behavioral descriptions used in the assessments. In this case, we approach the analysis of parental ratings through a special form of model for bivariate data which we will refer to as *psychometric models* (see Chapter 12 for examples).

Third, we consider a model of *rater bias*. Bias in this context is considered to be the tendency of an individual rater to overestimate or underestimate scores consistently. This tendency is a deviation from the mean of all possible raters in the rater group; no reference is made here to any external criterion such as a clinician's judgement. Neale and Stevenson (1989) considered the general problem of rater bias and the particular issues of parental biases in ratings of children. They presented a model in which the rating of a child's phenotype is considered to be a function both of the child's phenotype and of the bias introduced by the rater. In this way it is possible, when two parents rate each of their twin children, to conduct a behavior genetic analysis of the variation in the latent phenotype while allowing for variation due to rating biases. If the rater bias model adopted by Neale and Stevenson (1989) provides an adequate account of the ratings of children by their parents, it becomes possible to partition the variance in these parental ratings into their components due to reliable trait variance, due to parental bias , and due to unreliability or error in the particular rating of a particular child. The reliable trait variance can then be decomposed into its components due to genetic influences, shared environments, and individual environments. Since rater bias models represent restricted special cases for the parental ratings of more general psychometric and biometric models of the kind discussed by Heath *et al.*, (1989) and

McArdle and Goldsmith (1990) and in Chapter 12 of this volume, it is possible to compare the adequacy of bias models with the alternative bivariate psychometric and biometric models. Further, comparison of the biometric and psychometric models indicates how reasonable it is to assume that two raters are assessing the same phenotype in a child. As we move from the biometric to the psychometric to the bias models, our assumptions become more restrictive but, if appropriate, our analyses become more directly informative psychologically. Here we outline how an analysis of parental ratings using the bias model can be implemented simply using LISREL. We discuss the properties of the alternative models and illustrate their application with data from a twin study of child and adolescent behavior problems.

16.2   Models for Multiple Rating Data

16.2.1   Rater Bias Model

Figure 16.1 shows a path model for the ratings of twins by their parents, in which the phenotypes of a pair of twins (PT_1 and PT_2) are functions of additive genetic influence (A), shared environments (C) and non-shared environments (E). The ratings by the mother (MRT) and father (FRT) are functions of the twin's phenotype, the maternal (B_M) or paternal (B_F) rater bias, and residual errors (R_{1MRT}, etc).

If this model is correct, the following discriminations may be made:

1. the structural analysis of the latent phenotypes of the children can be considered independently of the rater biases and unreliability of the ratings;

2. the extent of rater biases and unreliability of ratings can be estimated;

3. the relative accuracy of maternal and paternal ratings can be assessed.

A simple implementation of the model in LISREL is achieved by defining the model by the following matrix equations:

$$
\begin{pmatrix} MRT_1 \\ MRT_2 \\ FRT_1 \\ FRT_2 \end{pmatrix} = \begin{pmatrix} b_m & 0 & 1 & 0 \\ b_m & 0 & 0 & 1 \\ 0 & b_f & \alpha & 0 \\ 0 & b_f & 0 & \alpha \end{pmatrix} \begin{pmatrix} B_M \\ B_F \\ PT_1 \\ PT_2 \end{pmatrix} \tag{16.1}
$$

$$
\begin{pmatrix} B_M \\ B_F \\ PT_1 \\ PT_2 \end{pmatrix} = \begin{pmatrix} 1 & 0 & 0 & 0 & 0 & 0 & 0 & 0 \\ 0 & 1 & 0 & 0 & 0 & 0 & 0 & 0 \\ 0 & 0 & a & c & e & 0 & 0 & 0 \\ 0 & 0 & 0 & 0 & 0 & a & c & e \end{pmatrix} \begin{pmatrix} B_M \\ B_F \\ A_1 \\ C_1 \\ E_1 \\ A_2 \\ C_2 \\ E_2 \end{pmatrix} \tag{16.2}
$$

$$
\eta = \Gamma\xi. \tag{16.3}
$$

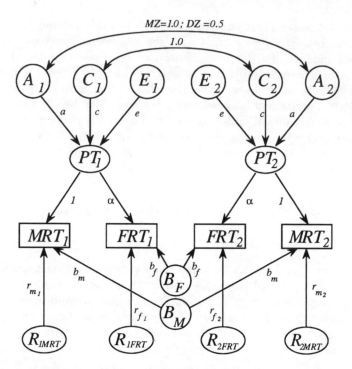

Figure 16.1: Model for ratings of a pair of twins (1 and 2) by their parents. Maternal and paternal observed ratings (MRT and FRT) are linear functions of the true phenotypes of the twins (PT), maternal and paternal rater bias (B_M and B_F), and residual error (R_{MRT} and R_{FRT}).

Then, the covariance matrix of the ratings is given by

$$\mathcal{E}\{\mathbf{yy'}\} = \mathbf{\Lambda}_y \mathbf{\Gamma \Phi \Gamma'} \mathbf{\Lambda}_y' + \mathbf{\Theta}_\epsilon \tag{16.4}$$

$$= \mathbf{\Gamma \Phi \Gamma'} + \mathbf{\Theta}_\epsilon \tag{16.5}$$

where $\mathbf{\Phi}$ contains the appropriate correlations between the B, A, C, and E latent variables, and the diagonal elements of $\mathbf{\Theta}_\epsilon$ are the residual variances in the model. Equations 16.4 and 16.5 are equivalent because $\mathbf{\Lambda}_y$ is an identity matrix. A LISREL script for this model is listed in Appendix H.1. In considering the rater bias model, and the other models discussed below, we should note that parameters need not be constrained to be equal when rating boys and girls and, as Neale and Stevenson (1988) pointed out, we need not necessarily assume that parental biases are equal for MZ and DZ twins' ratings. This latter relaxation of the parameter constraints allows us to consider the possibility that twin correlations differ across zygosities for reasons related to differential parental biases based on beliefs about their twins' zygosity.

16.2.2   Psychometric Model

Figure 16.2 shows a bivariate psychometric or 'common pathway' model. Implementation of this model in LISREL can be achieved by the approaches illustrated in

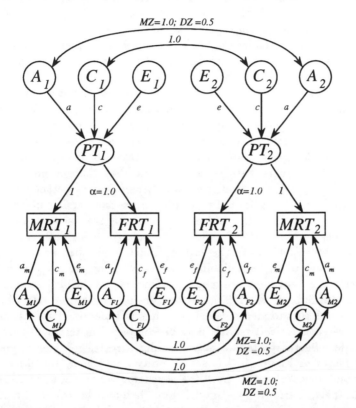

Figure 16.2: Psychometric or common pathway model for ratings of a pair of twins (1 and 2) by their parents. Maternal and paternal observed ratings (MRT and FRT) are linear functions of the latent phenotypes of the twins (PT), and rater specific variance (e.g., A_M, C_M and E_M).

Chapter 12 and in Heath *et al.* (1989) or McArdle and Goldsmith (1990). The psychometric model estimates, for each source of influence (A, C, and E) the variance for mothers' ratings, the variance for fathers' ratings and the covariance between these ratings. These estimates are subject to the constraints that the covariances are positive and neither individual rating variance can be less than the covariance between the ratings. The psychological implication of this psychometric model is that the mothers' and fathers' ratings are composed of consistent assessments of reliable trait variance, together with assessments of specific phenotypes uncorrelated between the parents.

There are some technical points to note with this model. First, bivariate data for MZ and DZ twins (of a given sex) yield 20 observed variances and covariances. However, only 9 of these have unique expectations under the classes of model we are considering, the remaining 11 being replicate estimates of particular expectations (e.g., the variance of maternal ratings of MZ twin 1, of MZ twin 2, of DZ twin 1 and of DZ twin 2 are four replicate estimates of the variance of maternal ratings in the population). Given this, we might expect our 9 parameter psychometric model to fit as well as any other 9 parameter model for bivariate twin data. However, there are some implicit constraints in our psychometric model. For example, the phenotypic covariance of mothers' and fathers' ratings cannot be greater than the variance of either type of rating. Such constraints may cause the model to fail in some circumstances even though the 9 parameter biometric model discussed below (Figure 16.3) may fit adequately[1]. The second technical point is that if we do not constrain the loadings of the common factor to be equal on the mothers' ratings and on the fathers' ratings, and assume that there is no specific genetic variance for either mothers' ratings or for fathers' ratings, then this variant of the psychometric model is formally equivalent to our version in the Neale and Stevenson bias model described above. In this case the "shared environmental" specific variances for the mothers' and fathers' ratings are formally equivalent to the maternal and paternal biases in the earlier model, while the "non-shared" specific variances are equal to the unreliability variance of the earlier parameterization. Thus, although the 9 parameter psychometric model and the bias model do not form a nested pair (Mulaik *et al.*, 1989), they represent alternative sets of constraints on a more general 10 parameter model (which is not identified with two-rater twin data) and these constrained models may be compared in terms of parsimony and goodness of fit. Furthermore, we may consider a restricted bias model in which the scaling factor in Figure 16.1 is set to unity and which, therefore, has 7 free parameters and is nested within both the psychometric model and the unrestricted bias model. This restricted bias model may therefore be tested directly against either the psychometric or the unrestricted bias models by a likelihood ratio chi-square.

16.2.3   Biometric Model

The final model to be considered is the biometric model shown in Figure 16.3, and again may be readily implemented using the procedure described in Chapter 12 and in Heath *et al.*, (1989) or McArdle and Goldsmith (1990). In this model there are two factors for each source of variance (A, C, and E). One factor is subscripted M, e.g., A_M, and loads on the maternal rating (MRT) and on the paternal rating (FRT). The other factor subscripted F, e.g., A_F, loads only on the paternal rating.

---

[1] There are in fact some other special cases such as scalar sex-limitation – where identical genetic or environmental factors may have different factor loadings for males and females — when the psychometric model may fit as well or better than the biometric model.

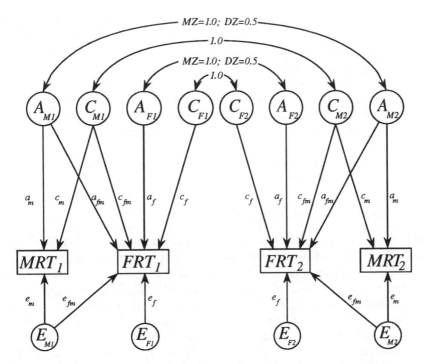

Figure 16.3: Biometric or independent pathway model for ratings of a pair of twins (1 and 2) by their parents. Maternal and paternal observed ratings (MRT and FRT) are linear functions of general (subscript M) and restricted (subscript F) genetic and environmental factors.

Thus, for each source of influence we estimate three factor loadings which enable us to reconstruct estimates of the contribution of this influence to the variance of maternal ratings, the variance of paternal ratings and the covariance between them. Which factor loads on both types of rating and which on only one is arbitrary. This type of model is referred to as a Cholesky model or decomposition or a triangular model and provides a standard general approach to multivariate biometrical analysis (see Chapter 12). This biometric model is a saturated unconstrained model for the nine unique expected variances and covariances (in the absence of sibling interactions or other influences giving rise to heterogeneity of variances across zygosities, cf. Heath *et al.*, 1989) and provides the most general approach to estimating the genetic, shared environmental and non-shared environmental components of variance and covariance. However, the absence of theoretically motivated constraints lessens the psychological informativeness of the model for the analysis of parental ratings. In this context, we may use the biometric model first to test the adequacy of the assumption that of the 20 observed variances and covariances for bivariate twin data of a given sex, 11 represent replicate estimates of the 9 unique structural expectations. Once again, sex differences in factor loadings (scalar sex limitation) may in principle lead to model failure for opposite sex data even though the biometric model is adequate for a given sex. In this case the non-scalar sex limitation model described in Heath *et al.* (1989) and Chapter 11 would be required. The bivariate biometric model provides a baseline for comparison of the adequacy of the psychometric and bias models. This comparison alerts us to the important possibility that mothers and fathers are assessing different (but possibly correlated) phenotypes as, for example, they might be if mothers and fathers were reporting on behaviors observed in different situations or without a common understanding of the behavioral descriptions used in the assessment protocol.

16.2.4   Comparison of Models

We have considered four alternative models for parental ratings of children's behavior. Each model is for bivariate twin data where the two variables are the special case of mothers' ratings and fathers' ratings of the children's behavior. The least restrictive model, the biometric model, provides a baseline for comparison with the psychologically more informative psychometric and bias models. The most restricted bias model may be formally tested by likelihood ratio chi-square against either the psychometric or the unrestricted bias models. However, these latter two are not themselves nested. The relationships between these models, without taking into account sex limitations, are summarized in Figure 16.4. In this figure the solid arrows represent the process of constraining a more general model to yield a more restrictive model; the model at the arrow head is nested within the model at the tail of the arrow and may be tested against it by a likelihood ratio chi square. The dashed arrows represent rotational constraints on the biometric model. The nine parameter psychometric model requires, for example, that the covariance between maternal and paternal ratings be no greater than the variance of either type of rating; in factor analytic terms this would require a constrained rotation of the biometric model solution. The ten parameter psychometric model, allowing α not equal to unity, still imposes the constraints that the contributions of the common influences to the variance of maternal ratings, the variance of paternal ratings, and the covariance between them be in the ratio $1 : \alpha^2 : \alpha$ for each source of influence. Thus, even though this model has 10 parameters (and hence is not identified for bivariate twin data) any of its solutions, arrived at by fixing one of the parameters to an arbitrary value, will again represent in factor analytic terms a constrained rotation of the biometric model.

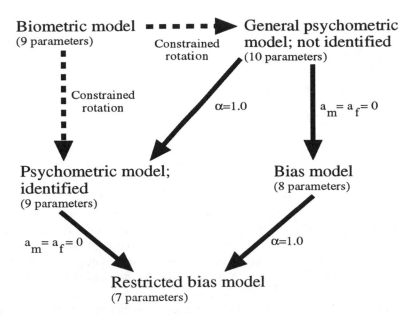

Figure 16.4: Diagram of the nesting of biometric, psychometric, and rater bias models.

16.3   Application to Data from the Child Behavior Checklist

16.3.1   Subjects and Methods

To illustrate the application of these models we consider an updated set of data first presented by Hewitt, *et al.*, (1990) and now based on 983 families where both parents rated each of their twin children using Achenbach's Child Behavior Checklist (CBC; Achenbach and Edelbrock, 1983). Details of the full study and its results are in preparation (Silberg *et al.*, 1992). For the full analysis, published in Hewitt *et al.* (1992), data from a population-based sample of 500 MZ twin pairs and 483 DZ twin pairs were considered and ratings were included irrespective of the biological or social relationship of the parent to the child. The children were Caucasian and ranged in age from 8 to 16 years. Ratings on 23 core items assessing children's internalizing behavior in both younger and older children and in either boys or girls were totalled to obtain an internalizing scale score for each child. The items contributing to this scale are listed in Appendix H.2.

For illustrative purposes in this chapter we just consider the "prepubertal" subsample of younger children aged 8-11 years. More detailed analyses, including older children, may be found in Hewitt *et al.* (1992). The scale scores were log-transformed to approximate normality and adjusted for linear regression on age and sex within age cohorts. The observed variances, covariances, and correlations of the resulting scores are given in Table 16.1 by zygosity and sex group.

16.3.2   Results of Model-Fitting

A summary of the adequacy of the models fitted to these data on younger children's internalizing problems is shown in Table 16.2. The illustrative program in Appendix H.1 runs the analysis for the bias model with 34 degrees of freedom.

As can be seen from Table 16.2, all three types of model give excellent fits to the data for younger children, with the psychometric model being preferred by Akaike's criterion. Thus, our first conclusion would be that to a very good approximation, mothers and fathers can be assumed to be rating the same phenotype in their children when using the Child Behavior Checklist, at least as far as these internalizing behaviors are concerned. This may not be so for other behaviors or assessment instruments and in each particular case the assumption ought to be tested by a comparison of models of the kind we have described. Although there are numerous submodels or alternative models that may be considered, (for example: no sex limitation; non-scalar sex-limitation; and setting non-significant parameters to zero), only a subset will be presented here for illustration.

Table 16.3 shows the parameter estimates for the full bias and psychometric models allowing for scalar sex limitation and, in the case of the biometric model, we have allowed for non-scalar sex-limitation[2] of the shared environmental influences specific to fathers' ratings ($\chi^2_{31} = 20.76$ for the model presented with the correlation between boys' and girls' effects of this kind estimated at 0.86 rather than unity). To show the relationship between the more parsimonious bias model and the full parameterization of the biometric model, in Table 16.4 we present the expected contributions of A, C, and E to the variance of mothers' ratings, fathers' ratings, and the covariances between mothers' and fathers' ratings. What Table 16.4 shows is that, providing the rater bias model is adequate, we can partition the environmental variance of mothers' and fathers' ratings into variance attributable to those effects consistently rated by both parents and those effects which either represent rater bias or residual unreliable environmental variance. In this particular case, while a univariate consideration of maternal ratings would suggest a heritability of 47% [$= .263/(.263 + .194 + .108)$], a shared environmental influence of 34%, and a non-shared environmental influence of 19%, it is clear that more than half of the shared environmental influence can be attributed to rater bias, and the major portion of the non-shared environmental influence to unreliability or inconsistency between ratings. The heritability of internalizing behaviors in young boys rated consistently by both parents may be as high as 70% [$= .269/(.269 + .077 + .036)$].

---

[2]This is to avoid estimated loadings of opposite sign in boys and girls – see Neale and Martin (1989) or Chapter 11 for LISREL formulations.

Table 16.1: Observed variance-covariance matrices (lower triangle) and twin correlations (above the diagonal) for parental ratings of internalizing behavior problems in five zygosity-sex groups (MZ female, N=96; MZ male, N=102; DZ female, N=102; DZ male, N=97; DZ male-female, N=103). All twins were between 8 and 11 years at assessment.

Zygosity/sex group		Twin 1		Twin 2	
MZ female		Mothers	Fathers	Mothers	Fathers
	MT1	.694	.47	.84	.46
	FT1	.312	.638	.37	.72
	MT2	.569	.238	.666	.45
	FT2	.308	.461	.293	.647
MZ male		Mothers	Fathers	Mothers	Fathers
	MT1	.675	.40	.74	.43
	FT1	.265	.652	.35	.77
	MT2	.513	.237	.714	.51
	FT2	.292	.513	.354	.676
DZ female		Mothers	Fathers	Mothers	Fathers
	MT1	.565	.41	.55	.29
	FT1	.241	.604	.25	.57
	MT2	.291	.137	.488	.52
	FT2	.171	.347	.285	.604
DZ male		Mothers	Fathers	Mothers	Fathers
	MT1	.621	.47	.70	.34
	FT1	.315	.719	.35	.73
	MT2	.434	.236	.623	.37
	FT2	.233	.531	.251	.743
DZ male-female		Mothers	Fathers	Mothers	Fathers
	MT1	.538	.26	.49	.18
	FT1	.162	.730	.17	.56
	MT2	.243	.102	.465	.37
	FT2	.103	.372	.191	.574

Table 16.2: Summary of models fitted to younger children's internalizing problems.

Model*	Fit statistics		
	df	χ^2	AIC
Restricted bias	36	30.07	-41.9
Bias	34	25.78	-42.2
Psychometric	32	20.71	-43.3
Biometric	32	20.95	-43.1

*All models allow scalar sex limitation of individual parameters. The solution avoiding effects of opposite sign in boys and girls by allowing for sex-limitation of shared environmental influences specific to fathers' ratings gives $\chi^2_{31} = 20.76$.

16.3.3   Discussion of CBC Application

The data we have analyzed are restricted to parental checklist reports of their twin children's behavior problems, without the benefit of self reports, teachers' reports or clinical interviews. As such, they are limited by the ability of parents to provide reliable and valid integrative assessments of their children, using cursorily defined concepts like 'Sulks a lot,' 'Worrying,' or 'Fears going to school.' It is clear from meta-analyses of intercorrelations of ratings of children by different types informants that while the level of agreement between mothers and fathers is often moderate (e.g., yielding correlations around .5 to .6) the level of agreement between parents and other informants (e.g., parent with child or parent with teacher) is modest and generally yields a correlation around 0.2 to 0.3 (Achenbach *et al.*, 1987). Thus, parental consistency in evaluating their children does not guarantee cross situational validity, although it does provide evidence that ratings of behavior observable by parents are not simply reflecting individual rater biases. In assessing the importance of the home environment on children's behavior this becomes a critical issue since studies of children's behavior based on ratings by a single individual in each family, e.g., the mother, confound the rater bias with the influence of the home environment. This may have the dual effect of inflating global estimates of the home environment's influence while at the same time either attenuating the relationship between objective indices of the environment and children's behavior (which is being assessed by a biased observer) or spuriously augmenting apparent relationships which are in fact relationships between environmental indices and maternal or paternal rating biases.

   An issue distinguishable from that of bias is that of behavior sampling or situational specificity. Thus maternal and paternal ratings of children may differ not because of the tendency of individual parents to rate children in general as more or less problematic (bias), but because they are exposed to different samples of

Table 16.3: Parameter estimates from the bias, psychometric, and biometric models for parental ratings of internalizing behaviors in younger children.

Bias model			Psychometric model			Biometric model		
Path	Boys	Girls	Path	Boys	Girls	Path	Boys	Girls
a	.519	.163	a	.370	.145	a_m	.513	.134
c	.277	.363	a_m	.338	-.027	a_{fm}	.261	.132
e	.189	.156	a_f	-.069	.281	a_f	.265	.286
a	.671	1.416						
b_m	.320	.545	c	.308	.449	c_m	.440	.659
b_f	.509	.473	c_m	.332	.479	c_{fm}	.225	.308
r_m^2	.074	.154	c_f	.437	.507	c_f	.490	.603
r_f^2	.175	.115						
			e	.176	.200	e_m	.328	.423
			em	.278	.372	e_{fm}	.096	.097
			ef	.386	.333	e_f	.414	.377

behavior. If this is so, then treating informants' ratings as if they were assessing a common phenotype, albeit in a biased or unreliable way, will be misleading. It is of considerable psychological importance to know whether different observers are being presented with different behaviors. The approach outlined in this chapter first enables us to examine the adequacy of the assumption that different informants are assessing the same behaviors and then, if that assumption is deemed adequate, to separate the contributions of rater bias and unreliability from the genetic and environmental contribution to the common behavioral phenotype. For our particular example, all the models fit our data adequately and the bias model, even in its restricted version, does not fit significantly worse than the psychometric or biometric models.

Although not presented here, there is some evidence that for externalizing behavior mothers and fathers cannot be assumed to be simply assessing the same phenotype with bias. In this context it is worth noting, however, that the adequacy of the assumption that parents are assessing the same phenotype in their children does not imply a high parental correlation (which may be lowered by bias and unreliability) and, conversely, even though parents may be shown to be assessing different phenotypes in their children to a significant degree the parental correlation in assessments may predominate over variance specific to a given parent. Our comparison of the bias with the psychometric and biometric models provides important evidence of the equivalence of the internalizing behaviors assessed by mothers and fathers using this instrument. This equivalence does not preclude bias or unreliability and the evidence presented in Table 16.4 provides a striking illustration of the impact of these sources of variation on maternal or paternal assessments. A

Table 16.4: The contributions to the phenotypic variances and covariance of mothers' and fathers' ratings of young boys' internalizing behavior.

Source	Biometric model			Bias model		
	Ratings		Cov (r)	Ratings		Cov (r)
	Mother	Father	M-F	Mother	Father	M-F
Additive genetic (A)	.268	.138	.134 (.70)	.269	.121	.181 (*1.0*)
Shared Env. (C)	.194	.291	.099 (.42)	.077	.035	.051 (*1.0*)
Bias	—	—	—	.102	.259	.000 (*.00*)
C + Bias	.194	.291	.099 (.42)	.179	.294	.051 (.22)
Random Env. (E)	.108	.181	.031 (.22)	.036	.016	.024 (*1.0*)
Residual	—	—	—	.074	.175	.000 (.00)
E + Residual	.108	.181	.031 (.22)	.110	.191	.024 (.17)
Phenotypic Total	.564	.609	.264 (.45)	.558	.606	.256 (.44)

Italicized numbers indicate parameters are fixed *ex hypothesi* in the rater bias model.

shared environmental component which might be estimated to account for 34% of variance if mothers' ratings alone were considered, may correspond to only 20% of the variance when maternal biases have been removed. Similarly, a non-shared environmental variance component of 19% of variance may correspond to 9% of variance in individual differences between children that can be consistently rated by both parents. Finally, once allowance has been made for bias and inconsistency or unreliability, the estimated heritability rises from 47% to 70% in this case.

We have not been concerned here to seek the most parsimonious submodel within each of the model types. We should be aware that although we have, for the younger children, presented the full models with sex limitation, differences between boys and girls are not necessarily significant (for example, although the biometric model without sex limitation fit our data significantly worse than the corresponding model allowing for sex limitation ($\chi^2_9 = 21.31$, $p < .05$), the overall fit without sex limitation is still adequate, $\chi^2_{41} = 42.26$). Furthermore, individual parameter estimates reported for our full models may not depart significantly from zero. Other limitations of the method are that it does not allow for interaction effects between parents and children[3] and, in our application, assumed the inde-

---

[3] However, if these effects were substantial and if MZ twins correlated more highly than DZ twins in their interactional style, the variance of parents' ratings should differ (Neale *et al.*, 1992).

pendence of maternal and paternal biases. The analysis of parental bias under this model requires that both parents rate each of two children. Distinguishing between correlated parental biases and shared environmental influences would require a third, independent, rater (e.g., a teacher); thus we cannot rule out a contribution of correlated biases to our estimates of the remaining shared family environmental influence.

The final caveat against overinterpretation of particular parameter estimates is that we have reported analyses for families in which both parents have returned a questionnaire and we have made no distinction between different biological or social parental statuses. Clearly, we anticipate that the inclusion and exclusion criteria are not neutral with respect to children's behavior problems and their perception by parents. However, we have illustrated that behavior genetic analyses are possible even when we have to rely on ratings by observers, providing that we have at least two degrees of relatedness among those being rated (e.g., MZ and DZ twins). Without an approach of this sort we have no way of establishing whether parents are assessing the same behaviors in their children and whether analyses will spuriously inflate estimates of the shared environment as much as parental biases inflate the correlations for pairs of twins independent of zygosity. Extension of the model to include other raters, for example, teachers, is straightforward.

Given sufficient sample size, these effects would lead to failure of these models.

Chapter 17

Assortment and Cultural Transmission

17.1 Introduction to the Twin–Parent Design

At the *First International Course on Twin Methodology*, it was recognized that the analysis of twin data alone has its limitations:

> *Although the main emphasis of this workshop is on the analysis of twin data alone, it is important to recognize that the analysis of genetic and environmental effects cannot end with twins. There are effects that cannot be resolved with data on twins by themselves including the effects of assortment and the shared environment. Furthermore, any model that we start to build with twin data has to predict the results for other kinship data or it is of very restricted value.* (Eaves et al., 1989b)

During the course these authors developed a model for analysis of data from twins and their parents that could be easily accommodated in the existing LISREL program (LISREL VI; Jöreskog and Sörbom, 1986). The model was restricted to a special case of both assortative mating and cultural inheritance in which only shared or common environment, what we have called C in this text, were involved. Because the process of assortative mating — "like marrying like" — was assumed to involve only C, the model was essentially one of *social homogamy*. In some situations this may well be a plausible model to adopt (Rao *et al.*, 1974; Morton, 1982) and it is the first model we describe in this chapter.

However, another plausible model for a number of behavioral traits is that assortative mating and cultural transmission are based on the phenotypes of the parents and not on any particular component of which the phenotype is comprised. For example, mate selection for stature is almost certainly determined by the visible phenotypes of the mates involved. It may also be the case for general intelligence, where it is the perception of the individual that may be important, rather than social background *per se* or knowledge of the genotype, such as may be gained by observing the individual's relatives. In this form of assortative mating, all components of the phenotype, A, C, and E, become correlated in a rather complex manner. Similarly, in cultural transmission, environmental influences in the present generation may stem from the parental phenotypes in the preceding generation.

The combined effects of *phenotypic assortative mating* and *cultural transmission* will obviously lead to a complex inter-relationship among genetic and environmental components, A, C, and E, across generations. Most important among these relationships is genotype-environment covariance; that is, A and C become correlated and inflate the phenotypic variance. The second model we describe attempts to take account of these relationships and assess their importance.

But whichever model one chooses to employ, it should be emphasized that the addition of parental data into a twin study is all that is needed to resolve the complexities of the models we describe. This is usually a relatively simple and inexpensive process for the investigator who plans to carry out a twin study. The very simple design of twins and their parents is, in effect, a crude substitute for the much more powerful design of adopted or separated individuals and, thus, may provide some preliminary indication of what these more expensive studies might yield.

17.2 Social Homogamy Model

The basic social homogamy model for resemblance between two parents and DZ twins is shown in Figure 17.1. Phenotypic values for mothers and fathers are represented by P_M and P_F and twins' phenotypes appear as P_{T1} and P_{T2}. Additive genetic and shared environmental variables (A and C) in the parent generation transmit to the genotypes and shared environment of the twins with paths $\frac{1}{2}$ and m or f, depending on the gender of the parent. Random environmental effects, E, are assumed not to transmit across generations. A, C, and E in both the parent and offspring generations determine phenotypic measurements with paths a, c, and e as in the conventional twin model.

In order to explain the total variance of A in the children's' generation, a residual term arising from genetic segregation, R_{AT}, is required with a fixed path $\sqrt{1/2}$ for each twin. Also, because the shared environmental influences affecting twins are unlikely to be completely explained by paths m and f, another residual term, R_{CT}, is needed to account for the total variance of C. This variable is weighted by the path coefficient r, which, when squared represents all shared environmental influences outside of the home ($r^2 = 1 - m^2 - f^2 - 2mf\mu$).

One of the most important features of this social homogamy model is the assumption that the spousal correlation is due entirely to assortment for the cultural environment. This process of assortative mating is represented in Figure 17.1 by the parameter μ. Although this is an arbitrary and controversial assumption (Rao

LISREL Variables

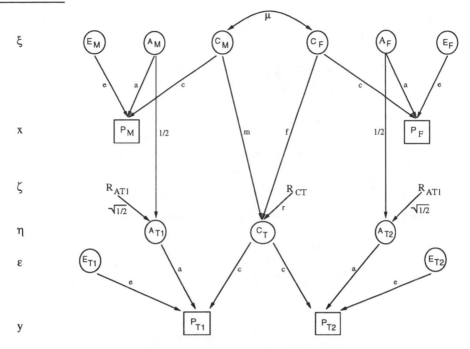

Figure 17.1: Cultural transmission and social homogamy.

et al., 1974), it greatly simplifies expression of the model in LISREL because it does not induce any complex interactions between model parameters which arise when assortment is assumed to occur on the basis of observed spousal attributes. Following the rules of path analysis (Li, 1975), we obtain the expectations for twins and parent-offspring resemblance in Table 17.1.

17.2.1   LISREL Formulation of the Model

Eaves *et al.* (1989b) have presented a LISREL formulation of the social homogamy model. In this specification, the observed parental variables (P_M, P_F) are given as x-variables and the twins' phenotypes as y-variables. Latent A and C variables of the parental generation are modeled as the LISREL variables ξ. Non-shared environment variables are models as residual variables, δ. In the twin generation, the genotypic (A) and shared environment (C) values are modeled as η variables, and within-twin environmental values (E) are specified as ϵ. Residual genetic (R_{AT}) and shared environment values (R_{CT}) are represented by ζ variables. These LISREL variables are shown in the margin of Figure 17.1.

Table 17.1: Expected correlations between relatives under social homogamy model of twins and parents.

Relationship	Algebraic Expression
MZ Twins	$a^2 + c^2$
DZ Twins	$1/2a^2 + c^2$
Spouses	$c^2\mu$
Mother-Offspring	$1/2a^2 + c^2(m + f\mu)$
Father-Offspring	$1/2a^2 + c^2(f + m\mu)$

The measurement model for the parental variables, **x**, is:

$$\begin{pmatrix} P_M \\ P_F \end{pmatrix} = \begin{pmatrix} a & c & 0 & 0 \\ 0 & 0 & a & c \end{pmatrix} \begin{pmatrix} A_M \\ C_M \\ A_F \\ C_F \end{pmatrix} + \begin{pmatrix} E_M \\ E_F \end{pmatrix}$$

or

$$\mathbf{x} = \mathbf{\Lambda}_x \boldsymbol{\xi} + \boldsymbol{\delta} \ .$$

This measurement model yields the (2×2) matrix of expected variances and covariances between the spouses' phenotypes:

$$\mathbf{\Sigma}_{\mathbf{x},\mathbf{x}} = \mathbf{\Lambda}_x \mathbf{\Phi} \mathbf{\Lambda}_x' + \mathbf{\Theta}_\delta,$$

where

$$\mathbf{\Phi} = \begin{pmatrix} 1 & 0 & 0 & 0 \\ 0 & 1 & 0 & \mu \\ 0 & 0 & 1 & 0 \\ 0 & \mu & 0 & 1 \end{pmatrix}$$

and

$$\mathbf{\Theta}_\delta = \begin{pmatrix} e^2 & 0 \\ 0 & e^2 \end{pmatrix}$$

Similarly, the measurement model for the (DZ) twin variables, **y**, is:

$$\begin{pmatrix} P_{T1} \\ P_{T2} \end{pmatrix} = \begin{pmatrix} a & c & 0 \\ 0 & c & a \end{pmatrix} \begin{pmatrix} A_{T1} \\ C_T \\ A_{T2} \end{pmatrix} + \begin{pmatrix} E_{T1} \\ E_{T2} \end{pmatrix}$$

$$\mathbf{y} \qquad = \qquad \mathbf{\Lambda}_{yDZ} \qquad \boldsymbol{\eta} \qquad + \qquad \boldsymbol{\epsilon}$$

Because the phenotypes of MZ twins are determined by a single genetic variable, the $\mathbf{\Lambda}_{yMZ}$ matrix differs slightly from that shown for DZ twins:

$$\mathbf{\Lambda}_{yMZ} = \begin{pmatrix} a & c & 0 \\ a & c & 0 \end{pmatrix}$$

The structural equation model relating the latent parent and twin variables is given by:

$$\begin{pmatrix} A_{T1} \\ C_T \\ A_{T2} \end{pmatrix} = \begin{pmatrix} .5 & 0 & .5 & 0 \\ 0 & m & 0 & f \\ .5 & 0 & .5 & 0 \end{pmatrix} \begin{pmatrix} A_M \\ C_M \\ A_F \\ C_F \end{pmatrix} + \begin{pmatrix} R_{A_{T1}} \\ R_{CT} \\ R_{A_{T2}} \end{pmatrix}$$

$$\eta \quad = \quad \mathbf{\Gamma} \quad \quad \xi \quad + \quad \zeta$$

These measurement and structural equation models generate the (2×2) expected covariance matrices between twins and parents and between members of a twin pair:

$$\begin{aligned} \mathbf{\Sigma}_{x,y} &= \mathbf{\Lambda}_x \mathbf{\Phi} \mathbf{\Gamma}' \mathbf{\Lambda}_y' \\ \mathbf{\Sigma}_{y,y} &= \mathbf{\Lambda}_y (\mathbf{\Gamma} \mathbf{\Phi} \mathbf{\Gamma}' + \mathbf{\Psi}) \mathbf{\Lambda}_y' + \mathbf{\Theta}_\epsilon, \end{aligned}$$

in which $\mathbf{\Psi}$ is a diagonal matrix of residual effects on the twins' latent variables

$$\mathbf{\Psi} = \begin{pmatrix} .5 & 0 & 0 \\ 0 & r^2 & 0 \\ 0 & 0 & .5 \end{pmatrix}$$

and $\mathbf{\Theta}_\epsilon$ is a diagonal matrix of unique environment effects

$$\mathbf{\Theta}_\epsilon = \begin{pmatrix} e^2 & 0 \\ 0 & e^2 \end{pmatrix} = \mathbf{\Theta}_\delta.$$

For the full social homogamy model, observed covariance matrices between MZ twins and parents and between DZ twins and parents form 2 (4×4) matrices. The model has 7 free parameters, including a, c, m, f, μ, e^2, and r^2. Degrees of freedom for the model, using the chi-squared statistic based on one of the fit functions in LISREL, are calculated as

$$df = \sum_{i=1}^{2} [p_i(p_i + 1)/2] - n \tag{17.1}$$

where p_i is the order of the MZ and DZ parent-offspring matrices and n is the number of free parameters estimated. In the present example, $p_i = 4$ and $n = 7$. Thus, the full model has $20 - 7 = 13$ degrees of freedom.

Eaves *et al.* (1989) applied this model to simulated parent-twin correlations which were derived from parameter values $a = .548, c = .775, m = .400, f = .100, \mu = .800, e^2 = .100$, and $r^2 = .766$. These values were recovered exactly from application of the model to the correlations, demonstrating that the model is identified. Although the data as such are of little interest, being simulated, it is important to consider that the simulated correlations are based upon a very large value for μ and substantial shared environment effects (c^2). The social homogamy model cannot account for data that deviate dramatically from those simulated, particularly in the case of small or absent c^2 effects. This issue will be described in more detail later in this chapter. The LISREL program for the social homogamy model is given in Appendix K.1.

17.3   Phenotypic Assortment Model

Models of phenotypic assortment originated in the classic work of Fisher (1918) and Wright (1921b, 1931, 1934). They were further developed by Jencks (1972), Eaves *et al.* (1978), Young *et al.* (1980), Fulker (1982), and Heath and Eaves (1985). The model we describe in this section assumes that the combined processes of cultural transmission and assortative mating have been going on for some generations and have reached a state of equilibrium. The implication of this equilibrium is that the interdependencies of the parameters in the model, what are formally referred to as model constraints, are constant across generations. To use a program such as LISREL 7 to take account of these constraints has proved to be extremely difficult — it may not even be possible. Heretofore, we have been forced to employ special purpose optimizers to solve the necessary equations. However, with the development of LISREL 8, which accommodates explicit algebraic constraints on the parameters in the model, the analysis of phenotypic assortative mating and cultural transmission can be performed with relatively little difficulty (Cardon *et al.*, 1991).

17.3.1   Reverse Path Analysis

The upper panel in Figure 17.2 shows the simple model of a behavioral phenotype upon which the present phenotypic assortment model is based. This model is the familiar model we have used throughout the text for the analysis of twin data, with the addition of genotype-environment covariation. Standardized latent variables of the additive genetic value, environmental value shared by twins, and random environmental value of an individual are represented by A, C, and E, respectively. The phenotypic measurement, P, is determined by these genetic, shared environment, and unique environment latent variables, respectively weighted by path coefficients a, c, and e, as in the classical twin design and in the social homogamy parent-twin model. The correlation, s, between the additive genetic and shared environmental values is induced by parental transmission of both genetic and environmental factors to their offspring. In the twin analyses presented throughout this text, including the social homogamy model described previously, we have assumed this correlation to be zero. The parent-twin model outlined in this section provides a means to explicitly test this assumption.

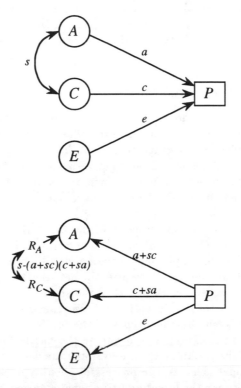

Figure 17.2: Equivalent path diagrams expressing relationships among additive genetic values (A), shared and unique environmental values (C, E) and phenotypic values (P): basic phenotypic model (top); reverse path diagram (bottom).

Application of path tracing rules to the diagram in Figure 17.2 generates the expression for phenotypic variance under genetic and cultural transmission

$$V_p = a^2 + c^2 + e^2 + 2asc \tag{17.2}$$

This expression is equivalent to that of the classical twin design but contains the additional term $2asc$ which inflates the variance because of genotype-environment covariance, s.

In order to accommodate the effects of assortative mating into this simple description of an individual's phenotype, we have to introduce the approach of reverse path analysis developed by Sewall Wright (1968). A reverse path model is shown

in the lower portion of Figure 17.2. This model provides an equivalent representation of the relationships among the latent and observed variables as the basic
phenotypic model. The method reverses the causal pathways between observed
and latent variables such that the standardized observed variable, P, *causes* the
genetic, shared environmental, and unique environmental variables. The residual
genetic (R_A) and shared environmental (R_C) effects are correlated in this specification to preserve the variable relationships shown in the traditional path model
of Figure 17.2.

17.3.2   Parameter Constraints

As noted previously, the combined effects of phenotypic assortative mating and
cultural transmission generate complex inter-relations among the genotypic and
environmental variables across generations. We have shown that the presence of
cultural transmission inflates the phenotypic variance; here we describe the effects
of phenotypic assortative mating on variance and covariance expectations, then
illustrate the combined effects of cultural transmission and phenotypic assortment
using reverse path models.

The reverse path specification greatly facilitates derivation of covariance expectations based on the effects of phenotypic assortative mating. To incorporate
assortment effects into the simple phenotypic model, Figure 17.2 may be specified
for two parents, with all sources of covariation between the parents encompassed
by a single path. This reverse path model of the spousal assortment correlation is
shown in the top portion of Figure 17.3. The assortment process is represented by
the parameter, μ, between the phenotypes of the mother (P_M) and father (P_F).

Because assortment is expected to occur on the basis of observed, phenotypic,
characteristics, all of the variables which determine the parental phenotypes become
correlated in this model. That is, the process of phenotypic assortative mating in-
duces correlations between the latent additive genetic values, shared environmental
values, and unique environmental values of spouses. These correlations, which are
illustrated in the bottom portion of Figure 17.3, may be derived on the basis of
model parameters a, c, e, s, and μ:

$$
\begin{aligned}
\alpha &= r_{E_M E_F} = e^2 \mu \\
\tau &= r_{E_M C_F} = r_{C_M E_F} = e(c + sa)\mu \\
\omega &= r_{E_M A_F} = r_{A_M E_F} = e(a + sc)\mu \\
\delta &= r_{A_M C_F} = r_{C_M A_F} = (a + sc)(c + sa)\mu \\
\gamma &= r_{A_M A_F} = (a + sc)^2 \mu \\
\epsilon &= r_{C_M C_F} = (c + sa)^2 \mu
\end{aligned}
\tag{17.3}
$$

These constrained quantities are embedded within the reverse path model of Figure 17.3, and, therefore, do not need to be explicitly specified for a model of reverse

paths. It is this feature of the reverse path model that permits simple formulation of the present parent-twin model in LISREL.

The effects of cultural transmission on familial resemblances between twins and parents are combined with those due to assortative mating in the path diagram shown in Figure 17.4. In this diagram, cultural transmission originates in the parental phenotypes and exerts influence on the shared environment of twins. Because the effects of cultural transmission stem from parental phenotypes (rather than parental environment (C) variables as in the social homogamy model), the twins' shared environment is impacted by all sources that determine the observed adult measurements; namely, A, C, and E. All such influences are contained in the model parameter z. For the present model, we have assumed that the transmission of cultural effects are equal for both parents (i.e., $m = f = z$), although this is not a formal requirement of the general model. The values of $\frac{1}{2}$ shown in Figure 17.4 represent contributions of additive genetic values from parents to offspring based upon Mendelian inheritance.

Application of path tracing rules to the diagram reveals that the expected correlation between a single twin's environment and genotype ($r_{AT,CT}$) is $z(1 + \mu)(a + sc)$. At equilibrium, this genotype-environment correlation is the same in both generations and, thus, equal to the model parameter s. This implies the parameter constraint

$$s = z(1 + \mu)(a + sc) \tag{17.4}$$

Expected correlations between relatives under this model of assortative mating and cultural transmission are shown in Table 17.2. These expectations are derived from Figure 17.4, although it is important to recognize that, strictly speaking, the figure is drawn for DZ twins. For derivation of MZ twin correlations, one of the twin genotype variables, A_{T2} for example, would be omitted from the diagram and the remaining genotype factor (A_{T1}) would be drawn as having paths a to the phenotypes of both twins, completely analogous to the diagram for the twin shared environment variable C_T. The relationships between these expected correlations and those expected from the classical twin design are that a^2 in the classical design is heritability under random mating and the classical c^2 is now partitioned into the effects of assortative mating, cultural transmission, genotype-environment covariation, and environmental effects shared by twins (Fulker, 1982).

17.3.3 LISREL 8 Specification of the Model

Cardon *et al.*, (1992) have presented a LISREL formulation of the phenotypic assortment and cultural transmission model. The model is made possible by the recently developed constrained optimization procedure in LISREL 8 (Jöreskog and Sörbom, 1992). This model is illustrated in Figure 17.5. Latent variables are expressed using the same notation as in Figure 17.4. In addition, R_{AM}, R_{AF}, R_{AT1}, R_{AT2}, and R_{CT} represent residual influences on the maternal, paternal, and twin genotypic variables, and the latent environmental variable shared by twins,

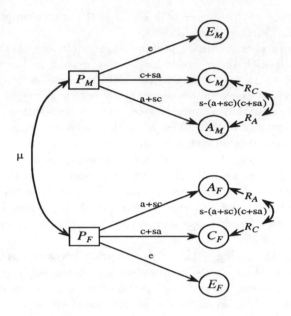

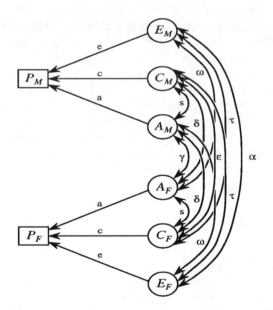

Figure 17.3: Model of assortative mating showing reverse path coefficients (top), and induced correlations among the variables (bottom).

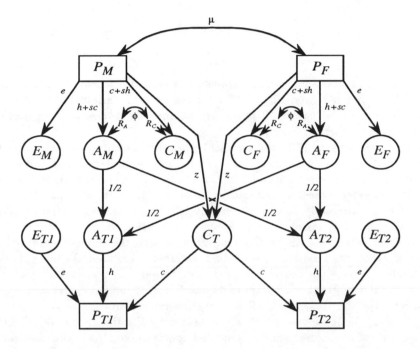

Figure 17.4: Reverse path diagram representing genetic and environmental transmission and assortative mating in twin families.

Table 17.2: Expected correlations between relatives under reverse path model of twins and parents.

Relationship	Algebraic Expression
MZ Twins	$a^2 + c^2 + 2asc$
DZ Twins	$1/2a^2[1 + (a + sc)^2\mu] + c^2 + 2asc$
Spouses	μ
Mother-Offspring	$[1/2a(a + sc) + cz](1 + \mu)$
Father-Offspring	$[1/2a(a + sc) + cz](1 + \mu)$

respectively. Parental shared and unique environmental latent variables (C and E) have been omitted from Figure 17.5 for clarity; the variables do not directly contribute to expected parent-offspring resemblances in reverse path expression of this phenotypic assortment model.

As shown in Figure 17.5, the parental phenotypic values are determined exclusively by the latent ξ variables $(\tilde{P}_M, \tilde{P}_F)$. This formulation has the effect of substituting the observed x variables in LISREL with the latent variables, ξ, which allows the observed parental relationship to be directly estimated as a covariance between the ξ variables.[1] In the present model the estimated covariance between the ξ variables is the unstandardized spousal correlation, μ.

Genotypic values of both parents and offspring and the children's shared environmental values are modeled as the latent variables, η. Parental genotypic values are caused, in reverse path specification, by the "observed" ξ variables. The shared environmental and genotypic values of twins, C_T, A_{T1}, and A_{T2}, respectively, are caused by culturally transmitted effects (z) from the parental phenotypes and from parental genotypic influences which are weighted by the theoretical value, $1/2$.

Observed twin measurements are modeled as y variables. As in the classical twin design, these are determined by the latent genetic variables A_{T1} and A_{T2} and by the shared environmental latent variable C_T. Random environmental variables, E_{T1} and E_{T2}, also influence observed twin measurements but do not affect correlations between twins.

The appropriate measurement model for the parental variables is

$$\begin{pmatrix} P_M \\ P_F \end{pmatrix} = \begin{pmatrix} 1 & 0 \\ 0 & 1 \end{pmatrix} \begin{pmatrix} \tilde{P}_M \\ \tilde{P}_F \end{pmatrix}$$
$$\mathbf{x} \qquad = \qquad \mathbf{\Lambda}_x \qquad \xi$$

The matrix of expected covariances between spouses' phenotypes, $\mathbf{\Sigma}_{x,x}$ is deter-

---

[1] This is similar to the FIxed-x option in LISREL, see Jöreskog and Sörbom (1989), pp. 24-25.

LISREL Variables

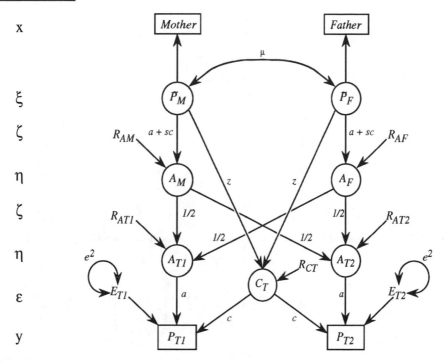

x

ξ

ζ

η

ζ

η

ε

y

Figure 17.5: LISREL model of parental transmission and assortative mating in twin families.

mined by this measurement model:

$$\boldsymbol{\Sigma}_{\mathbf{x,x}} = \boldsymbol{\Lambda}_x \boldsymbol{\Phi} \boldsymbol{\Lambda}'_x$$
$$= \mathbf{I}\boldsymbol{\Phi}\mathbf{I}$$
$$= \boldsymbol{\Phi}$$

where

$$\boldsymbol{\Phi} = \left(\begin{array}{cc} V_{\tilde{P}_M} & \mu \\ \mu & V_{\tilde{P}_F} \end{array} \right)$$

The LISREL structural equation relating latent variables of parents to those of their children is

$$
\begin{pmatrix} A_M \\ A_F \\ A_{T1} \\ C_T \\ A_{T2} \\ \eta \end{pmatrix} = \begin{pmatrix} 0 & 0 & 0 & 0 & 0 \\ 0 & 0 & 0 & 0 & 0 \\ .5 & .5 & 0 & 0 & 0 \\ 0 & 0 & 0 & 0 & 0 \\ .5 & .5 & 0 & 0 & 0 \end{pmatrix} \begin{pmatrix} A_M \\ A_F \\ A_{T1} \\ C_T \\ A_{T2} \\ \eta \end{pmatrix}
$$
$$
\mathbf{B}
$$

$$
+ \begin{pmatrix} a+sc & 0 \\ 0 & a+sc \\ 0 & 0 \\ z & z \\ 0 & 0 \end{pmatrix} \begin{pmatrix} \tilde{P}_M \\ \tilde{P}_F \end{pmatrix} + \begin{pmatrix} R_{A_M} \\ R_{A_F} \\ R_{A_{T1}} \\ R_{C_T} \\ R_{A_{T2}} \end{pmatrix}
$$
$$
\mathbf{\Gamma} \qquad\qquad \boldsymbol{\xi} \qquad\qquad \boldsymbol{\zeta}
$$

which is incorporated into the measurement model for the (DZ) twins' variables:

$$
\begin{pmatrix} P_{T1} \\ P_{T2} \end{pmatrix} = \begin{pmatrix} 0 & 0 & a & c & 0 \\ 0 & 0 & 0 & c & a \end{pmatrix} \begin{pmatrix} A_M \\ A_F \\ A_{T1} \\ C_T \\ A_{T2} \end{pmatrix} + \begin{pmatrix} E_{T1} \\ E_{T2} \end{pmatrix}
$$
$$
\mathbf{y} \qquad = \qquad \mathbf{\Lambda}_{yDZ} \qquad\qquad \boldsymbol{\eta} \qquad + \qquad \boldsymbol{\epsilon}
$$

As in the case of the social homogamy model, the $\mathbf{\Lambda}_y$ matrices differ between the two types of twins because of the difference in genotypic resemblance between MZ and DZ twin pairs. The form of the $\mathbf{\Lambda}_y$ matrix for MZ twins is given by

$$
\mathbf{\Lambda}_{yMZ} = \begin{pmatrix} 0 & 0 & a & c & 0 \\ 0 & 0 & a & c & 0 \end{pmatrix}
$$

The expected covariance matrices between twins and parents and between members of a twin pair are calculated using the parameter matrices just described. These are given in LISREL notation as

$$
\begin{aligned}
\mathbf{\Sigma_{x,y}} &= \mathbf{\Lambda}_x \mathbf{\Phi} \mathbf{\Gamma}' (\mathbf{I} - \mathbf{B}')^{-1} \mathbf{\Lambda}_y' \\
\mathbf{\Sigma_{y,y}} &= \mathbf{\Lambda}_y (\mathbf{I} - \mathbf{B})^{-1} (\mathbf{\Gamma} \mathbf{\Phi} \mathbf{\Gamma}' + \mathbf{\Psi})(\mathbf{I} - \mathbf{B}')^{-1} \mathbf{\Lambda}_y' + \mathbf{\Theta}_\epsilon
\end{aligned}
$$

in which $\mathbf{\Psi}$ is a diagonal matrix of residual effects on the latent variables of twins and parents, $\mathbf{\Theta}_\epsilon$, is a diagonal matrix of random environmental effects. The $\mathbf{\Theta}_\epsilon$ and $\mathbf{\Psi}$ matrices appear as

$$
\mathbf{\Theta}_\epsilon = \begin{pmatrix} e^2 & 0 \\ 0 & e^2 \end{pmatrix}
$$

and

$$\Psi = \begin{pmatrix} 1 - (a+sc)^2 & 0 & 0 \\ 0 & 1 - (a+sc)^2 & 0 \\ 0 & 0 & .5[1-(a+sc)^2\mu] \\ 0 & 0 & 0 \\ 0 & 0 & 0 \end{pmatrix}$$

$$\begin{pmatrix} 0 & 0 \\ 0 & 0 \\ 0 & 0 \\ 1-2z^2(1+\mu) & 0 \\ 0 & .5[1-(a+sc)^2\mu] \end{pmatrix}$$

It is important to recognize that the expressions for the variance/covariance matrices are similar to those listed for the social homogamy model described earlier in this chapter, yet include $(I-B)$ terms which were absent in the previous model. The $(I-B)$ were omitted from the social homogamy expectations because the **B** matrices were assumed to be **0** (i.e., $I-B = I-0 = I$).

17.3.4   Employing Constraints in LISREL

The free and constrained parameters in the path model of phenotypic assortment and cultural transmission are listed in Table 17.3. It can be seen that there are five free parameters in the model: $a+sc$, c, μ, z, and e^2. By allowing these particular parameters to be free, the constraints necessary for model identification may be imposed on other parameters with little difficulty.

The constraint on parameter a represents a derivation of the constraint listed in 17.4 that arises from genotype-environment correlation (s) induced by phenotypic assortative mating. Equation 17.4 can be written as

$$a + sc = a + z(1+\mu)(a+sc)c$$

or

$$a = (a+sc)[1 - cz(1+\mu)] \tag{17.5}$$

which transforms the constraint on s to a similar constraint imposed on a. Equation 17.4 is transformed in this manner in order to eliminate the implicit constraint on s [s is on both sides of 17.4]. Because $a+sc$ is a free parameter in the model the constraint in 17.5 is explicit, thus ensuring accurate function derivatives in LISREL. Although expression of the genotype-environment constraint in this manner eliminates the constrained s parameter from model, the value of s still may be examined in model applications, since s is calculated explicitly by LISREL in a matrix of covariances between the η latent variables. Jöreskog and Sörbom (1989) have described the form of this covariance matrix as $Cov(\eta\eta') = \Pi\Phi\Pi + \Psi^*$, where $\Pi = (I-B)^{-1}\Gamma$ and $\Psi^* = (I-B)^{-1}\Psi(I-B')^{-1}$. The parameter s is given

Table 17.3: Free (F) and constrained (C) parameters in LISREL specification of phenotypic assortment model.

Parameter	Status	Algebraic Constraint	LISREL Constraint
a	C	$(a+sc)[1-cz(1+\mu)]$	$\gamma_{1,1}[1-\lambda_{y_{1,4}}\gamma_{4,1}(1+\phi_{2,1})]$
V_p	C	c^2+e^2+	$\lambda_{y_{1,4}}^2+\theta_{\epsilon_{1,1}}+$
		$(a+sc)^2[1-c^2z^2(1+\mu)^2]$	$\gamma_{1,1}^2[1-\lambda_{y_{1,4}}^2\gamma_{4,1}^2(1+\phi_{2,1})^2]$
ψ_1	C	$1-(a+sc)^2$	$1-\gamma_{1,1}^2$
ψ_2	C	$1-(a+sc)^2$	$1-\gamma_{1,1}^2$
ψ_3	C	$1/2[1-\mu(a+sc)^2]$	$1/2(1-\phi_{2,1}\gamma_{1,1}^2)$
ψ_4	C	$1-2z^2(1+\mu)$	$1-2\gamma_{4,1}^2(1+\phi_{2,1})$
ψ_5	C	$1/2[1-\mu(a+sc)^2]$	$1/2(1-\phi_{2,1}\gamma_{1,1}^2)$
$a+sc$	F		
c	F		
μ	F		
z	F		
e^2	F		

in this matrix as the covariance of latent variables A_T and C_T ($\text{Cov}\eta,\eta_{(3,2)}$), which defines the genotype-environment covariance in standardized form. Calculation of this quantity reveals an equivalent algebraic expression to that listed in 17.4; thus, no information is lost by this constraint transformation.

The constraint imposed on the phenotypic variance (V_p) listed in Table 17.3 arises from the expectation of V_p under the effects of phenotypic assortative mating and cultural transmission shown in 17.2. This constraint is derived by modeling a^2 as the square of 17.5 and calculating the term $2asc$ using 17.4 and 17.5:

$$a^2 = [(a+sc)(1-cz(1+\mu))]^2 \qquad (17.6)$$
$$= (a+sc)^2 - 2cz(a+sc)^2(1+\mu) + c^2z^2(a+sc)^2(1+\mu)^2$$

and

$$2asc = 2(a+sc)[1-cz(1+\mu)]z(1+\mu)(a+sc)c \qquad (17.7)$$
$$= 2[cz(a+sc)^2(1+\mu) - c^2z^2(a+sc)^2(1+\mu)^2]$$

Thus,

$$V_p = c^2+e^2+a^2+2asc \qquad (17.8)$$
$$= c^2+e^2+(a+sc)^2[1-c^2z^2(1+\mu)^2]$$

using 17.6 and 17.7.

For this model of phenotypic assortment and cultural transmission all latent variables have been required to have unit variance in order to ensure appropriate scaling of the model parameters. In LISREL, this requires additional constraints on all η variables. These constraints, listed as $\psi_1 \cdots \psi_5$ in Table 17.3, are calculated as quantities of latent variable variation unexplained by other parameters in the model.

As indicated previously, the constrained correlations between parental genotypes and environments induced by assortative mating are unnecessary under this reverse path model. However, all the values needed for calculation of the $\alpha, \tau, \omega, \delta, \gamma$, and ϵ coefficients listed in 17.3 have been specified in the model. Therefore, the derived values may be calculated easily following application of the model to a particular data set using the parameter estimates generated by LISREL.

As in the social homogamy model, observed twin-parent variances and covariances form 2 (4×4) matrices. Using equation 17.1 with $p_i = 4$ and $n = 5$, the full phenotypic assortment model is shown to have $20 - 5 = 15$ degrees of freedom.

17.3.5 Writing the Constraints in LISREL

Jöreskog and Sörbom (1992) have presented a detailed description of the expressions required for specification of linear and non-linear constraints in LISREL 8. We now briefly review these rules of specification in the context of the present application.

Constraints are written in the LISREL input file on a CO line. Mathematical operators to be used on the CO line follow the general format of the FORTRAN programming language, addition: +, subtraction: –, multiplication: *, and exponentiation: **. Notice that division is only permitted through the use of negative exponents. Continuation statements for long constraint expressions are specified by a C at the end of a line. Only free parameters can appear on the right hand side of an equation (i.e., constraints cannot be recursive or implicit). Parentheses cannot be used anywhere in a CO line except for reference to matrix elements. For example, CO PS(1,1) = LY(2,1)+LY(3,1) is permitted, but CO PS(1,1) = (LY(2,1)+LY(3,1))**2 is not.

Using these rules to express constraints, all those listed in Table 17.3 may be specified in LISREL. It is useful to consider a few examples of the LISREL specification. The simplest constraint in Table 17.3 is that for ψ_1. This constraint appears as:

```
CO PS(1,1) = 1 - GA(1,1)**2
```

The other constraints shown in the table are slightly more complicated because they have been presented in factored form using parentheses. For example, the constraint $\psi_3 = \frac{1}{2}(1 - \phi_{2,1}\gamma_{1,1}^2)$ would be written in the LISREL file as:

```
CO PS(3,3) = .5 - .5*PH(2,1)*GA(1,1)**2
```

and the constraint on a would be specified as:

```
CO LY(1,3) = GA(1,1) - GA(1,1)*LY(1,4)*GA(4,1) - C
   GA(1,1)*LY(1,4)*GA(4,1)*PH(2,1)
```

using the continuation specifier C.

An important consideration in LISREL's handling of constraints is that specification of constrained parameters for multiple groups must be explicit in all groups. For example, to equate the a constraints for both MZ and DZ twin families, the LISREL CO line for a listed above needs to be written for both the MZ and DZ groups. Indeed, all occurrences of a constrained parameter must be explicitly specified; a constraint cannot be imposed upon a parameter and then equated to another parameter by use of the EQuality statement or by the INvariant command on the MOdel card.

We present the LISREL input file for the twin-parent constrained model in Appendix K.2. This model is for use with sample covariance matrices to fit the model by maximum likelihood. Cardon *et al.*, (1991) have presented an additional LISREL formulation of this model that can be used to fit it as a correlation structure to sample correlations matrices by weighted least squares (WLS), which requires an estimate of the asymptotic covariance matrix of the sample correlations such as that which may be obtained by PRELIS.

17.4   Illustration of Twin-Parent Models

In order to illustrate the LISREL parent-twin models, they were applied to questionnaire data from the Fear Survey Schedule II (FSS-II; Geer 1965) administered to 144 MZ twin families and 106 DZ twin families. A full description of the sample and of data ascertainment has been presented by Rose and Ditto (1983). The specific measure analyzed here is a composite of items assessing fear of meeting people, attending public events, and feelings of self-consciousness, labelled "fear of social criticism" in an earlier analysis of these data by Neale and Fulker (1984). Sample correlation matrices and observed variances from the MZ and DZ families are presented in Table 17.4.

We initially describe the results from application of the phenotypic assortment model to these data, then discuss results from the social homogamy model and the differences in outcomes from the models.

17.4.1   Phenotypic Assortment Model Results

Free, constrained, and derived parameter estimates resulting from application of the full model are given in Table 17.5, together with the standard errors of the estimates. The non-significant chi-square value indicates an adequate fit of the model to the data ($\chi^2_{15} = 14.05, p = .52$). All free parameters in the model are

Table 17.4: Observed twin-parent correlations for fear of social criticism (MZ: upper triangle; DZ: lower triangle; variances on diagonals).

	Twin 1	Twin 2	Mother	Father	
	.95	.54	.08	.28	Twin 1
		.89	.21	.18	Twin 2
Twin 1	1.21		1.11	.11	Mother
Twin 2	.29	1.03		.90	Father
Mother	.23	.16	.91		
Father	.13	.09	.21	1.08	

significantly different from zero with the exception of z, suggesting negligible effects of cultural transmission and an absence of genotype-environment correlation.

The negative estimate of z reflects the fact that observed parent-twin resemblance is lower than that expected from estimates of heritability obtained from the twins. Data in which estimates of genetic effects from parent offspring resemblance are smaller than those obtained from MZ/DZ twin comparisons, such as the data presently examined, will often yield negative estimates of cultural transmission in order to compensate for the apparent differences in genetic effects between the various familial relationships. Because the negative estimate of z appears non-significant in the full model, we fit a reduced LISREL model to the data in which the effects of cultural transmission on fear of social criticism were omitted.

The reduced model was specified by eliminating all portions of constraint equations having the term z. Specifically, the constraint on ψ_4 was omitted and the LISREL parameter PS(4,4) fixed at 1.0, the phenotypic variance constraints (V_p) were reduced by removing terms in the equations containing the parameter GA(4,1), and the constraints on a were relaxed [LY(1,3) and LY(2,5) for DZ twins; LY(1,3) and LY(2,3) for MZ twins]. It is important to recognize that elimination of cultural transmission, z, from the model is necessarily accompanied by elimination of genotype-environment covariance, s (see equation 17.4). Thus, relaxation of the a constraints LISREL requires that the parameters corresponding to a be equated to those representing $a + sc$ [DZ twins: EQ GA(1,1) LY(1,3) LY(2,5); MZ twins: EQ GA(1,1,1) LY(1,3) LY(2,3)].

Parameter estimates from the reduced LISREL model are presented in Table 17.5 with those obtained from the fit of the full model. The reduced model fits the data well ($\chi^2_{16} = 16.40, p = .43$) and is not significantly different from the full model (comparison $\chi^2_1 = 2.35, p > .10$). Parameter estimates indicate that genetic and shared environmental influences account for a considerable portion of the phenotypic variation, 32% and 19%, respectively, and that nearly 50% of the

Table 17.5: Parameter estimates from full and reduced phenotypic assortment models of twin family resemblance for fear of social criticism.

Parameter	Free Parameters Model Full	Reduced	Parameter	Constrained Parameters Model Full	Reduced
$a + sc$	.69(.07)	.57(.05)	a	.79	.57
c	.32(.12)	.44(.08)	V_p	1.01	1.00
μ	.15(.06)	.15(.06)	ψ_1	.52	.67
z	-.40(.37)	–	ψ_2	.52	.67
e^2	.44(.05)	.49(.05)	ψ_3	.46	.48
			ψ_4	.62	1.00
			ψ_5	.46	.48
			s	-.32	–
			δ	.01	.04
			γ	.07	.05
			ϵ	.00	.03
			α	.07	.07
			τ	.01	.05
			ω	.07	.06

Note: Standard Errors in Parentheses

total variance may be attributed to environmental factors unshared by twins. The effects of phenotypic assortative mating on fear of social criticism appear moderate ($\mu = .15$).

These results illustrate the advantage of analyzing parent and twin data over analyses using the classical twin design. For these fear of social criticism data, the classical twin design would yield a^2, c^2, and e^2 estimates of .50, .04, and .46, respectively. In comparison to the present parent-twin model, the classical a^2 estimate appears to be an overestimate of the proportion of observed variance attributable to genetic factors, whereas the estimate of c^2 in the classical design appears underestimated. The addition of parental data to that of twins is all that is needed to elucidate the sources of these biases.

17.4.2   Social Homogamy Model Results

Application of the full social homogamy model to the fear of social criticism data generated a χ^2_{13} value of 15.03, which suggests an adequate fit to the data ($p = .31$). However, the LISREL application required over 200 iterations to converge and parameter estimates indicate that the social homogamy formulation is ill-conditioned as regards these data. The parameter estimates from this model are shown in Table 17.6, although we note that these estimates should not be taken at all seriously because of problems encountered by LISREL. These problems are discussed presently.

Table 17.6: Parameter estimates from full social homogamy model of twin family resemblance for fear of social criticism.

Parameter	Estimate
a	.781
c	.026
e^2	.412
m	-.844
f	-.691
μ	263.565
r^2	-305.362

As may be seen in Table 17.6, estimates of the classical twin-design parameters appear reasonable: $a = .78$, $c = .03$, and $e^2 = .41$, yet other parameter estimates are completely unrealistic, particularly $\mu = 263.57$ and $r^2 = -305.36$! The primary problem in this application is that the social homogamy model requires substantial c^2 effects and spousal correlations from the data in order to provide a feasible solution, but the fear of social criticism correlations do not conform to these model requirements.

The expected correlation between spouses ($r_{PM,PF}$) is given in Table 17.1 as $c^2\mu$. Upon rearrangement, this expectation yields the expression for μ, the correlation between spouses' environments:

$$\mu = \frac{r_{PM,PF}}{c^2} \qquad (17.9)$$

Because μ is a correlation, bounded by ± 1.0, it can be seen from 17.9 that the spousal correlation must be less than or equal to the environmental effects to provide a reasonable estimate of μ. If $r_{PM,PF} > c^2$, μ exceeds 1.0 and the problem becomes non-feasible. At the other extreme, if shared environmental effects are absent from the data, the assortment parameter is undefined ($\mu = r_{PM,PF}/0$).

We noted previously that a classical twin-design analysis of the present data would yield a c^2 estimate of .04. The weighted average of the spousal correlations in these data is $\approx .17$. Simple comparison or these correlations suggests that μ exceeds its boundary ($r_{PM,PF}/c^2 = .17/.04 = 4.25$). Indeed, in the LISREL application, c^2 was estimated to be .00068, thus necessitating an extremely large μ estimate to account for the spousal correlation of $c^2\mu \approx .17$.

In this application, the large μ value further compounds the problem in LISREL. We have stated that residual twin environmental effects are modeled as $r^2 = 1 - m^2 - f^2 - 2mf\mu$ in the social homogamy specification. For the fear of social criticism data, the last term in this equation is very large because of the large μ estimate, which results in an unrealistic r^2 value < 0.0. In short, the full social homogamy model and the fear of social criticism data are incompatible.

These results should not be interpreted as evidence against the general utility of the social homogamy model for analysis of twin-parent data. Rather, they serve to show that the social homogamy model is designed for specific types of data — primarily those which are substantially influenced by environmental effects. In these domains the social homogamy specification has proved to be quite informative (e.g., Rao et al., 1982). What is interesting, however, is that we are able to choose between models using LISREL, not on the basis of χ^2 statistics, but on the internal consistency of the outcomes. Clearly for these data one model is much more plausible that the other.

17.5   Summary

In this chapter we have presented two twin-parent models which may be easily formulated in LISREL: a social homogamy specification including one form of cultural transmission and a model of phenotypic assortative mating including an alternative form of cultural transmission. In the development and application of the models to data concerning fear of social criticism we have attempted to illustrate the point made by Eaves et al. (1989) that extension of the classical twin design to include parental measurements can be used to elucidate sources of variation which are confounded in analyses of twin data alone. In addition, the applications have illustrated that the social homogamy and phenotypic assortment models are not interchangeable in terms of expectations or outcomes.

The social homogamy model represents a simple method for analyzing twin-parent data. The LISREL formulation is easy to implement and may be carried out using any extant version of the LISREL package. The social homogamy model provides valuable information about cultural and genetic determinants of behavior when applied to variables that may be strongly influenced from environmental factors, such as social class, religion, and geography (Morton, 1982). The social homogamy model also is extremely useful for analysis of variables in which assortative mating does not occur on the basis of observed traits, for example, spousal correlations for lipid concentrations (Rao et al., 1982).

Although slightly more difficult to implement in LISREL, the phenotypic assortment model represents a more general and numerically robust method for examination of twin and parent data than the social homogamy specification. The model is quite useful for analysis of behavioral traits in which mate selection is determined by the visible characteristics of the trait, such as stature or perhaps general intelligence. In addition, the model aids in exploring environmental effects on twins which arise from the general characteristics of their parents and provides a means by which correlations between genetic and environmental sources of variation may be examined.

We would like to emphasize that whichever model one chooses to employ, the addition of parental data to twin measurements is all that is needed to resolve the model complexities. The inclusion of such data allows one to disentangle sources of variation that are confounded in the classical twin design and explicitly assess the roles of mate selection and cultural transmission in the determination of human behaviors.

We conclude this chapter by noting that the linear and nonlinear constrained optimization procedure, which made possible the present formulation of the phenotypic assortment model, has only recently been incorporated into LISREL. The simplicity and efficiency of the constrained optimization procedure is certain to be valuable for application of the many biometrical models of various kinships which have previously required considerable time, effort, and expertise in computer programming. In principle, multivariate extensions of the designs described in this chapter could be implemented in LISREL, although the specification of constraints would be very complex. Perhaps future developments of the LISREL program will make these extensions feasible.

Chapter 18

Future Directions

Throughout this volume it has been our intention to lay the groundwork for future research by building simple models and operationalizing them via matrix algebra and LISREL scripts, which are available not only as hard copy in the appendices to this volume, but also as public domain software on Internet. We hope that placing these tools in the hands of the research community will maximize the quality and the quantity of analysis of human variation in as many areas as possible. A second hope is that researchers will be able to modify the prescribed models so that they test the most salient hypotheses in their field of study with maximum statistical rigor. To facilitate this process we shall (i) review the range of the existing approaches; and (ii) discuss strategies for extending them to new data structures. While a full description of these further methods cannot be given here, we aim to provide references to the relevant literature where available, and to indicate which software (if any) may be suitable for the application.

18.1 Issues Addressed in This Volume

We discussed the intended scope of this book in some detail in Chapter 1, particularly in Section 1.4 in which the general types of genetic and environmental effects were described. Here we review the utility of using LISREL to implement these models and to test hypotheses.

18.1.1 Linear Modeling

Our exclusive focus has been on *linear models* which suppose that the relationship between genotype, environment, and phenotype is extremely simple: for a given change in genotypic or environmental value there will be a corresponding change in the phenotype value. The amount of this change is constant, regardless of the values of the other variables in the system. Many would argue (and we would agree) that the functional relationships between many behavioral variables eventually will prove to be more complex. Yet linear models provide an excellent starting point for understanding individual differences, *because* of their simplicity, not in spite of it. Simple models are highly prized in science (Popper, 1961); they are easy to falsify, easy to communicate, and may predict most efficiently. For non-linear relationships such as cubic, logistic or cumulative normal functions, linear models may characterize most of the variance in the system, and make useful predictions of other phenomena, despite being incorrect. Some may argue that phenomena as complex as human behavior would seem *a priori* unlikely to be generated by simple linear models. While this may be the case for certain variables, we should note that recent work on cellular automata (see Wolfram, 1986) and chaos theory (Hao, 1984; Casti, 1989) indicates that very complex behavior can arise from very simple models.

One of the advantages of using linear models is that there are several ways in which they can be expressed in a mathematically complete form. The first is as a set of linear equations, for example:

$$y_1 = aA_1 + eE_1$$
$$y_2 = aA_2 + eE_2.$$

While complete, this expression becomes tedious when there are many variables in the system. The use of matrix algebra to refer to entire sets of linear equations is a natural extension of this approach; thus we may write:

$$y = \Gamma \xi.$$

A third method is to use a complete graph of the system, the path diagram. This procedure has been used extensively in this book, and for many people is a very efficient medium for conveying the basic structure of a model, in which case the path coefficients are usually drawn as letters. A second application of these graphics (though not used here) is to communicate model fitting results with a path diagram by placing parameter estimates on the paths. Version 8 of LISREL has incorporated this feature, printing t-values and standard errors on the paths in addition to the parameter estimates, and allowing sub-models to be fitted by deleting selected paths from diagram shown on the computer screen. This feature also has been usefully extended in the RAMPATH software (McArdle and Boker, 1990) in which the values of parameter estimates are divided by their standard errors and these quotients may be used to adjust the thickness of the lines. Although the result is not always aesthetically pleasing, it does provide a means for rapidly finding the salient aspects of the data, and we would encourage the binding of such interactive graphical devices to model-fitting software.

Non-linear models are becoming more common in modern psychometrics. For example, Kenny and Judd (1975) describe two-variable models for the effects not only of latent variables X and Y but also for those of X^2 and XY. A similar treatment in a genetic context has been described by Molenaar *et al.* (1990). These models imply certain non-linear constraints among the parameters describing the variances and covariances of the latent variables, which Kenny and Judd showed could be applied in the COSAN program (Fraser, 1988). Hayduk (1987) has shown how these models may be fitted using LISREL 6, though the treatment is far from simple. More complex models such as these become very difficult to fit using the commercial packages. The advent of LISREL 8 with its constraint functions will simplify this approach, but judging by the example using non-linear constraints to model assortative mating and cultural transmission (Chapter 17) the methods will not be easy to modify nor simple to generalize for multivariate data.

18.1.2 Univariate Genetic Analysis

Quite clearly the LISREL model is useful for univariate analysis of twin data. The simple uniform structure of the data makes them ideal for the regular multigroup structure that LISREL offers. The general formulation for η-variables is convenient for testing for the effects of sibling interaction (see Chapter 10). It also would be very straightforward to include other types of pairs of collateral relatives such as cousins, half-siblings, twins or siblings separated at birth, and so on. Although we have not examined these relationships in this book, such data could be used to resolve the effects of shared environment and non-additive genetic effects, and are therefore extremely valuable as a first step away from the classical twin study. However, unlike twins, these other relationships do not always occur as pairs, which introduces an additional complication to their analysis (see Section 18.2.2 below).

Univariate genetic analysis with LISREL is not limited to the ideal but elusive normally-distributed variable. If we are prepared to assume that there is a continuous normal distribution of liability underlying measurements on a less regular scale, then the use of polychoric correlation matrices with an appropriate weight matrix is asymptotically correct. These methods do require large samples, preferably more than 200 pairs in each group (Jöreskog and Sörbom, 1988). Furthermore, as we have seen in Chapter 9, the loss of power with dichotomous variables can be considerable, with quite large samples being unable to reject models of either completely environmental or completely genetic covariance between relatives.

In the early days of biometrical model fitting, tests for homogeneity of means between groups were usually performed prior to covariance analysis. Today they are often forgotten in the rush to test the hypotheses that were the *raison d'être* of the twin study in the first place. Nevertheless, tests of means can provide important clues to the effects of sampling biases. For example, if the process of MZ twinning involved neurological deficits that affected cognitive performance, then one would expect a lower mean IQ for MZ than DZ twins. Ideally one would like to control for these effects before proceeding with genetic analysis. Fortunately, it is possible to test for mean differences between groups within LISREL (Section 8.7; see McArdle, 1986), thus unifying these two parts of data analysis.

The same types of mean tests are desirable for the analysis of discontinuous data. Consider the example of handedness. Suppose that a large proportion of MZ twin pairs exhibited "mirror-imaging" in which the pairs had opposite handedness. Given that only about 10% of individuals in most populations exhibit left-handedness (McManus, 1980; Annette, 1978) the mirror-imaging phenomenon should lead to increased rates of left-handedness in MZ twins, which would be manifested by a different threshold between MZ and DZ twins. Group differences in thresholds are not easy to test with the PRELIS-LISREL combination. PRELIS allows constraints within a group (so Twin 1 would have the same threshold as Twin 2) but not across groups. For the same reason, fitting models of sibling interaction, which predict group differences in total variance, to ordinal data is not practical with PRELIS and LISREL. With these problems it may be better to fit to the raw data, which may be summarized as a contingency table (see Sections 18.3.2 and 18.2.1 below).

18.1.3 Multivariate Genetic Analysis

In Chapters 12, 13, and 16 we showed how a variety of multivariate models may be fitted to data collected from twins. In basic multivariate genetic analysis, several different models may be used to decompose or simplify each source of variation. One type of model is the triangular or Cholesky decomposition which completely characterizes the covariance structure of the source of variance in question (see Section 12.4.2). The second type of model consists of (i) one or more general factors that affect all variables, and (ii) specific factors that affect only one variable (Section 12.3.4). A third type is the 'latent phenotypes' model in which genetic and environmental factors act through a common latent variable to produce variation and covariation in the observed variables. While these models are simple enough to implement when the number of variables is small, it becomes tedious (and hence error-prone) to change a model for, say 10 variables, to one for 11 variables. In addition, as we expand our analyses to include more and more variables, we run the risk of reducing our sample size since there is usually some chance that data will not be available for any particular item or variable. LISREL does not offer a method of dealing with incomplete data of this type, other than listwise deletion of incomplete cases which can lead to drastic decreases in the effective sample size. Nevertheless, initially at least, LISREL provides a powerful system for multivariate genetic analysis. Those wishing to work with large numbers of variables may turn to a formal programming language such as FORTRAN of C, or use the recently developed Mx package (Section 18.3.2).

18.1.4 Analysis of Repeated Measures

In Chapters 14 and 15 we described models for data collected from the same individuals on more than one occasion. The tremendous power of these data lies in the use of the *a priori* definition of causal processes: that for A to cause B, A must occur before B. Thus, data collected on one variable at several time points might be seen as a long causal chain, in which the direction of causation is *known*. Unlike multivariate data, we can immediately eliminate all causal processes except those going forward in time. We cannot eliminate the possibility of a general factor, so analyses of repeated measures typically incorporate both general factors and occasion-to-occasion transmission. Modeling these processes is relatively straightforward in LISREL, and univariate longitudinal data analysis does not impose too great a hardship when the number of occasions is increased. However, extending the models to repeated measures of more than one variable is quite demanding with LISREL, as it becomes difficult to add or delete variables for analysis.

The structure of longitudinal data shares certain characteristics with multivariate data, and our modeling is subject to similar limitations. We can discriminate between two basic forms of repeated measures data:

- *Single occasion* where repeated measures of the same variable are made during the same testing session, interview or questionnaire, e.g., heart rate at one minute intervals during exercise

- *Multiple occasion* where repeated measures are made on several different occasions, e.g., two waves of questionnaires, or annual laboratory visits.

The problem of missing data often may be *less* acute for single occasion repeated measures than it is for general multivariate data. Typically, missing data arise because a subject is unwilling or unable to answer or take part in a particular test. For repeated measures of the same test on the same occasion, subjects are likely to take part in all or none of the assessments. Although boredom and fatigue may increase the chance of missing data after several trials, most studies are designed not to suffer from this type of attrition. For multiple occasion repeated measures, however, the problem of missing data often is *more* acute than it is for general multivariate data, simply because subjects may be unwilling or unable to attend more than one occasion. The problem of missing data is discussed below in Section 18.2.2.

18.1.5 Measurement

Measurement is fundamental to science, so it is no surprise to find that it plays a key role in the use of twins and family members to study human variation. In Chapter 2 we described methods for obtaining suitable data summaries of both continuous and ordinal data. It should be clear that the PRELIS-LISREL combination is extremely useful for data sets incorporating either continuous or ordinal variables or both. We note (see Section 9.3) that there is a great loss of statistical power when dealing with categorical variables, so investigators are urged to obtain continuous, normally distributed data whenever possible. Ideally, such data should come from homogeneous items loading on the same dimension. Yet in practice, this may be difficult or impossible to achieve, especially in the first genetic study in any particular area. It is not possible to discriminate between the 'psychometric factors' model and the 'biometric factors model' (Chapter 16) without genetically informative data, yet conventional factor analysis tacitly assumes a psychometric factor or latent phenotype model. Thus, although genetically uninformative studies of unrelated individuals may be used to construct scales that in turn give rise to factor loadings which may be used to derive normally distributed factor scores for each individual, this scale may itself be heterogeneous, containing, for example, some genetic items and some shared environment items. These considerations have given rise to the development of genetic factor analysis (Heath *et al* 1989a)..

While we have considered ordinal and continuous variables, it is less clear how to deal with categorical variables that cannot be ordered reasonably. For example, although one could order the data from an item such as "How often do you play sports," and compute the polychoric correlation for twin resemblance of athletic interest, it is not so obvious how to deal with an item like "What is your favorite sport?" Intrinsically we don't have an interval or ratio scale for sport preference, so there is no way to rank, e.g. soccer, above or below tennis[1]. Nevertheless, we might observe that MZ twins are more often concordant for sport preference than DZ twins, and might wish to quantify this difference. There are a variety of measures of association for such data; one used by Eaves *et al.* (1990) in the context of religious affiliation is the U statistic (Goodman and Kruskal, 1979). However, the relationship between the model and the mathematics used to derive the measure of association is less straightforward than usual. In many analyses we are simply using the central limit theorem to predict that variables are normally distributed because variation arises from the additive action of a large number of factors, genetic or environmental in origin. When we use the U statistic, we lose this parametric assumption. Were the analysis of categorical data to become an area of broad interest, additional methodological work would be required — preferably including simulation of data under precisely defined mathematical models, followed by estimation in the hope of recovering the true model with some fidelity.

18.2   Issues Beyond LISREL

One of the primary reasons that LISREL is popular is because it saves time. The user does not require extensive knowledge of optimization software, nor of how to compute the particular loss function desired. Instead, he or she may focus effort on precise specification of the linear model for the data, and on the results of the analysis. By restricting the matrix specification for the model to one form (Equation 6.4) the great numerical advantage of having explicit first and second derivatives of the

---

[1] We might rank sports for the amount of stamina required, and thus make an ordinal ranking, but there is no guarantee that this is the factor used by the subject to select this particular sport. Here we simply wish to study the choice itself, irrespective of possible scalings that could be applied.

fitting function is obtained (Jöreskog, 1973; Hayduk, 1987, pp. 155-156). These derivatives are valuable not simply because they increase the speed of optimization (compared to using numerical estimates of the derivatives), but also because they permit accurate calculation of standard errors and modification indices [2]. Again the user saves time because there is no need to learn how to compute these quantities, nor is there a need to learn a programming language to calculate them. The same applies for the wide variety of goodness-of-fit statistics available in LISREL. Use of the β-test version of LISREL 8 reveals a wide array of goodness-of-fit indices, which are subject to periodic critical review (e.g. Browne and Cudeck, 1988; Marsh *et al.* 1988; Bollen 1989, Mulaik *et al* 1989; Kaplan, 1990). There is some controversy over which is the best, some preferring indices that are independent of sample size, some favoring parsimony and so on. This is not the place for a review of these methods; they have been used sparingly in genetic modeling perhaps because of the stronger theoretical basis for the revision and comparison of models. The situation may change however, as more multivariate models become popular and a larger number of multivariate datasets are assembled. Model selection based on Akaike's Information Criterion (AIC; Akaike, 1987) seems often to concur with the preference of experienced researchers. Even for relatively large studies, the confidence intervals of the χ^2 and related statistics are often frighteningly large, so a tad more caution would seem wise when drawing substantive conclusions, however exciting they may be.

A very wide class of models is encompassed by the LISREL model. Perhaps the key element to its generality is the $(\mathbf{I} - \mathbf{B})^{-1}$ component of the formulation. Within $\mathbf{B}$ it is possible to specify both recursive and non-recursive elements to any degree (as shown by McArdle and McDonald, 1984). Thus, a model incorporating 1000 different variables in one long causal chain could be handled within the $\mathbf{B}$ matrix. The only limitations are computer workspace and user patience in setting up the model. The computer workspace issue was critical for many years within the MS-DOS environment, making models with as few as 17 latent variables too large for available memory. Fortunately with the advent of 386 hardware technology, this restriction has been lifted; DOS extender versions of PRELIS and LISREL are now available, which will make use of memory above the 640K limit imposed by hardware and software designers in the 1970's. In addition, LISREL is available for several mainframes, and versions for certain workstation platforms are being developed. In principle, therefore, we can fit any linear model using LISREL. However, in practice we may encounter data structures that are not readily accommodated within the LISREL package. We may also develop models that are awkward to implement with LISREL, or time-consuming to change from an application with n

---

[2]LISREL will calculate the expected decrease in χ^2 that could be obtained by freeing any of the fixed elements in the component matrices in the model. We have not emphasized this approach because in studies of relatives the parameters of interest would normally be freed simultaneously for all relatives in all groups, subject to equality constraints (e.g. all four c paths for MZ and DZ twins). The expected improvement in fit from such a respecification cannot be estimated using modification indices in LISREL.

variables to another with $n + 1$ variables.

18.2.1   Ascertainment and Selection Effects

The applications described in this book tacitly assume that the data have been collected from groups (usually pairs) of relatives sampled at random from the population. While this seems to be the most widely used approach for collecting genetically informative data, it is not always the most efficient. For rare disorders it is likely to be more efficient to ascertain affected individuals and then examine their relatives. As long as we are regular and consistent in our method of ascertainment, it is usually possible to derive an appropriate statistical correction in order to compute the likelihood. We shall not give an exhaustive description of these techniques here, but simply try to demonstrate the principles involved.

Power calculations have shown that the error of a tetrachoric correlation calculated from a 2×2 contingency table is much greater than the error of a correlation calculated from a continuous variable (see Section 9). The loss of power associated with this change of measurement corresponds approximately to a three-fold increase in required sample sizes when the threshold divides the population into two equal parts. Further power loss occurs as the threshold diverges from the mean. For example, suppose we fit a false model of common and specific environmental effects, with no additive genetic effects, when the true model comprises 50% additive genetic, 0% shared environment, and 50% specific environment effects. Using equal numbers of MZ and DZ twin pairs, the sample sizes required for 90% power to reject the false model (at the .05 significance level) are: 428 for a continuous variable, 1,326 for a two-category measure with 50% of the population in each category, 3,659 for 10% above threshold, and 40,085 for 1% above threshold. However, if we have a precise estimate of the threshold, we can use proband ascertained samples and avoid measuring the majority of subjects that lie in the concordant normal cell of the contingency table. For thresholds at 50%, 10%, and 1%, the corresponding total numbers of twin pairs required become 1,325, 453, and 396, respectively. Thus, for studies directed at the analysis of a single outcome with prevalence of less than 50%, proband ascertainment can be very efficient.

If data have been collected from a non-randomly sampled population, covariances calculated from the observed sample will be biased (Martin and Wilson, 1982; Neale et al., 1989). However, it is often possible to correct for the effects of ascertainment. Conceptually, as we omit certain classes of subjects from observation, the likelihood of observing the remaining individuals increases. Mathematically, correction for ascertainment involves dividing the likelihood by the proportion of the population remaining after ascertainment. We obtain this proportion by subtracting the proportions in all omitted classes from the total population proportion (i.e., 1.0). For example, in pairs of relatives selected because individual 1 is above threshold, the proportion omitted is

$$
\begin{aligned}
L_{\tilde{A}} &= \int_{-\infty}^{t}\int_{-\infty}^{t} \phi(v_1, v_2)\, dv_2 dv_1 + \int_{-\infty}^{t}\int_{t}^{\infty} \phi(v_1, v_2)\, dv_2 dv_1 \\
&= \int_{-\infty}^{t} \phi(v_1)\, dv_1
\end{aligned}
\tag{18.1}
$$

The likelihood corrected for ascertainment would be simply the likelihood as obtained before, but divided by $1 - L_{\tilde{A}}$. In general, supposing that we have excluded more than one class of subjects from measurement, we should correct the likelihood function for the non-random sampling by dividing it by $1 - \sum_{i=1}^{k} \tilde{a}_i$ where k is the number of missing cells, $\tilde{a}_i$. For this particular example, we have assumed *complete ascertainment* because all pairs with at least one affected individual have been obtained.

Another common ascertainment scheme is called *single ascertainment*. Essentially, the investigator finds a collection of probands (e.g., from hospital records) and assesses their relatives. Assuming that none of the probands is also a relative (i.e., there is no double ascertainment) then effectively two cells have been omitted from the contingency table — if the proband is unaffected then neither affected nor normal relatives will be observed. Single ascertainment and complete ascertainment define two extremes of a continuum of possible ascertainment schemes[3]:

1. $\pi \to 0$: A sample of probands is ascertained and there is no additional probability of ascertaining concordant pairs. *'Single Incomplete Ascertainment'*

2. $\pi \to 1$: Exhaustive search is conducted to ascertain every affected person in a population. *'Complete Ascertainment'*

3. $0 < \pi < 1$: There is some increased probability of ascertainment for concordant pairs, a proportion of which are ascertained more than once. *'Multiple Incomplete Ascertainment'*

The first two situations translate to specifying one of the discordant groups as either missing (1), or not (2). Representation of the third situation may be achieved by separating the data into two groups, one where there is single incomplete ascertainment, and one where there is complete ascertainment. The relative magnitude of these groups confers information about the parameter π.

Although it is fairly simple to write software to fit models to these data, it becomes more difficult to handle multivariate ordinal data. As the number of variables increases, we are faced with the "curse of dimensionality" because numerical integration of the truncated multivariate normal becomes very cpu-intensive. However, if ascertainment is based on one ordinal measure, and any additional variables of interest are continuous, then no such practical limitation is encountered. In practise there seems to be no way to deal with these data within the LISREL-PRELIS

---

[3]We use the term π to represent the probability of ascertaining concordant pairs.

package. As an alternative we may look towards writing our own code in FOR-
TRAN or C, or to using the Mx package.

18.2.2   Unbalanced Data Structures

Unlike the analysis of data collected from single population of unrelated individuals, the analysis of genetically informative data is fraught with problems that lead
to missing data. We encountered such data in Section 8.8, in which some twin
pairs were discordant for participation in the study. LISREL's multigroup features
seem to have been developed for the purpose of testing for heterogeneity of covariance or mean structures between different populations measured on the same set of
variables. Yet almost immediately in genetic analysis we are faced with data that
do not conform to this regular structure. In Section 8.8 we used a combination
of dummy variables and adjustments of the degrees of freedom in order to accommodate the different group sizes. This is practical in LISREL, and allows some
preliminary tests of the effects of sampling bias, if not for testing of models thereof
(Neale and Eaves, 1992). However, as our pedigree structures grow, to include for
example sibships of different size or twins and other relatives, the number of group
types increases and the practicality of using LISREL to fit models to these data
diminishes. These problems are exacerbated when we wish to analyze multivariate
or longitudinal data.

A further difficulty arises when the sample size of groups with certain patterns
of missing data become small. For data that are expensive to collect, we would
not wish to omit them from analysis, but might easily find that the sample size
was less than the number of variables measured, leading to a a non-positive definite
observed covariance matrix. One way to circumvent this obstacle is to use moment,
rather than covariance, matrices. Another approach is to fit directly to the raw
data by maximum likelihood (see Chapter 7, page 141). LISREL allows one to
read in raw data but it uses *listwise deletion* so that if data on any variable is
missing, that case (subject, twin pair, or family) will be excluded from analysis.
Apart from being wasteful of data, this method is open to question if the missing
data are not missing at random. If those cases so removed were not a random
sample, the remaining observations excluding them would no longer be random,
and parameter estimates and tests of significance would therefore be biased (see
Little and Rubin (1987) for a thorough discussion of bias due to missing data).
Again for a solution to these problems we may write our own FORTRAN or C
code, or use Mx.

So what happens when our studies are extensive in several ways? What if we
have a large number of subjects forming large pedigrees, who may be measured on a
large number of occasions on a large number of variables? While this scenario might
seem like a behavioral geneticist's fantasy, several data sets of this type already
exist. One has been collected in Virginia from approximately 30,000 twins and
their relatives on a variety of health-related items (Truett *et al.*, 1992). Another

concerns weight and measures of cardiac function collected in Norway as part of a national screening (Tambs *et al.*, 1991). Such data sets put the greatest demand on our computing resources, both hardware and software. At the time of writing, there seems to be no practical and statistically 'correct' ways of handling these data sets. In theory, maximum likelihood is appropriate for continuous multivariate normal data, but in practice the optimization of the likelihood function is prohibitively slow for these vast data sets, especially if the whole data set cannot be held in memory.

The approach adopted by Truett *et al.* is to compute correlations between all possible pairs of relatives of a given type. This procedure gives too much weight to those observations from large pedigrees, since the same individual will appear several times within the same statistic (for example a sibship of size 5 will contribute 10 pairs to the correlation). However, if the sibling correlation is the same regardless of sibship size, which is to be expected under most models of gene and environment action (except sibling interaction), then the correlations obtained from this procedure should be unbiased. Their precision cannot be considered to be as great as the apparent sample size, because one individual may contribute to more than one pair. A further problem is that the correlations are not independent of one another, because, for example, the same individual who contributes to a sibling correlation may also contribute to a parent-offspring correlation and an uncle-niece correlation and so on. One possible solution would be to estimate the correlations and their variance-covariance matrix once by maximum likelihood, and then use these statistics for weighted least-squares estimation. Another may be to try to get close to the solution by using the correlations, and then switch to maximum likelihood estimation for the final few iterations. More complete exploration of these methods is desirable, but cannot be addressed in this introductory text.

18.2.3 Data-Specific Models

We now turn to a class of problems that has received scant attention in this book or in the mathematical genetics literature to date. We call them "data-specific models" because certain measured variables are used to fix parameters of the model. In fact, throughout this text we have been employing this method to identify genetic models based on twin data. Effectively, we measure the zygosity of the twin pairs and use this to fix the correlation between the genotypes at 1.0 or 0.5, according to whether the twins are MZ or DZ. We will describe how this principle can be extended to provide solutions to a number of related problems.

Suppose that we wish to test the hypothesis that there is reciprocal sibling interaction for alcohol use. At first glance we might think to use the methods outlined in Chapter 10 of this volume. But suppose we are looking at an adult sample, consisting of some pairs that have been cohabiting for the past 20 years, and some who have been living apart, with little contact between cotwins since the age of 18. Under these circumstances, the basic sibling interaction model assumes that all interaction took place prior to the time of separation. In our data the presence of twins who separated at age 18 will have diluted the effects of any subsequent interaction in those still cohabiting. The natural next step would be to split the twin pairs into four groups: MZ cohabiting, DZ cohabiting, MZ separated, and DZ separated, and fit a model with two sibling interaction parameters, one for the cohabiting groups and one for the separated groups. If these two parameters could be equated then we would conclude that the available data do not reject the hypothesis of no sibling interaction relevant to alcohol consumption taking place after age 18. We could fit this type of model in LISREL.

Unfortunately, in the real world we are often faced with more than the simple two-class discrimination just described. For example, it would be quite possible to encounter pairs with anything from 0 to 40 years of cohabitation since the age of 18 years. When we have a continuous measure of cohabitation, how might we examine sibling interaction? This is difficult because as we encounter an increasing number of cohabitation values, our sample size becomes smaller for each particular value observed. Finally, we are faced with data in which each pair has its own unique value and thus *each pair requires its own model*. Hopper and Mathews (1983) described the theory behind analysis of this type of data but there seems to be no packaged software available for models of this type. For the time being we would recommend either (i) ordering the data into a sufficiently small number of categories to leave at least moderate sample sizes within each category, or (ii) developing FORTRAN programs, perhaps in conjunction with the FISHER library of routines, specifically for the problem at hand.

It seems likely that data-specific models will be appropriate in a variety of different contexts. Although the discrete measure of gender seems reasonable for analysis, since existing techniques are capable of resolving genotype × sex interaction, it is quite possible that continuous measures related to gender could become the focus of research. Such measures could include psychological tests of masculinity/femininity (Bem, 1974), or Follicle Stimulating Hormone response to a challenge dose of Luteinizing Hormone, or even the number of cells in a particular region of the hypothalamus. The same applies to genotype × environment interaction, where we may wish to study the effects of life events on depression. A simple dichotomy of 'has had' versus 'has not had' life events rapidly becomes unsatisfactory if we want to find answers to questions such as "Which life events increase vulnerability to depression and by how much?" or "Do the effects of life events cumulate in a linear fashion, or is there a life-event threshold above which depression is almost certain?" We can represent models for continuous G×E interaction graphically, as shown in Figure 18.1. The key difference between this diagram and a regular path diagram is the substitution of an observed variable for a path coefficient at two places in the figure. The observed modifier variables E_1 and E_2 are drawn in boxes rotated 45 degrees, but they function just as if they were path coefficients. Thus, the effects of an individual's sensitivity to the environment are modified by his or her measured environmental index E_i.

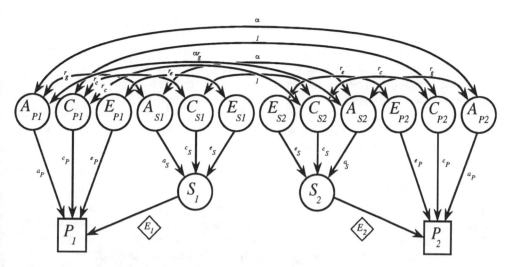

Figure 18.1: Path model for genotype-environment interaction, showing observed phenotypes of a pair of relatives (P_1 and P_2), their additive genetic, common and specific environmental sources of variance in the phenotype (A_{Pi}, C_{Pi} and E_{Pi}, respectively). Also shown are latent sensitivity variables with their respective components of variation (S_1 with A_{S1}, C_{S1}, E_{S1}). α is fixed at 1.0 for MZ and at .5 for DZ twins or siblings. Note that the observed environmental indices (E_1 and E_2) function as path coefficients in this model.

A further general area for data-specific models concerns data that arc *necessarily* missing. For example, we cannot observe age at onset of (or severity of symptoms of) schizophrenia in persons free of the disease. Thus, it would seem difficult to assess the relationship of these putative indices to disease liability. Yet this obviously is another case for twin and family methodology. If relatives correlate in liability to disease (they often do, especially MZ twins), and if our putative index is related to the disease phenotype, then we would expect differences between the means and higher moments of concordant pairs and those of discordant pairs (Neale *et al.*, 1989). We require likelihood methods applied to each distinct pair of relatives especially when the putative index is a consequence rather than a cause of disease liability. The same is true of models for age at onset based on survival analysis (Meyer and Eaves, 1988; Meyer *et al.*, 1991) and of models for comparative ratings (Eaves *et al.*, 1991).

It seems probable that as mathematical genetics develops, there will be an increasing demand for data-specific models. Some general approach to computing likelihood functions would be highly desirable, unlocking the door to broad domains of biometrical modeling that remain as yet untapped (see e.g., Murray, 1989).

18.3   Software: Convenience vs. Generality

In this section we briefly review some of the alternatives to using LISREL for modeling genetically informative data. A thorough description of these techniques would fill another volume; here we wish only to outline the advantages and disadvantages of the different methods. Our aims in this outline are twofold: (i) to guide the advanced user in the right general direction for applications beyond what has been presented so far, and (ii) to inspire software developers to produce tools that will be of maximum use to genetic epidemiology.

18.3.1   FORTRAN and C Languages

The most flexible way of controlling a computer is through its own *machine code*, wherein every instruction that the computer can understand may be used directly. These instructions are simply numeric codes for moving data in and out of memory, and performing elementary operations such as addition and multiplication. Most computers have an *assembler* which uses mnemonics to represent various instructions, thus making programming in machine code somewhat easier than using all the numeric codes themselves. However, there is a price to pay for the functionality of the low level assembler language, which is the very heavy programming demand for even simple operations, like printing out a number, obtaining $\sin(x)$, or adding two matrices. The basic strategy here would be to write general subroutines for each function that could be called as required from the main program. In the early days of computing, it was recognized that higher level languages which could take direct advantage of collections of machine code subroutines would be advantageous, and so languages such as FORTRAN[4] were born. It became unnecessary for the user to learn assembler or machine code, as long as the high level language retained the minimum set of functions required to compute the answer to the problem at hand.

The two languages most often used in genetic modeling are FORTRAN and C. Each has its stalwart supporters, and there has been considerable debate over the relative merits of each language. No doubt the dispute over FORTRAN and C will continue to rage for many years, even though both languages may mutate beyond recognition during the process. We do not wish to reiterate the content of this controversy, but simply to try to determine which language is better for the purpose of fitting the type of genetic models described here. The current FORTRAN standard, FORTRAN 77 (which stands for FORmula TRANslation, 1977 version)[5], contains a large library of scientific functions — such as those found on a good scientific calculator. The C language, on the other hand, includes

---

[4]To create a working program, most high level languages have to go through a two-stage process of (i) *compiling* to create one or more intermediate *object modules* and (ii) *linking* to combine different objects to form an *executable image*.

[5]The 1977 FORTRAN standard is soon to be replaced by FORTRAN 90, but the new compiler is not available at the time of writing.

a much smaller set of such functions 'by default', but a very large set of these are available in the public domain. The choice of C versus FORTRAN is really one of personal preference, since there exists a public domain FORTRAN to C translation utility (F2C), which incorporates libraries of C functions exactly parallel to those available in FORTRAN.

Given equivalent libraries of elementary mathematical functions, we can consider higher level algorithms and subroutines available for each language. Here we believe FORTRAN to be superior to C for the variety and quality of available numerical libraries. Two such libraries are of particular note: Numerical Algorithms Group (NAG, 1990) and IMSL (IMSL, 1987). Both contain efficient routines for constrained and unconstrained optimization, numerical quadrature, and matrix functions. At the time of writing, the C version of the NAG library is partly complete, so the scales may tip towards C in the near future. At present, C retains some lower level superiority, particularly in the area of memory handling, and is therefore better suited to certain applications. There is also the possibility of writing mixed code (LISREL is in fact written this way), incorporating both C and FORTRAN subroutines. Many — though by no means all — compilers will produce object modules that are compatible for linking across languages. Unfortunately mixed code is less easy to transport from one machine to another, so we would recommend programming in one language as a general rule. Despite our cumulated years of programming in FORTRAN, the best language for the future may well turn out to be C. Both languages have the flexibility to deal with the most complicated data analytic scenarios imaginable. The remaining barriers are only data collection, storage, computational speed, and one's own ingenuity.

We note that using FORTRAN or C to fit certain models restricts the range of possible model builders quite drastically — this is one of the reasons we have chosen to use LISREL throughout this book. Debugging FORTRAN is a skill that requires much experience which is not common among biomedical researchers. Even experienced programmers make subtle errors which are not easily detected by colleagues. So, while FORTRAN and C have inherent flexibility, they are very much "experts only" tools, which leave much of the programming task to the user (Hopper, 1988).

18.3.2 Alternative Packages

From the preceding discussion it is clear that existing programs for structural equation modeling do not meet all the requirements of statistical genetic analysis. On the other hand, writing applications in a commercially available command language facilitates communication with other researchers (as attested to by the popularity of the LISREL and EQS programs) and greatly simplifies detection of programming errors. Better still, the use of the same general software in a variety of applications decreases the probability of errors in code segments which are shared by the different applications. Here we review briefly the advantages and disadvantages of several of the more widely available programs.

FISHER

FISHER (Lange *et al.*, 1988) is a library of FORTRAN subroutines that may be linked with the user's own FORTRAN code to fit models to almost any data structure. FISHER contains subroutines for optimization and for computing the likelihood of a given set of vectors of observations, which can save considerable time and effort in programming. There is still some loss of freedom associated with using certain modules in the library; for example, if data are missing for one observation of an individual, the whole case is dropped (Hopper, 1988).

By using FISHER we may be able to solve some of the problems outlined in Section 18.2 above. Certainly this is the case if we view FISHER as an extension of the FORTRAN language which, as we have noted above, is capable of solving almost any conceivable problem in genetic studies. On what problems, however, will use of the package really save time for the user? From a brief inspection, it seems that at least some of the data-specific models could be handled quite easily within FISHER (Hopper, 1988; Rose *et al.*, 1990) . For those experienced with FORTRAN, FISHER can be a boon.

COSAN

On the positive side, COSAN (COvariance Structure ANalysis; McDonald, 1978, 1980; Fraser, 1988) allows for non-linear constraints; its role in advancing both linear and non-linear structural equation modeling has been especially significant (e.g., Kenny and Judd, 1984). The user can implement constraints by providing FORTRAN subroutines which calculate the constraints and their partial derivatives with respect to the function being minimized. Unfortunately, for genetic purposes, COSAN is difficult to endorse because it does not permit analysis of multiple groups. Furthermore, the particular form of the COSAN model:

$$\Sigma = \mathbf{F}_1 \ldots \mathbf{F}_n \mathbf{C} \mathbf{F}'_n \ldots \mathbf{F}'_1 \,, \tag{18.2}$$

where $\mathbf{F}_i$ may be specified as an inverse matrix, is somewhat cumbersome for dealing with the repetitive structures often found in genetic applications.

RAM

The remaining packages described here do not require programming in a structured language like FORTRAN or C. This can yield significant savings in time to compile and debug, and for new users, time to learn programming. One of the earliest programs designed specifically to simplify input is the RAM program (Reticular Action Model; McArdle and McDonald 1984), which has a delightful method of defining models. The program recognizes that there are two basic types of relationship between variables in a path model: causal and correlational. These are represented with the character combinations <- and <->, so valid statements might read:

```
B<->A
C<-A
C<-B
D<-B
```

The program also has facilities for interfacing with the SAS procedure CALIS, and with the LISREL, Mx, and RAMPATH packages [RAMPATH is a software package for drawing path diagrams (McArdle and Boker, 1990)]. Sadly, the program is restricted to single group models, and by itself cannot fit models to genetically informative data. However, through the interfaces with LISREL and Mx, multigroup functionality can be achieved.

RAMONA

Designed by one of the leaders of statistical theory, Browne's program RAMONA (Browne, 1990) bases its input structure on that of RAM; RAMONA in fact stands for RAM Or Near Approximation. Again this program does not have immediate multigroup facilities and is, therefore, rather limited for fitting genetic models. Nevertheless, RAMONA has some redeeming features, particularly in that it employs the most modern measures of goodness-of-fit such as the Root Mean Square Error of Approximation (RMSEA; Steiger and Lind, 1980) and the Expected Cross-Validation Index (Browne and Cudeck, 1990), together with their standard errors. It also permits correct analysis of correlation matrices, which are so often treated incorrectly (Cudeck, 1989).

EQS

Bentler's program, EQS (Bentler, 1989), has recently added multiple group options. Specification of models does not require matrix algebra, but relies on specifying structural relations with command syntax such as:

```
V1 = .5*F1 + E1;
```

where V is an observed variable, F is a latent variable, and E is an error term. Like RAMPATH, this is a succinct way to represent a model, particularly when many of the paths between variables are zero and may be omitted from the specification. A similar form of command language, SIMPLIS, is under development for use in LISREL. However, EQS, like LISREL, imposes the restriction that the number of observed variables has to be the same in each group. EQS does allow non-linear constraints and, therefore, may be of use when fitting models to data on parents and twins. Unfortunately, what works well for the univariate case can become rather cumbersome when extended to multivariate situations.

CALIS

The recent addition to the SAS package, CALIS (SAS, 1990, pp. 292-365) is more flexible in model specifications (allowing Σ to be a sum of equations of the COSAN format), but also is limited to a single group. While the model flexibility is a significant improvement, further flexibility in model specification with a more general matrix algebra interpreter would be better still. Among other features, CALIS has the advantage of being able to understand input in a number of formats, most notably those of RAM, EQS, and COSAN, though not LISREL. There are also facilities for linear and non-linear constraints. Unfortunately, like several other packages, only one group is permitted, so CALIS is of little practical use for genetic applications.

LISCOMP

LISCOMP (Muthen, 1987) is a LISREL-based command language that allows model-fitting to truncated observed variables and to contingency tables. The program has facilities for multiple groups in the same style as LISREL, and can simulate and then analyze data for Monte-Carlo studies. Although early versions of the code were problematic, many of the bugs have been fixed and some use of the program already has been made in genetic applications (Waller and Reise, 1992). LISCOMP's ability to handle threshold models for contingency tables makes it almost unique among publicly available packages.

EZPATH

We mention EZPATH (Steiger, 1989) because it forms part of the popular SYSTAT package for microcomputers. It has a very simple to use graphical interface, and will handle data sets within SYSTAT very easily. Again this program is limited to single groups so it is of little value for genetic applications.

One useful feature that would be welcome in twin and family methodology is the calculation of confidence intervals for goodness-of-fit indices. Currently many studies are drawing substantive inferences from rather small differences in statistics such as the Akaike's Information Criterion. Some knowledge of the probability that two such statistics are actually different would be most welcome.

Mx

Mx is a recent addition to the family of structural equation modeling programs (Neale, 1991). It is perhaps rather ironic that although both path analysis and maximum likelihood theory were developed by geneticists, structural modeling packages were not designed for use with genetic data. Mx goes some way towards rectifying this situation. Written by the first author of this text, it has been expressly designed to meet many of the specific demands of modeling genetically informative data. Models are built using matrix formulae that can be specified in any way the user likes, and the program provides facilities for boundary, linear, and non-linear constraints. Summary statistics, contingency tables, and raw data may be used to fit models with a variety of fit functions, including user-defined.

Whereas LISREL provides a very useful analytical and didactic tool for most straightforward genetic applications, Mx is designed specifically to accommodate the complex data structures and models that are surfacing as researchers probe deeper into more subtle genetic issues and as family studies with variable designs proliferate. The convenience with which Mx handles multivariate applications, including longitudinal multivariate models, the simple treatment of missing data and unbalanced pedigrees, the facilities for threshold and ascertainment models, and other features useful in genetic applications make the package a valuable companion to LISREL for analysis of twin and family data. With the increasing interest in the twin methodology workshops, we are entertaining the idea of writing a second volume of this text to address more advanced genetic applications in Mx.

18.3.3 Summary

In Table 18.1 we show a summary of the characteristics of different software packages for structural equation modeling. The list of packages is doubtless incomplete, but the more well-known programs are present. These characteristics are chosen because of their relevance to genetic applications; other criteria would most definitely tell a different story.

Obviously, any software package is temporary because it depends on rapidly changing hardware to run it. In addition, software itself changes quickly to meet new demands from users and to take advantage of computer system upgrades. We emphasize that this book, though oriented towards LISREL applications, should be used as a guide to fitting models using software with which the user feels most comfortable. One imagines that in a few short years we will be fitting models by clicking and dragging mice, and that learning detailed command languages will be aided by graphical interfaces, context-sensitive help, and menu-driven selection — a far cry indeed from the card punches and line-printers with which most of the contributors to this book began computing! We hope that the lasting value of this book will be in the models and their generalizations rather than the techniques of using a particular software package.

Table 18.1: Summary of characteristics of different software packages.

Feature	FISHER	COSAN	LISREL7	LISREL8	LISCOMP	RAMONA	EQS	CALIS	Mx	EZPATH
Multiple groups	•		•	•	•		•		•	
Boundary constraints	•		•				•	•	•	
Non-linear constraints	•	•	•				•	•	•	
Threshold models					•				•	
Programming required	•	•								
Missing data									•	
Unbalanced pedigrees	•		○	○	○		○		•	
Ascertainment					•				•	
Multivariate convenience									•	
Data-specific models	•									
Sophisticated goodness-of-fit statistics			•			•	•	•	○	•
Graphical interface			•			○			○	•

Full and partial implementation of features are denoted by • and ○, respectively.

Appendix A

List of Participants

Bryan Adams
Department of Social Sciences
The City University
Northampton Square
London EC1V OHB
Great-Britain Tel: 44 71 253 4399 ext 4525
Fax: 44 71 253 2296
Email: b.d.adams@uk.ac.city

David Allison
Obesity Research Center
Columbia University School of Medicine
411 West 114th St, #3D
New York, NY 10025
U.S.A.
Tel: 1 212 523 3570
Fax: 1 212 523 3571

Christopher Amos
Family Studies Section
National Cancer Institute
EPN 439
Bethesda, Maryland 20892
U.S.A.
Tel: 1 301 496 4375
Fax: 1 301 496 9146
Email: nfnia3m@nihcu

Andrey Anokhin
Institut für Humangenetik
Heidelberg
Im Neuenheimer Feld 328
D-6900 Heidelberg
Deutschland
Tel: 49 62 21 56 38 88
Fax: 49 62 21 56 53 32

Michael Bailey
Department of Psychology
Northwestern University
2029 Sheridan Road
Evanston, Illinois 60208
U.S.A.
Tel: 1 708 491 7429
Fax: 1 708 491 7859
Email: mbailey@nuacvm.acns.nwu.edu

Robert Blizard
Academic Department of Psychiatry
Royal Free Hospital School of Medicine
Pond Street, Hampstead
London NW3 2QG
Great-Britain
Tel: 44 71 403 6870
Fax: 44 71 433 3917
Email: bob@uk.ac.lon.rfhsm.ux

Dorret I. Boomsma*
Department of Psychonomics
Free University Amsterdam
De Boelelaan 1111
1081 HV Amsterdam
Netherlands
Tel: 31 20 548 5044
Fax: 31 20 642 6275
Email: dorret@psy.vu.nl

Julia Braungart
Center for Development and Health Genetics
Pennsylvania State University
S-211 Henderson Building
University Park, Pennsylvania 16802
U.S.A.
Tel: 1 814 865 7135
Fax: 1 814 863 4768
Email: jxb29@psuvm

Kazima Bulayeva
Genetics of Human Adaptation
N.I. Vavilov Institute of General Genetics
Gubkin st.3
(095) 117809 Moscow B-333
USSR
Tel: 7 095 135 50 76
Fax: 7 095 135 12 89

Lon R. Cardon*
Institute of Behavioral Genetics
University for Colorado
Campus Box 447
Boulder, Colorado 80309
U.S.A.
Tel: 1 303 492 2843
Fax: 1 303 492 8063
Email: cardon@ibg.colorado.edu

Carine Carels
Department of Dentistry
Catholic University Leuven
Kapucijnenvoer 7, St. Rafaël
B-3000 Leuven
Belgium
Tel: 32 16 21 24 39
Fax: 32 16 21 24 40

Benedetta Casini
The Mendel Institute
International Society of Twin Studies
Piazza Galeno 5
00162 Roma
Italy
Tel: 31 6 844 0964/ 31 6 537 1484

Stacey Cherny
Institute for Behavioral Genetics
University of Colorado
Campus Box 447
Boulder, Colorado 80309
U.S.A.
Tel: 1 303 492 2826
Fax: 1 303 492 8063
Email: cherny@ibg.colorado.edu

Howard Chilcoat
Dept. of Mental Hygiene
Johns Hopkins School of Hygiene & Public Health
rm. 880 Hampton House
612 N Broadway
Baltimore MD 21205
U.S.A.
Tel: 1 303 955 3910
Fax: 1 301 955 9088
Email: chilcoat@jhuhyg

Gloria Dal Colletto
Instituto de Ciencias Biomedicas
University of Sao Paulo
Av. Prof. Lineu Prestes, 2415, C. Postal 4365
CEP 05508 Sao Paulo SP
Brazil
Tel: 55 11 210 2122 ext 564
Fax: 55 11 813 0845
Email: glodalco@brusp.ansp.br

Sylvia De Bie
Centre of Human Genetics
State University Gent
De Pintelaan 185
B-9000 Gent
Belgium
Tel: 32 91 40 36 03
Fax: 32 91 40 49 70

Fatma Demircioglu
Department of Internal Medicine
Gazi University School of Medicine
G M K Bul 18/5 Demirtepe
06440 Ankara
Turkey
Tel: 90 4 212 48 31
Fax: 90 3233 1209

Catherine Derom
Center for Human Genetics
Catholic University Leuven
Herestraat 49
B-3000 Leuven
Belgium
Tel: 32 16 21 58 65
Fax: 32 16 21 59 92
Email: hekabo@blekul13

Robert Derom*
Centre of Human Genetics
Catholic University of Leuven
Herestraat 49
B-3000 Leuven
Belgium
Tel: 32 16 21 58 65
Fax: 32 16 21 59 92
Email: hekabo@blekul13

Dianne De Visser
Department of Psychophysiology
Vrije Universiteit
De Boelelaan 1111
1081 HV Amsterdam
Netherlands
Tel: 31 20 548 7324
Fax: 31 20 642 6275
Email: diannev@psy.vu.nl

Conor V. Dolan*
Department of Psychology
University of Amsterdam
Roetersstraat 15
1010 WB Amsterdam
Netherlands
Tel: 31 20 525 6735
Fax: 31 20 525 6710
Email: peter_mo@sara.nl

Lindon J. Eaves*
Department of Human Genetics
Medical College of Virginia
Box 3
Richmond, Virginia 23298
U.S.A.
Tel: 1 804 371 8754
Fax: 1 804 371 8761
Email: eaves@vcuruby

Abdessadek El Ahmadi
Faculté de Psychologie
Dpt. de Statistique appliquée
Université de Liège Bât. 32
4000 Liege
Belgium
Tel: 32 41 56 20 11
Email: u012302@bliulg11

Deborah Finkel
Department of Psychology
University of Minnesota
75 East River Rd.
Minneapolis, Minnesota 55455
U.S.A.
Tel: 1 612 625 7534
Fax: 1 612 626 2079
Email: eqz6571@ca.acs.umn.edu

David W. Fulker*
Institute for Behavioral Genetics
University of Colorado
Campus Box 447
Boulder, Colorado 80309
U.S.A.
Tel: 1 303 492 2840
Fax: 1 303 492 8063
Email: fulker@abacus.colorado.edu

Kurt Geldhof
Center of Human Genetics
Catholic University Leuven
Herestraat 49
B-3000 Leuven
Belgium
Tel: 32 16 29 42 27

Lucienne Geurts
Department of Psychology
University of Amsterdam
Roetersstraat 15
1018 WB Amsterdam
Netherlands
Tel: 31 20 525 6734
Fax: 31 20 525 6710

Jackie Gillis
Department of Psychology
University of Colorado
Campus Box 447, IBG
Boulder, Colorado 80309
U.S.A.
Tel: 1 303 492 2817
Fax: 1 303 492 8063
Email: gillis@abacus.colorado.edu

Jennifer Harris
Department of Environmental Hygiene
The Karolinska Institute
Box 60400
S-104 01 Stockholm
Sweden
Tel: 46 8 728 7484
Fax: 46 8 31 39 61
Email: jennifer.harris.hy@kicom.ki.se

Andrew C. Heath*
Department of Psychiatry
Washington University School of Medicine
4940 Audubon Ave.
St. Louis, Missouri 63110
U.S.A.
Tel: 1 314 367 7746
Fax: 1 314 361 8288
Email: andrew@wupsych1.wustl.edu

Kauko Heikkilä
Department of Public Health
University of Helsinki
Haartmaninkatu 3
00290 Helsinki
Finland
Tel: 358 0 434 6364
Fax: 358 0 434 6456
Email: heikkila@cc.helsinki.fi

Scott Hershberger
Human Development and Family Studies
Pennsylvania State University
S-110 Henderson / College of Health
University Park, Pennsylvania 16802
U.S.A.
Tel: 1 814 863 6147
Fax: 1 814 863 4768
Email: slh10@psuvm

John K. Hewitt*
Department of Human Genetics
Medical College of Virginia
Box 3
Richmond, Virginia 23298
U.S.A.
Tel: 1 804 371 8754
Fax: 1 804 371 8761
Email: hewitt@vcuruby

Karl G. Jöreskog*
Department of Statistics
University of Uppsala
P.O.Box 513
S-75120 Uppsala
Sweden
Tel: 46 18 181165
Fax: 46 18 554422
Email: stakg@seudac21

Judith Koopmans
Department of Psychonomics
Vrije Universiteit
De Boelelaan 1111
1081 HV Amsterdam
Netherlands
Tel: 31 20 548 7399
Fax: 31 20 642 6275
Email: judith@psy.vu.nl

Einar Kringlen
Department of Psychiatry
Oslo University
Box 85
Vindern, N-0319 Oslo 3
Norway
Tel: 47 2 14 65 90

Isabelle Lauweryns
Department of Dentistry
Catholic University Leuven
Kapucijnenvoer 7, St. Rafaël
B-3000 Leuven
Belgium
Tel: 32 16 21 24 39
Fax: 32 16 21 24 40

Birgit Ljungquist
University of Health & Care
Institute of Gerontology
Brunnsgatan 30
S-553 17 Jönköping
Sweden
Tel: 46 36 10 49 00
Fax: 46 36 10 49 16

Dasen Luo
Department of Psychology
Case Western Reserve University
10900 Euclid Avenue
Cleveland, Ohio 44106
U.S.A.
Tel: 1 216 368 2686
Fax: 1 216 368 4891

Alison Macdonald
Genetics Section,Institute of Psychiatry
University of London
De Crespigny Park, Denmark Hill
London SE5 8AF
Great-Britain
Tel: 44 71 703 5411 ext 3416
Fax: 44 71 703 5796
Email: amacdona@uk.ac.lon.psych.ux

Pamela Madden
Clinical Psychobiology Branch
National Institute of Mental Health
RM 4S-239, 9000 Rockville Pike
Bethesda, Maryland 20892
U.S.A.
Tel: 1 301 496 2141
Fax: 1 301 496 5439

Hermine Maes
Institute of Physical Education
Catholic University Leuven
Tervuursevest 101
B-3001 Heverlee
Belgium
Tel: 32 16 20 14 31/ 32 16 21 58 66
Fax: 32 16 20 14 60/ 32 16 21 59 97
Email: hermine@aski.ilo.kuleuven.ac.be

Izabela Makalowska
Institute of Anthropology
Poznan University
Fredry 10
61-701 Poznan
Poland
Tel: 48 61 52 30 15
Fax: 48 61 53 55 35

Sergei Malykh
Genetic Psychophysiology
Inst. of General and Educational Psychology
pr. Marxa 20 "V"
103009 Moscou
USSR
Tel: 7 095 202 93 63
Fax: 7 095 292 65 11

Nicholas G. Martin*
Queensland Institute
for Medical Research
300 Herston Road
Brisbane, Queensland 4029
Australia
Tel: 61 7 362 0278
Fax: 61 7 362 0111
Email: qmrmartin@uqvax.cc.uq.oz.au

Godelieve Masuy-Stroobant
Institut de Demographie
Collège J. Leclercq
1 Pl. Montesquieu, bte 17
B-1348 Louvain-la-Neuve
Belgium
Tel: 32 10 47 29 51
Fax: 32 10 47 29 97

Jack McArdle
Department of Psychology
University of Virginia
102 Gilmer Hall
Charlottesville, Virginia 22903
U.S.A.
Tel: 1 804 924 0656/ 1 804 589 5909
Fax: 1 804 924 7185
Email: jjm@virginia

Shirley McGuire
Center for Developmental and Health Genetics
Pennsylvania State University
S-211 Henderson Building
University Park, Pennsylvania 16802
U.S.A.
Tel: 1 814 865 7135
Fax: 1 814 863 4768
Email: sam115@psuvm

Wim Meulemans
Center for Human Genetics
Catholic University Leuven
Herestraat 49
B-3000 Leuven
Belgium
Tel: 32 16 21 58 65
Fax: 32 16 21 59 97
Email: hekabo@blekul13

Joanne M. Meyer*
Department of Human Genetics
Medical College of Virginia
Box 3
Richmond, Virginia 23298
U.S.A.
Tel: 1 804 371 8754
Fax: 1 804 371 8761
Email: meyer@vcuruby

Geert Mortier
Pediatric Department
State University Gent
De Pintelaan 185
B-9000 Gent
Belgium
Tel: 32 91 40 35 92/ 32 91 74 79 99

Walter E. Nance*
Department of Human Genetics
Medical College of Virginia
Box 33
Richmond, Virginia 23298
U.S.A.
Tel: 1 804 786 9632
Fax: 1 804 786 3760
Email: nance@vcuruby

Michael C. Neale*
Department of Human Genetics
Medical College of Virginia
Box 3
Richmond, Virginia 23298
U.S.A.
Tel: 1 804 371 8754
Fax: 1 804 371 8761
Email: neale@vcuruby

Jenae Neiderhiser
Center for Development and Health Genetics
Pennsylvania State University
S-211 Henderson Building
University Park, Pennsylvania 16802
U.S.A.
Tel: 1 814 865 7135
Fax: 1 814 863 4768
Email: jmn101@psuvm

Nancy Pedersen
Department of Environmental Hygiene
The Karolinska Institute
Box 60400
S-104 01 Stockholm
Sweden
Tel: 46 8 728 7418
Fax: 46 8 31 41 24
Email: nancy_pedersen.hy@kicom.ki.se

Daniel Pérusse
Department of Human Genetics
Medical College of Virginia
Box 3, MCV Station
Richmond, Virginia 23298
U.S.A.
Tel: 1 804 371 8754
Fax: 1 804 371 8761
Email: dperusse@vcuvax

Stephen Petrill
Department of Psychology
Case Western Reserve University
10900 Euclid Avenue
Cleveland, Ohio 44106
U.S.A.
Tel: 1 216 321 8713
Fax: 1 216 368 4891
Email: sxp12%po@cwru.edu

Kay Phillips
Louisville Twin Study
University of Louisville
CDU, HSC, MDR - 111
Louisville, Kentucky 40292
U.S.A.
Tel: 1 502 588 1086
Fax: 1 502 588 7013
Email: dkphil01@ulkyvx.bitnet

Andrew Pickles
Child Psychiatry,Institute of Psychiatry
University of London
De Crespigny Park, Denmark Hill
London SE5 8AF
Great-Britain
Tel: 44 71 703 5411 ext 3481
Fax: 44 71 708 5800
Email: apickles@uk.ac.lon.psych.ux

Monica Pittaluga
The Mendel Institute
International Society of Twin Studies
Piazza Galeno 5
00162 Roma
Italy
Tel: 31 6 844 0964/ 31 6 411 2056

Carol Prescott
Department of Human Genetics
Medical College of Virginia
Box 3, MCV Station
Richmond, VA 23298
U.S.A.
Tel: 1 804 371 8754
Fax: 1 804 371 8761
Email: cprescott@vcuvax

Rumi Kato Price
Department of Psychiatry
Washington University School of Medicine
4940 Audubon Ave.
St. Louis, Missouri 63110
U.S.A.
Tel: 1 314 362 2430
Fax: 1 314 362 2470

Timothy Rebbeck
Population Science
Fox Chase Cancer Center
7701 Burholme Avenue
Philadelphia, Pennsylvania 19111
U.S.A.
Tel: 1 215 728 3118
Fax: 1 215 728 3574
Email: rebbeck@fccc.edu

Lawrence Rodriguez
Institute for Behavioral Genetics
University of Colorado at Boulder
Campus Box 447
Boulder, Colorado 80309-0447
U.S.A.
Tel: 1 303 492 0933
Fax: 1 303 492 8063
Email: rodriguez_l@ibg.colorado.edu

Katarzyna Rutkowska
Medical Academy
University of Gdansk
Kolberga 6 D/28
81 - 881 Sopot
Poland
Tel: 48 58 51 86 41
Fax: 48 58 20 19 78

Judy L. Silberg*
Department of Human Genetics
Medical College of Virginia
Box 3
Richmond, Virginia 23298
U.S.A.
Tel: 1 804 371 8754
Fax: 1 804 371 8761
Email: jsilberg@vcuruby

Emily Simonoff
Child Psychiatry,Institute of Psychiatry
University of London
De Crespigny Park, Denmark Hill
London SE5 8AF
Great-Britain
Tel: 44 71 703 5411
Fax: 44 71 708 5800

Ingunn Skre
Department of Psychology
Oslo University
P.O.Box 1094
Blindren, N-0317 Oslo
Norway
Tel: 47 2 85 53 64

Harold Snieder
Department of Psychophysiology
Vrije Universiteit
De Boelelaan 1111
1081 HV Amsterdam
Netherlands
Tel: 31 20 548 3858
Fax: 31 20 642 6275
Email: harold@psy.vu.nl

Giovanna Sorrentino
Department of Neurological Science
Universita di Firenze
Viale Morgagni 85
50134 Firenze
Italy
Tel: 39 55 427 7536
Fax: 39 55 41 36 03

Thérèse Stroet
Department of Psychophysiology
Vrije Universiteit
De Boelelaan 1111
1081 HV Amsterdam
Netherlands
Tel: 31 20 548 5029
Fax: 31 20 642 6275
Email: therese@psy.vu.nl

Eva Susanszky
Department of Human Genetics and Teratology
National Institute of Hygiene
Gyali ut 2-6
Budapest 1097
Hungary
Tel: 36 1 133 5773
Fax: 36 1 133 5773

Kristian Tambs
National Institute of Public Health
Geitmyrsvn. 75
N-0462 Oslo 4
Norway
Tel: 47 2 35 60 20 ext 387
Fax: 47 2 35 36 05

Martine Thomis
Institute of Physical Education
Catholic University Leuven
Tervuursevest 101
B-3001 Heverlee
Belgium
Tel: 32 16 21 58 66
Fax: 32 16 21 59 97
Email: hekabo@blekul13

William Thompson
Department of Psychology
University of Virginia
102 Gilmer Hall
Charlottesville, Virginia 22903
U.S.A.
Tel: 1 804 982 4756
Fax: 1 804 924 7185
Email: wwt2f@virginia.edu

Kim Truett
Department of Human Genetics
Medical College of Virginia
Box 3, MCV Station
Richmond, Virginia 23298
U.S.A.
Tel: 1 804 371 8754
Fax: 1 804 371 8761
Email: ktruett@vcuvax

Dilek Ural
Department of Dentistry
Catholic University Leuven
Kapucijnenvoer 7, St. Rafaël
B-3000 Leuven
Belgium
Tel: 32 16 21 23 01
Fax: 32 16 21 24 80

Caroline Van Baal
Department of Psychophysiology
Vrije Universiteit
De Boelelaan 1111
1081 HV Amsterdam
Netherlands
Tel: 31 20 548 5087
Fax: 31 20 642 6275
Email: caroline@psy.vu.nl

Nathalie Van Cauwenberghe
Department of Dentistry
Catholic University Leuven
Kapucijnenvoer 7, St. Rafaël
B-3000 Leuven
Belgium
Tel: 32 16 21 24 39
Fax: 32 16 21 24 40

Jan Van Den Broeck
Center for Human Genetics
Catholic University Leuven
Herestraat 49
B-3000 Leuven
Belgium
Tel: 32 16 21 58 68
Fax: 32 16 21 59 97
Email: hekabo@blekul13

Tony Vernon
Department of Psychology
University of Western Ontario
Social Science Centre
London, Ontario N6A 5C2
Canada
Tel: 1 519 661 3682
Fax: 1 519 661 3961
Email: vernon@vaxr.sscl.uwo.ca

Richard Viken
Department of Psychology
Indiana University
Psychology Building
Bloomington, Indiana 47405
U.S.A.
Tel: 1 812 855 1697
Fax: 1 812 855 4691
Email: viken@iubacs

Robert Vlietinck**
Centre of Human Genetics
Catholic University of Leuven
Herestraat 49
B-3000 Leuven
Belgium
Tel: 32 16 21 58 66
Fax: 32 16 21 59 92
Email: hekabo@blekul13

Niels Waller
Department of Psychology
University of California-Davis
Davis, California 95616
U.S.A.
Tel: 1 916 752 4459
Fax: 1 916 752 2087
Email: ngwaller@ucdavis

Keith Whitfield
Institute for Behavioral Genetics
University of Colorado
Campus Box 447
Boulder, Colorado 80309
U.S.A.
Tel: 1 303 492 2826
Fax: 1 303 492 8063
Email: whitfield@ibg.colorado.edu

Appendix B

The Greek Alphabet

Uppercase	Lowercase	Name
A	α	alpha
B	β	beta
Γ	γ	gamma
Δ	δ	delta
E	ϵ	epsilon
Z	ζ	zeta
H	η	eta
Θ	θ	theta
I	ι	iota
K	κ	kappa
Λ	λ	lambda
M	μ	mu
N	ν	nu
Ξ	ξ	xi (or ksi)
O	o	omicron
Π	π	pi
P	ρ	rho
Σ	σ	sigma
T	τ	tau
Υ	υ	upsilon
Φ	ϕ	phi
X	χ	chi
Ψ	ψ	psi
Ω	ω	omega

Appendix C

LISREL Scripts for Univariate Models

C.1 Path Coefficients Model

The following LISREL 7 script represents a univariate genetic model fitted to covariance matrices for two twin groups: 1) MZ pairs reared together, and 2) DZ pairs reared together.

```
Analysis of Australian BMI data-young female MZ twins pairs
;
; Univariate genetic models fitted to two like-sex groups
;
; Reference: Heath A.C., Neale M.C., Hewitt J.K., Eaves L.J.,
;    Fulker D.W.  Testing structural equation models for twin
;    data using LISREL.  Behavior Genetics 19:9-36,1989.
;
; Structural equation: P1 = a A + c C + e E + d D
;    where A is additive genetic deviation
;          C is shared environmental deviation
;          E is unique environmental deviation
;          D is dominance genetic deviation
;          P1 is phenotype of twin (P2 that of cotwin)
;
; Data are Body-mass index data, estimated as 7 x log(wt/ht2),
; where wt is weight in kg, ht is height in meters
;
DA NG=2 NI=2 NO=534 MA=CM
LA
```

```
BMI-Tw1 BMI-Tw2
CM SY
0.7247
0.5891 0.7915
MO NY=2 NE=2 NK=8 GA=FU,FI LY=ID PH=SY,FI BE=ZE PS=ZE TE=ZE
LK
A1 C1 E1 D1 A2 C2 E2 D2
LE
P1 P2
MA PH
1
0 1
0 0 1
0 0 0 1
1 0 0 0 1
0 1 0 0 0 1
0 0 0 0 0 0 1
0 0 0 1 0 0 0 1
; elements of GAmma are
; a c e d 0 0 0 0
; 0 0 0 0 a c e d
;
; To fit a c e model:
;PA GA
;1 1 1 0 0 0 0 0
;0 0 0 0 1 1 1 0
; To fit a d e model:
PA GA
1 0 1 1 0 0 0 0
0 0 0 0 1 0 1 1
; To fit a e model:
;PA GA
;1 0 1 0 0 0 0 0
;0 0 0 0 1 0 1 0
; To fit c e model:
;PA GA
;0 1 1 0 0 0 0 0
;0 0 0 0 0 1 1 0
; To fit e model:
;PA GA
;0 0 0 1 0 0 0 0
;0 0 0 0 0 0 0 1
EQ GA(1,1) GA(2,5)
```

```
EQ GA(1,2) GA(2,6)
EQ GA(1,3) GA(2,7)
EQ GA(1,4) GA(2,8)
START .6 ALL
OU TM=1200 ND=4 NS
;
; Here comes the second group
;
YOUNG FEMALE DZ PAIRS
DA NI=2 NO=328 MA=CM
LA
BMI-tw1 BMI-tw2
CM SY
0.7786
0.2461 0.8365
MO GA=IN PS=IN LY=IN PH=SY,FI TE=IN BE=IN
LK
A1 C1 E1 D1 A2 C2 E2 D2
LE
P1 P2
MA PH
1
0 1
0 0 1
0 0 0 1
.5 0 0 0 1
0 1 0 0 0 1
0 0 .0 0 0 0 1
0 0 0 .25 0 0 0 1
OU ND=5 NS SE ad=off SC
```

C.2   Variance Components Model

This LISREL 8 script fits a variance components model to twin covariances on BMI. It is a two group problem, for MZ and DZ pairs reared together.

```
Analysis of Australian BMI data-young male MZ twins pairs
DA NG=2 NI=2 NO=251 MA=CM
LA
BMI-Tw1 BMI-Tw2
CM SY
0.5971
0.4475 0.5692
```

```
MO NY=2 NE=2 NK=8 GA=FU,FI LY=ID PH=SY,FI BE=ZE PS=ZE TE=ZE
LK
E1 C1 A1 D1 E2 C2 A2 D2
LE
P1 P2
PA PH
2
0 0
0 0 3
0 0 0 4
0 0 0 0 2
0 0 0 0 0 0
0 0 3 0 0 0 3
0 0 0 4 0 0 0 4
ST 0.25 PH(1,1) PH(3,3) PH(4,4)
MA GA
1.0 1.0 1.0 1.0 0.0 0.0 0.0 0.0
0.0 0.0 0.0 0.0 1.0 1.0 1.0 1.0
OU TM=1200 ND=5 NS
YOUNG MALE DZ PAIRS
DA NI=2 NO=184 MA=CM
LA
BMI-tw1 BMI-tw2
CM SY
0.7191
0.2447 0.8179
MO GA=IN PS=IN LY=IN PH=IN TE=IN BE=IN
LK
E1 C1 A1 D1 E2 C2 A2 D2
LE
P1 P2
EQ PH(1,1,1) PH(1,1) PH(5,5)
EQ PH(1,2,2) PH(2,2) PH(6,6) PH(6,2)
EQ PH(1,3,3) PH(3,3) PH(7,7)
EQ PH(1,4,4) PH(4,4) PH(8,8)
CO PH(7,3)=0.5*PH(1,7,3)
CO PH(8,4)=0.25*PH(1,8,4)
OU TM=1200 ND=5 NS PC IT=500 AD=OFF SC RS
```

C.3   Model for Means and Covariances

The following LISREL 8 script estimates path coefficients for like-sex twins under
the univariate genetic model, incorporating estimation of means.

Analysis of Australian BMI data-older female MZ twins pairs
;
; Univariate genetic models fitted to two like-sex groups
;
; Reference: Heath A.C., Neale M.C., Hewitt J.K., Eaves L.J.,
;   Fulker D.W. Testing structural equation models for twin
;   data using LISREL. Behavior Genetics 19:9-36,1989.
;
; Structural equation: P1 = a A + c C + e E + d D
;   where A is additive genetic deviation
;   C is shared environmental deviation
;   E is unique environmental deviation
;   D is dominance genetic deviation
;   P1 is phenotype of twin (P2 that of cotwin)
;
; Data are Body-mass index data, estimated as 7 x log(wt/ht2),
; where wt is weight in kg, ht is height in meters
;
DA NG=2 NI=2 NO=637 MA=CM
LA
BMI-Tw1 BMI-Tw2
CM SY
0.9759
0.6656 0.9544
ME
0.9087 0.8685
MO NY=2 NE=2 NK=8 GA=FU,FI LY=ID PH=SY,FI BE=ze C
    PS=ZE TE=ZE TY=FI AL=ZE KA=ZE
LK
A1 C1 E1 D1 A2 C2 E2 D2
LE
P1 P2
MA PH
1
0 1
0 0 1
0 0 0 1
1 0 0 0 1
0 1 0 0 0 1
0 0 0 0 0 0 1
0 0 0 1 0 0 0 1
PA GA
1 0 1 0 0 0 0 0

```
0 0 0 0 1 0 1 0
; elements of GAmma are
; a c e d 0 0 0 0
; 0 0 0 0 a c e d
;
; To fit a c e model:
;PA GA
;1 1 1 0 0 0 0 0
;0 0 0 0 1 1 1 0
; To fit a d e model:
PA GA
1 0 1 1 0 0 0 0
0 0 0 0 1 0 1 1
; To fit a e model:
;PA GA
;1 0 1 0 0 0 0 0
;0 0 0 0 1 0 1 0
; To fit c e model:
;PA GA
;0 1 1 0 0 0 0 0
;0 0 0 0 0 1 1 0
; To fit e model:
;PA GA
;0 0 0 1 0 0 0 0
;0 0 0 0 0 0 0 1
EQ GA(1,1) GA(2,5)
EQ GA(1,2) GA(2,6)
EQ GA(1,3) GA(2,7)
EQ GA(1,4) GA(2,8)
START .6 ALL
FR TY(1)
EQ TY(1) TY(2)
ST 1 ty(1)
OU TM=1200 ND=4 NS
;
; Here comes the second group
;
OLDER FEMALE DZ PAIRS
DA NI=2 NO=380 MA=CM
LA
BMI-tw1 BMI-tw2
CM SY
0.915
```

```
0.3124 1.042
ME
0.8102 0.8576
MO GA=IN PS=IN LY=IN PH=SY,FI TE=IN BE=IN TY=FI
LK
A1 C1 E1 D1 A2 C2 E2 D2
LE
P1 P2
MA PH
1
0 1
0 0 1
0 0 0 1
.5 0 0 0 1
0 1 0 0 0 1
0 0 0 0 0 0 1
0 0 0 .25 0 0 0 1
EQ TY(1,1) TY(1) TY(2)
OU ND=5 NS SE ad=off SC it=50
```

C.4   Univariate Genetic Model for Twin pairs and Singles

This script is fits the simple univariate genetic model (incorporating means) to BMI data from like-sex female twins in which (a) both twins in the pair responded to the survey; (b) the cotwin did not cooperate.

```
Analysis of Australian BMI data-older female MZ twins pairs
;
; Univariate genetic models fitted to two like-sex groups
;
; Reference: Heath A.C., Neale M.C., Hewitt J.K., Eaves L.J.,
;    Fulker D.W.  Testing structural equation models for twin
;    data using LISREL.  Behavior Genetics 19:9-36,1989.
;
; Structural equation: P1 = a A + c C + e E + d D
;    where A is additive genetic deviation
;          C is shared environmental deviation
;          E is unique environmental deviation
;          D is dominance genetic deviation
;          P1 is phenotype of twin (P2 that of cotwin)
```

```
;
; Data are Body-mass index data, estimated as 7 x log(wt/ht2),
; where wt is weight in kg, ht is height in meters
;
; This version includes means, to provide a check on sampling
;  representativeness, i.e., testing equality of means
;  between MZs and DZs as well as between 1st and 2nd twins
;
DA NG=4 NI=2 NO=637 MA=CM
LA
BMI-Tw1 BMI-Tw2
CM SY
0.9759
0.6656 0.9544
ME
0.3408 0.351
MO NY=2 NE=2 NK=8 GA=FI LY=ID PH=FI PS=ZE TE=FI TY=FI AL=ZE KA=ZE
LK
A1 C1 E1 D1 A2 C2 E2 D2
LE
P1 P2
MA PH
1
0 1
0 0 1
0 0 0 1
1 0 0 0 1
0 1 0 0 0 1
0 0 0 0 0 0 1
0 0 0 1 0 0 0 1
; elements of GAmma are
; e c h d 0 0 0 0
; 0 0 0 0 e c h d
;
; To fit e c h model:
;PA GA
;1 1 1 0 0 0 0 0
;0 0 0 0 1 1 1 0
;To fit e h d model:
PA GA
1 0 1 1 0 0 0 0
0 0 0 0 1 0 1 1
; To fit e h model:
```

```
;PA GA
;1 0 1 0 0 0 0 0
;0 0 0 0 1 0 1 0
;To fit e c model:
;PA GA
;1 1 0 0 0 0 0 0
;0 0 0 0 1 1 0 0
; To fit e model (obsessional types only)
; 1 0 0 0 0 0 0 0
; 0 0 0 0 1 0 0 0
EQ GA(1,1) GA(2,5)
EQ GA(1,2) GA(2,6)
EQ GA(1,3) GA(2,7)
EQ GA(1,4) GA(2,8)
START .5 GA(1,1)-GA(2,8)
; estimating mean for MZ pairs
FR TY(1)
EQ TY(1) TY(2)
ST 0.3 TY(1)
OU TM=1200 ND=5 NS
OLDER FEMALE DZ PAIRS
DA NI=2 NO=380 MA=CM
LA
BMI-tw1 BMI-tw2
CM SY
0.915
0.3124 1.042
ME
0.4444 0.4587
MO GA=IN PS=IN LY=IN PH=SY,FI TE=FI BE=IN TY=FI AL=IN KA=IN
LK
A1 C1 E1 D1 A2 C2 E2 D2
LE
P1 P2
MA PH
1
0 1
0 0 1
0 0 0 1
.5 0 0 0 1
0 1 0 0 0 1
0 0 0 0 0 0 1
0 0 0 .25 0 0 0 1
```

```
; no heterogeneity of means
EQ TY(1,1,1) TY(1) TY(2)
; heterogeneity of means
;FR TY(1)
;EQ TY(1) TY(2)
;ST 0.4 TY(1)
OU NS AD=OFF
OLDER FEMALE MZ PAIRS WHOSE COTWIN DID NOT RESPOND
DA NI=2 NO=44 MA=CM
LA
BMI-tw1 Dummy
CM SY
1.1461
0.0     1.0
ME
0.6852 0.0
MO GA=IN PS=IN LY=IN PH=SY,FI TE=FI BE=IN TY=FI AL=IN KA=IN
LK
A1 C1 E1 D1 A2 C2 E2 D2
LE
P1 P2
MA PH
1
0 1
0 0 1
0 0 0 1
0 0 0 0 0
0 0 0 0 0 0
0 0 0 0 0 0 0
0 0 0 0 0 0 0 0
; no heterogeneity of means
EQ TY(1,1,1) TY(1)
FR TY(2)
ST 0.8 TY(2)
FR TE(2,2)
ST 1.0 TE(2,2)
; heterogeneity of means
;FR TY(1)
;EQ TY(1) TY(2)
;ST 0.4 TY(1)
OU NS AD=OFF
OLDER FEMALE DZ PAIRS WHOSE COTWIN DID NOT RESPOND
DA NI=2 NO=62 MA=CM
```

```
LA
BMI-tw1 Dummy
CM SY
1.7357
0.0     1.0
ME
1.0168 0.0
MO GA=IN PS=IN LY=IN PH=SY,FI TE=FI BE=IN TY=FI AL=IN KA=IN
LK
A1 C1 E1 D1 A2 C2 E2 D2
LE
P1 P2
MA PH
1
0 1
0 0 1
0 0 0 1
0 0 0 0 0
0 0 0 0 0 0
0 0 0 0 0 0 0
0 0 0 0 0 0 0 0
; no heterogeneity of means
EQ TY(1,1,1) TY(1)
FR TY(2)
ST 0.0 TY(2)
FR TE(2,2)
ST 1.0 TE(2,2)
; heterogeneity of means
;FR TY(1)
;EQ TY(1) TY(2)
;ST 0.4 TY(1)
OU TM=1200 ND=5 NS SE TV PC IT=500 AD=OFF SC EF RS
```

C.5   Age-correction Model

This LISREL script is the basic model *without* age effects described in Section 8.11.
Modifications to the script to incorporate age effects are described in Section 8.11
on page 184. The model is fit to conservatism data from Australian female twins.

```
CONSERVATISM: Australia 1980 - MZ FEMALES
DA NG=2 NI=3 NO=941 MA=CM
LA
age con1 con2
```

```
SE
con1 con2/
CM
 179.522
  63.463     143.361
  66.167      97.159     141.530
MO NY=2 NE=2 NK=6 GA=FU,FI LY=ID PH=SY,FI TE=ZE PS=ZE BE=ZE
LE
con1 con2
LK
A1 C1 E1 A2 C2 E2
PA GA
1 1 1 0 0 0
0 0 0 1 1 1
EQ GA(1,1) GA(2,4)
EQ GA(1,2) GA(2,5)
EQ GA(1,3) GA(2,6)
MA PH
1.
0. 1.
0. 0. 1.
1. 0. 0. 1.
0. 1. 0. 0. 1.
0. 0. 0. 0. 0. 1./
ST 5.0 ALL
OU NS AD=OFF SC
FEMALE DZ PAIRS POLYCHORICS
DA NO=548
LA
age con1 con2
SE
con1 con2/
CM
 168.343
  66.365     141.840
  76.316      88.083     157.763
MO GA=IN PH=SY,FI
MA PH
1.
0. 1.
0. 0. 1.
.5 0. 0. 1.
0. 1. 0. 0. 1.
```

```
0. 0. 0. 0. 0. 1./
OU
```

Appendix D

LISREL Script for Power Calculation

D.1 ACE Model for Power Calculations

The LISREL 7 script below fits the univariate ACE model to simulated twin co-variances. The application is described in Section 9.2.

```
Power calculations with classical twin design: MZ twins
DA NG=2 NI=2 NO=1000 MA=CM
CM
1.000 0.5 1.000
LA
MZ-1 MZ-2
SE
 1 2/
MO NY=2 NE=2 NK=6 LY=ID GA=FU,FR BE=ZE PH=FI PS=ZE TE=ZE
PA GA
1 1 1 0 0 0
0 0 0 1 1 1
EQ GA(1,1) GA(2,4)
EQ GA(1,2) GA(2,5)
EQ GA(1,3) GA(2,6)
VA 1. PH(1,1) PH(2,2) PH(3,3) PH(4,4) PH(5,5) PH(6,6)
VA 1. PH(4,1) PH(5,2)
ST 0.3 GA(1,1)-GA(2,6)
OU NS ND=2 AD=OFF
Power calculations for classical twin design: DZ twins
DA NO=1000 MA=CM
```

```
CM
1.000 0.350 1.000
LA
DZ-1 DZ-2
SE
 1 2/
MO NY=2 NE=2 NK=6 LY=IN GA=IN BE=IN PH=FI PS=IN TE=IN
VA 1.0 PH(1,1) PH(2,2) PH(3,3) PH(4,4) PH(5,5) PH(6,6)
VA 1.0 PH(5,2)
VA 0.5 PH(4,1)
OU NS ND=2 AD=OFF
```

Appendix E

LISREL Scripts for Multivariate Models

E.1 Genetic Factor Model

The following LISREL script fits the genetic common factor model as described in Chapter 12 for additive (A), common environmental (C), and non-shared environment (E) effects to arithmetic computation data from Australian female twins. The data comprise assessments taken once before (T0) and three times after (T1 — T3) a standard dose of alcohol. Measure specific non-shared environment effects are modeled as squared quantities in the Θ_ϵ matrix.

```
Arithmetic Computation : Number Correct - MZ FEMALES
DA NG=2 NI=8 NO=43
LA
Tw1-T0 Tw1-T1 Tw1-T2 Tw1-T3 Tw2-T0 Tw2-T1 Tw2-T2 Tw2-T3
CM
   .259664D+03    .209325D+03    .259939D+03    .209532D+03    .220755D+03
.245235D+03
   .221610D+03    .221491D+03    .221317D+03    .249298D+03    .211678D+03
.200684D+03
   .191937D+03    .196068D+03    .283802D+03    .166020D+03    .187932D+03
.164335D+03
   .177413D+03    .193615D+03    .249487D+03    .184389D+03    .191922D+03
.182497D+03
   .188341D+03    .213771D+03    .220240D+03    .262092D+03    .179332D+03
.188079D+03
   .180813D+03    .195734D+03    .218767D+03    .224939D+03    .230575D+03
.270928D+03
```

```
MO NY=8 NE=6 LY=FU,FI PS=FI TE=DI,FR
LE
A1 C1 E1 A2 C2 E2
PA LY
1 1 1 0 0 0
1 1 1 0 0 0
1 1 1 0 0 0
1 1 1 0 0 0
0 0 0 1 1 1
0 0 0 1 1 1
0 0 0 1 1 1
0 0 0 1 1 1
EQ LY 1,1 LY 5,4
EQ LY 2,1 LY 6,4
EQ LY 3,1 LY 7,4
EQ LY 4,1 LY 8,4
EQ LY 1,2 LY 5,5
EQ LY 2,2 LY 6,5
EQ LY 3,2 LY 7,5
EQ LY 4,2 LY 8,5
EQ LY 1,3 LY 5,6
EQ LY 2,3 LY 6,6
EQ LY 3,3 LY 7,6
EQ LY 4,3 LY 8,6
EQ TE 1 TE 5
EQ TE 2 TE 6
EQ TE 3 TE 7
EQ TE 4 TE 8
VA 1 PS 1,1 PS 2,2 PS 3,3 PS 4,4 PS 5,5 PS 6,6
VA 1 PS 4,1 PS 5,2
ST 5.0 ALL
OU NS AD=OFF
Arithmetic Computation : Number Correct - DZ FEMALES
DA NO=44
LA
Tw1-T0 Tw1-T1 Tw1-T2 Tw1-T3 Tw2-T0 Tw2-T1 Tw2-T2 Tw2-T3
CM
   .297917D+03    .232357D+03    .229414D+03    .231170D+03    .213544D+03
.247423D+03
   .236979D+03    .214943D+03    .225486D+03    .274943D+03    .670523D+02
.790291D+02
   .951977D+02    .932791D+02    .281959D+03    .730122D+02    .919974D+02
.102842D+03
```

```
     .120643D+03   .257657D+03   .359701D+03   .490507D+02   .628626D+02
.754841D+02
     .105886D+03   .240163D+03   .295774D+03   .326934D+03   .661126D+02
.777743D+02
     .907304D+02   .103362D+03   .227552D+03   .273660D+03   .263839D+03
.281088D+03
MO LY=IN TE=IN PS=FI
LE
A1 C1 E1 A2 C2 E2
VA 1 PS 1,1 PS 2,2 PS 3,3 PS 4,4 PS 5,5 PS 6,6
VA 0.5 PS 4,1
VA 1 PS 5,2
OU
```

E.2   Genetic Factor Model Using x Variables

This script fits the genetic common factor model of Appendix E.1 to arithmetic computation data, modeling only additive (A) and non-shared environmental (E) effects. Observed measures are modeled as x variables and *all* parameters (including specific variances) are estimated in Λ_x.

```
Arithmetic Computation : Number Correct - MZ FEMALES
DA NG=2 NI=8 NO=43
LA
Tw1-T0 Tw1-T1 Tw1-T2 Tw1-T3 Tw2-T0 Tw2-T1 Tw2-T2 Tw2-T3
CM
     .259664D+03   .209325D+03   .259939D+03   .209532D+03   .220755D+03
.245235D+03
     .221610D+03   .221491D+03   .221317D+03   .249298D+03   .211678D+03
.200684D+03
     .191937D+03   .196068D+03   .283802D+03   .166020D+03   .187932D+03
.164335D+03
     .177413D+03   .193615D+03   .249487D+03   .184389D+03   .191922D+03
.182497D+03
     .188341D+03   .213771D+03   .220240D+03   .262092D+03   .179332D+03
.188079D+03
     .180813D+03   .195734D+03   .218767D+03   .224939D+03   .230575D+03
.270928D+03
MO NX=8 NK=12 LX=FU,FI PH=FI TD=ZE
LK
A1 A2 E1 T1U1 T1U2 T1U3 T1U4 E2 T2U1 T2U2 T2U3 T2U4
PA LX
1 0 1 1 0 0 0 0 0 0 0 0
```

```
1 0 1 0 1 0 0 0 0 0 0 0
1 0 1 0 0 1 0 0 0 0 0 0
1 0 1 0 0 0 1 0 0 0 0 0
0 1 0 0 0 0 0 1 1 0 0 0
0 1 0 0 0 0 0 1 0 1 0 0
0 1 0 0 0 0 0 1 0 0 1 0
0 1 0 0 0 0 0 1 0 0 0 1
EQ LX 1,1 LX 5,2
EQ LX 2,1 LX 6,2
EQ LX 3,1 LX 7,2
EQ LX 4,1 LX 8,2
EQ LX 1,3 LX 5,8
EQ LX 2,3 LX 6,8
EQ LX 3,3 LX 7,8
EQ LX 4,3 LX 8,8
EQ LX 1,4 LX 5,9
EQ LX 2,5 LX 6,10
EQ LX 3,6 LX 7,11
EQ LX 4,7 LX 8,12
VA 1 PH 1,1 PH 2,2 PH 3,3 PH 4,4 PH 5,5 PH 6,6 PH 7,7 PH 8,8
VA 1 PH 9,9 PH 10,10 PH 11,11 PH 12,12
VA 1 PH 1,2
ST 5.0 ALL
OU NS AD=OFF
Arithmetic Computation : Number Correct - DZ FEMALES
DA NO=44
LA
Tw1-T0 Tw1-T1 Tw1-T2 Tw1-T3 Tw2-T0 Tw2-T1 Tw2-T2 Tw2-T3
CM
   .297917D+03   .232357D+03   .229414D+03   .231170D+03   .213544D+03
.247423D+03
   .236979D+03   .214943D+03   .225486D+03   .274943D+03   .670523D+02
.790291D+02
   .951977D+02   .932791D+02   .281959D+03   .730122D+02   .919974D+02
.102842D+03
   .120643D+03   .257657D+03   .359701D+03   .490507D+02   .628626D+02
.754841D+02
   .105886D+03   .240163D+03   .295774D+03   .326934D+03   .661126D+02
.777743D+02
   .907304D+02   .103362D+03   .227552D+03   .273660D+03   .263839D+03
.281088D+03
MO LX=IN PH=FI
LK
```

```
A1 A2 E1 T1U1 T1U2 T1U3 T1U4 E2 T2U1 T2U2 T2U3 T2U4
VA 1 PH 1,1 PH 2,2 PH 3,3 PH 4,4 PH 5,5 PH 6,6 PH 7,7 PH 8,8
VA 1 PH 9,9 PH 10,10 PH 11,11 PH 12,12
VA 0.5 PH 1,2
OU
```

E.3 Bivariate Genetic Factor Model

The LISREL script below adds a genetic "alcohol" factor to the common factors for A and E in Appendix E.2. Genetic effects on the three arithmetic computation measurements taken after alcohol administration load on the alcohol factor.

```
Arithmetic Computation: Number Correct - MZ FEMALES
DA NG=2 NI=8 NO=43
LA
Tw1-T0 Tw1-T1 Tw1-T2 Tw1-T3 Tw2-T0 Tw2-T1 Tw2-T2 Tw2-T3
CM
   .259664D+03   .209325D+03   .259939D+03   .209532D+03   .220755D+03
.245235D+03
   .221610D+03   .221491D+03   .221317D+03   .249298D+03   .211678D+03
.200684D+03
   .191937D+03   .196068D+03   .283802D+03   .166020D+03   .187932D+03
.164335D+03
   .177413D+03   .193615D+03   .249487D+03   .184389D+03   .191922D+03
.182497D+03
   .188341D+03   .213771D+03   .220240D+03   .262092D+03   .179332D+03
.188079D+03
   .180813D+03   .195734D+03   .218767D+03   .224939D+03   .230575D+03
.270928D+03
MO NX=8 NK=14 LX=FU,FI PH=FI TD=ZE
LK
A1 Aalc1 A2 Aalc2 E1 T1U1 T1U2 T1U3 T1U4 E2 T2U1 T2U2 T2U3 T2U4
PA LX
1 0 0 0 1 1 0 0 0 0 0 0 0 0
1 1 0 0 1 0 1 0 0 0 0 0 0 0
1 1 0 0 1 0 0 1 0 0 0 0 0 0
1 1 0 0 1 0 0 0 1 0 0 0 0 0
0 0 1 0 0 0 0 0 0 1 1 0 0 0
0 0 1 1 0 0 0 0 0 1 0 1 0 0
0 0 1 1 0 0 0 0 0 1 0 0 1 0
0 0 1 1 0 0 0 0 0 1 0 0 0 1
EQ LX 1,1 LX 5,3
EQ LX 2,1 LX 6,3
```

```
EQ LX 3,1 LX 7,3
EQ LX 4,1 LX 8,3
EQ LX 2,2 LX 6,4
EQ LX 3,2 LX 7,4
EQ LX 4,2 LX 8,4
EQ LX 2,2 LX 3,2
EQ LX 4,2 LX 2,2
EQ LX 1,5 LX 5,10
EQ LX 2,5 LX 6,10
EQ LX 3,5 LX 7,10
EQ LX 4,5 LX 8,10
EQ LX 1,6 LX 5,11
EQ LX 2,7 LX 6,12
EQ LX 3,8 LX 7,13
EQ LX 4,9 LX 8,14
VA 1 PH 1,1 PH 2,2 PH 3,3 PH 4,4 PH 5,5 PH 6,6 PH 7,7
VA 1 PH 8,8 PH 9,9 PH 10,10 PH 11,11 PH 12,12 PH 13,13
VA 1 PH 14,14 PH 1,3 PH 2,4
ST 5.0 ALL
OU NS AD=OFF
Arithmetic Computation: Number Correct - DZ FEMALES
DA NO=44
LA
Tw1-T0 Tw1-T1 Tw1-T2 Tw1-T3 Tw2-T0 Tw2-T1 Tw2-T2 Tw2-T3
CM
   .297917D+03    .232357D+03    .229414D+03    .231170D+03    .213544D+03
.247423D+03
   .236979D+03    .214943D+03    .225486D+03    .274943D+03    .670523D+02
.790291D+02
   .951977D+02    .932791D+02    .281959D+03    .730122D+02    .919974D+02
.102842D+03
   .120643D+03    .257657D+03    .359701D+03    .490507D+02    .628626D+02
.754841D+02
   .105886D+03    .240163D+03    .295774D+03    .326934D+03    .661126D+02
.777743D+02
   .907304D+02    .103362D+03    .227552D+03    .273660D+03    .263839D+03
.281088D+03
MO LX=IN PH=FI
LK
A1 Aalc1 A2 Aalc 2E1 T1U1 T1U2 T1U3 T1U4 E2 T2U1 T2U2 T2U3 T2U4
VA 1 PH 1,1 PH 2,2 PH 3,3 PH 4,4 PH 5,5 PH 6,6 PH 7,7 PH 8,8
VA 1 PH 9,9 PH 10,10 PH 11,11 PH 12,12 PH 13,13 PH 14,14
VA 0.5 PH 1,3 PH 2,4
```

OU

E.4   Genetic Cholesky Model

The LISREL 7 script below fits a cholesky decomposition model to four skin-fold measures. Triangular cholesky matrices are fit only for additive genetic, **A**, and within-family environment, **E**, effects, and the entire model uses only the x variables in LISREL.

```
Cholesky Model for Skinfold Measurements: MZ males
DA NG=2 NI=8 NO=84
LA
Bicep1 Subsca1 Supra1 Tricep1 Bicep2 Subsca2 Supra2 Tricep2
CM
.1285
.1270  .1759
.1704  .2156  .3031
.1035  .1101  .1469  .1041
.0982  .1069  .1491  .0824  .1233
.0999  .1411  .1848  .0880  .1295  .1894
.1256  .1654  .2417  .1095  .1616  .2185  .2842
.0836  .0907  .1341  .0836  .1010  .1134  .1436 .1068
MO NX=8 NK=16 LX=FU,FI PH=FI TD=ZE
LK
T1A1 T1A2 T1A3 T1A4 T1E1 T1E2 T1E3 T1E4 T2A1 T2A2 T2A3 T2A4
T2E1 T2E2 T2E3 T2E4
PA LX
1 0 0 0 1 0 0 0 0 0 0 0 0 0 0 0
1 1 0 0 1 1 0 0 0 0 0 0 0 0 0 0
1 1 1 0 1 1 1 0 0 0 0 0 0 0 0 0
1 1 1 1 1 1 1 1 0 0 0 0 0 0 0 0
0 0 0 0 0 0 0 0 1 0 0 0 1 0 0 0
0 0 0 0 0 0 0 0 1 1 0 0 1 1 0 0
0 0 0 0 0 0 0 0 1 1 1 0 1 1 1 0
0 0 0 0 0 0 0 0 1 1 1 1 1 1 1 1
EQ LX 1,1 LX 5,9
EQ LX 2,1 LX 6,9
EQ LX 3,1 LX 7,9
EQ LX 4,1 LX 8,9
EQ LX 2,2 LX 6,10
EQ LX 3,2 LX 7,10
EQ LX 4,2 LX 8,10
EQ LX 3,3 LX 7,11
```

```
EQ LX 4,3 LX 8,11
EQ LX 4,4 LX 8,12
EQ LX 1,5 LX 5,13
EQ LX 2,5 LX 6,13
EQ LX 3,5 LX 7,13
EQ LX 4,5 LX 8,13
EQ LX 2,6 LX 6,14
EQ LX 3,6 LX 7,14
EQ LX 4,6 LX 8,14
EQ LX 3,7 LX 7,15
EQ LX 4,7 LX 8,15
EQ LX 4,8 LX 8,16
VA 1 PH 1,1 PH 2,2 PH 3,3 PH 4,4 PH 5,5 PH 6,6 PH 7,7 PH 8,8 PH 9,9
VA 1 PH 10,10 PH 11,11 PH 12,12 PH 13,13 PH 14,14 PH 15,15 PH 16,16
VA 1 PH 1,9 PH 2,10 PH 3,11 PH 4,12
ST 0.5 ALL
OU NS AD=OFF
Cholesky Model for Skinfold Measurements: DZ males
DA NO=33
LA
Bicep1 Subsca1 Supra1 Tricep1 Bicep2 Subsca2 Supra2 Tricep2
CM
.1538
.1999   .3007
.2266   .3298   .3795
.1285   .1739   .2007   .1271
.0435   .0336   .0354   .0376   .1782
.0646   .0817   .0741   .0543   .2095   .3081
.0812   .0901   .0972   .0666   .2334   .3241   .3899
.0431   .0388   .0376   .0373   .1437   .1842   .2108  .1415
MO LX=IN PH=FI
LK
T1A1 T1A2 T1A3 T1A4 T1E1 T1E2 T1E3 T1E4 T2A1 T2A2 T2A3 T2A4
T2E1 T2E2 T2E3 T2E4
VA 1 PH 1,1 PH 2,2 PH 3,3 PH 4,4 PH 5,5 PH 6,6 PH 7,7 PH 8,8 PH 9,9
VA 1 PH 10,10 PH 11,11 PH 12,12 PH 13,13 PH 14,14 PH 15,15 PH 16,16
VA 0.5 PH 1,9 PH 2,10 PH 3,11 PH 4,12
OU
```

E.5   Independent Pathway Model

This script fits the multivariate "independent pathway model" to Australian twin
data on asthma, hayfever, dust allergy, and eczema. The data are ordinal, thus,

polychoric correlations are modeled, using asymptotic weight matrices provided by PRELIS.

```
ASTHMA,HAYFEVER,DUST ALLERGY,ECZEMA: Australian MZ females
DA NG=2 NI=8 NO=1232 MA=PM
LA
asthma1 hayfvr1 dustal1 eczema1 asthma2 hayfvr2 dustal2 eczema2
MO NE=8 NK=22 NY=8 GA=FI,FU PH=SY,FI LY=ID PS=ZE TE=ZE
PM
1.000
 .556    1.000
 .573     .758    1.000
 .273     .264     .309    1.000
 .592     .366     .398     .232    1.000
 .411     .593     .451     .145     .549    1.000
 .434     .421     .518     .192     .640     .770    1.000
 .087     .196     .193     .589     .145     .122     .218    1.000
AC FI=ahdemzf.acv
LK
eatopy1 eatopy2 aatopy1 aatopy2 datopy1 datopy2
has1 hha1 hdu1 hec1 has2 hha2 hdu2 hec2
eas1 eha1 edu1 eec1 eas2 eha2 edu2 eec2
PA GA
1 0 1 0 1 0 1 0 0 0 0 0 0 0 1 0 0 0 0 0 0 0
1 0 1 0 1 0 0 1 0 0 0 0 0 0 0 1 0 0 0 0 0 0
1 0 1 0 1 0 0 0 1 0 0 0 0 0 0 0 1 0 0 0 0 0
1 0 1 0 1 0 0 0 0 1 0 0 0 0 0 0 0 1 0 0 0 0
0 1 0 1 0 1 0 0 0 0 1 0 0 0 0 0 0 0 1 0 0 0
0 1 0 1 0 1 0 0 0 0 0 1 0 0 0 0 0 0 0 1 0 0
0 1 0 1 0 1 0 0 0 0 0 0 1 0 0 0 0 0 0 0 1 0
0 1 0 1 0 1 0 0 0 0 0 0 0 1 0 0 0 0 0 0 0 1
EQ GA 1 1 GA 5 2
EQ GA 2 1 GA 6 2
EQ GA 3 1 GA 7 2
EQ GA 4 1 GA 8 2
EQ GA 1 3 GA 5 4
EQ GA 2 3 GA 6 4
EQ GA 3 3 GA 7 4
EQ GA 4 3 GA 8 4
EQ GA 1 5 GA 5 6
EQ GA 2 5 GA 6 6
EQ GA 3 5 GA 7 6
EQ GA 4 5 GA 8 6
EQ GA 1 7 GA 5 11
```

```
EQ GA 2 8 GA 6 12
EQ GA 3 9 GA 7 13
EQ GA 4 10 GA 8 14
EQ GA 1 15 GA 5 19
EQ GA 2 16 GA 6 20
EQ GA 3 17 GA 7 21
EQ GA 4 18 GA 8 22
MA PH
1.
0. 1.
0. 0. 1.
0. 0. 1. 1.
0. 0. 0. 0. 1.
0. 0. 0. 0. 1. 1.
0. 0. 0. 0. 0. 0. 1.
0. 0. 0. 0. 0. 0. 0. 1.
0. 0. 0. 0. 0. 0. 0. 0. 1.
0. 0. 0. 0. 0. 0. 0. 0. 0. 1.
0. 0. 0. 0. 0. 0. 1. 0. 0. 0. 1.
0. 0. 0. 0. 0. 0. 0. 1. 0. 0. 0. 1.
0. 0. 0. 0. 0. 0. 0. 0. 1. 0. 0. 0. 1.
0. 0. 0. 0. 0. 0. 0. 0. 1. 0. 0. 0. 1.
0. 0. 0. 0. 0. 0. 0. 0. 0. 0. 0. 0. 0. 0. 1.
0. 0. 0. 0. 0. 0. 0. 0. 0. 0. 0. 0. 0. 0. 0. 1.
0. 0. 0. 0. 0. 0. 0. 0. 0. 0. 0. 0. 0. 0. 0. 0. 1.
0. 0. 0. 0. 0. 0. 0. 0. 0. 0. 0. 0. 0. 0. 0. 0. 0. 1.
0. 0. 0. 0. 0. 0. 0. 0. 0. 0. 0. 0. 0. 0. 0. 0. 0. 0. 1.
0. 0. 0. 0. 0. 0. 0. 0. 0. 0. 0. 0. 0. 0. 0. 0. 0. 0. 0. 1.
0. 0. 0. 0. 0. 0. 0. 0. 0. 0. 0. 0. 0. 0. 0. 0. 0. 0. 0. 0. 1.
0. 0. 0. 0. 0. 0. 0. 0. 0. 0. 0. 0. 0. 0. 0. 0. 0. 0. 0. 0. 0. 1./
ST 0.3 ALL
OU NS AD=OFF DF=-12 IT=120
ASTHMA,HAYFEVER,DUST ALLERGY,ECZEMA: DZ Females
DA NO=751
LA
asthma1 hayfvr1 dustal1 eczema1 asthma2 hayfvr2 dustal2 eczema2
MO GA=IN PH=SY,FI
PM
1.000
 .524     1.000
 .588      .749     1.000
 .291      .314      .279     1.000
 .262      .170      .041      .139     1.000
```

```
 .129      .318      .262      .093      .395     1.000
 .079      .171      .214      .019      .684      .723     1.000
 .217      .114      .087      .313      .254      .218      .276     1.000
AC FI=ahdedzf.acv
LK
eatopy1 eatopy2 aatopy1 aatopy2 datopy1 datopy2
has1 hha1 hdu1 hec1 has2 hha2 hdu2 hec2
eas1 eha1 edu1 eec1 eas2 eha2 edu2 eec2
MA PH
1.
0. 1.
0. 0. 1.
0. 0. .5 1.
0. 0. 0. 0. 1.
0. 0. 0. 0. .25 1.
0. 0. 0. 0. 0. 0. 1.
0. 0. 0. 0. 0. 0. 0. 1.
0. 0. 0. 0. 0. 0. 0. 0. 1.
0. 0. 0. 0. 0. 0. 0. 0. 0. 1.
0. 0. 0. 0. 0. 0. .5 0. 0. 0. 1.
0. 0. 0. 0. 0. 0. 0. .5 0. 0. 0. 1.
0. 0. 0. 0. 0. 0. 0. 0. .5 0. 0. 0. 1.
0. 0. 0. 0. 0. 0. 0. 0. 0. .5 0. 0. 0. 1.
0. 0. 0. 0. 0. 0. 0. 0. 0. 0. 0. 0. 0. 0. 1.
0. 0. 0. 0. 0. 0. 0. 0. 0. 0. 0. 0. 0. 0. 0. 1.
0. 0. 0. 0. 0. 0. 0. 0. 0. 0. 0. 0. 0. 0. 0. 0. 1.
0. 0. 0. 0. 0. 0. 0. 0. 0. 0. 0. 0. 0. 0. 0. 0. 0. 1.
0. 0. 0. 0. 0. 0. 0. 0. 0. 0. 0. 0. 0. 0. 0. 0. 0. 0. 1.
0. 0. 0. 0. 0. 0. 0. 0. 0. 0. 0. 0. 0. 0. 0. 0. 0. 0. 0. 1.
0. 0. 0. 0. 0. 0. 0. 0. 0. 0. 0. 0. 0. 0. 0. 0. 0. 0. 0. 0. 1.
0. 0. 0. 0. 0. 0. 0. 0. 0. 0. 0. 0. 0. 0. 0. 0. 0. 0. 0. 0. 0. 1./
OU
```

E.6   Common Pathway Model

The following script fits the "common pathway model" to ordinal data on asthma,
hayfever, dust allergy, and eczema from the Australian twin sample. Asymptotic
weight matrices and polychoric correlations were obtained from PRELIS.

```
Common pathway model: Asthma, Hayfever, Dust allergy, Eczema
; MZ Females
DA NG=2 NI=8 NO=1232 MA=PM
LA
```

```
ASTHMA1 HAYFEVR1 DUSTAL1 ECZEMA1 ASTHMA2 HAYFEVR2 DUSTAL2 ECZEMA2
SE
1 5 2 6 3 7 4 8 /
MO NE=10 NK=24 NY=8 GA=FI,FU PH=SY,FI BE=FU,FI LY=FU,FI TE=ZE PS=ZE
PM FI=AHDEMZF.COR
AC FI=AHDEMZF.ACV
LE
A1 A2 H1 H2 D1 D2 E1 E2 ATOPY1 ATOPY2
LK
HATOPY1 HATOPY2 CATOPY1 CATOPY2 DATOPY1 DATOPY2 EATOPY1 EATOPY2
HA1 HA2 EA1 EA2 HH1 HH2 EH1 EH2
HD1 HD2 ED1 ED2 HE1 HE2 EE1 EE2
VA 1 LY 1 1 LY 2 2 LY 3 3 LY 4 4 LY 5 5 LY 6 6 LY 7 7
VA 1 LY 8 8
FR BE 1 9 BE 2 10 BE 3 9 BE 4 10 BE 5 9 BE 6 10 BE 7 9
FR BE 8 10
EQ BE 1 9  BE 2 10
EQ BE 3 9  BE 4 10
EQ BE 5 9  BE 6 10
EQ BE 7 9  BE 8 10
PA GA
0 0 0 0 0 0 0 0 1 0 1 0 0 0 0 0 0 0 0 0 0 0 0 0
0 0 0 0 0 0 0 0 0 1 0 1 0 0 0 0 0 0 0 0 0 0 0 0
0 0 0 0 0 0 0 0 0 0 0 0 1 0 1 0 0 0 0 0 0 0 0 0
0 0 0 0 0 0 0 0 0 0 0 0 0 1 0 1 0 0 0 0 0 0 0 0
0 0 0 0 0 0 0 0 0 0 0 0 0 0 0 0 1 0 1 0 0 0 0 0
0 0 0 0 0 0 0 0 0 0 0 0 0 0 0 0 0 1 0 1 0 0 0 0
0 0 0 0 0 0 0 0 0 0 0 0 0 0 0 0 0 0 0 0 1 0 1 0
0 0 0 0 0 0 0 0 0 0 0 0 0 0 0 0 0 0 0 0 0 1 0 1
1 0 0 0 1 0 0 0 0 0 0 0 0 0 0 0 0 0 0 0 0 0 0 0
0 1 0 0 0 1 0 0 0 0 0 0 0 0 0 0 0 0 0 0 0 0 0 0
VA 1 GA 9 7
EQ GA 9 1 GA 10 2
EQ GA 9 3 GA 10 4
EQ GA 9 5 GA 10 6
EQ GA 9 7 GA 10 8
EQ GA 1 9 GA 2 10
EQ GA 1 11 GA 2 12
EQ GA 3 13 GA 4 14
EQ GA 3 15 GA 4 16
EQ GA 5 17 GA 6 18
EQ GA 5 19 GA 6 20
EQ GA 7 21 GA 8 22
```

```
EQ GA 7 23 GA 8 24
MA PH
1
1 1
0 0 1
0 0 1 1
0 0 0 0 1
0 0 0 0 1 1
0 0 0 0 0 0 1
0 0 0 0 0 0 0 1
0 0 0 0 0 0 0 0 1
0 0 0 0 0 0 0 0 1 1
0 0 0 0 0 0 0 0 0 0 1
0 0 0 0 0 0 0 0 0 0 0 1
0 0 0 0 0 0 0 0 0 0 0 0 1
0 0 0 0 0 0 0 0 0 0 0 0 1 1
0 0 0 0 0 0 0 0 0 0 0 0 0 0 1
0 0 0 0 0 0 0 0 0 0 0 0 0 0 0 1
0 0 0 0 0 0 0 0 0 0 0 0 0 0 0 0 1
0 0 0 0 0 0 0 0 0 0 0 0 0 0 0 0 1 1
0 0 0 0 0 0 0 0 0 0 0 0 0 0 0 0 0 0 1
0 0 0 0 0 0 0 0 0 0 0 0 0 0 0 0 0 0 0 1
0 0 0 0 0 0 0 0 0 0 0 0 0 0 0 0 0 0 0 0 1
0 0 0 0 0 0 0 0 0 0 0 0 0 0 0 0 0 0 0 0 1 1
0 0 0 0 0 0 0 0 0 0 0 0 0 0 0 0 0 0 0 0 0 0 1
0 0 0 0 0 0 0 0 0 0 0 0 0 0 0 0 0 0 0 0 0 0 1 /
ST 0.7 ALL
OU RS NS AD=OFF SC IT=150 DF=-12
COMMON PATHWAY MODEL: DZ Females FOR AHDE 1980
DA NO=751
LA
A1 H1 D1 E1 A2 H2 D2 E2
SE
1 5 2 6 3 7 4 8 /
MO GA=IN PH=SY,FI BE=IN PS=IN LY=IN
PM FI=AHDEDZF.COR
AC FI=AHDEDZF.ACV
LE
A1 A2 H1 H2 D1 D2 E1 E2 ATOPY1 ATOPY2
LK
HATOPY1 HATOPY2 CATOPY1 CATOPY2 DATOPY1 DATOPY2 EATOPY1 EATOPY2
HA1 HA2 EA1 EA2 HH1 HH2 EH1 EH2
HD1 HD2 ED1 ED2 HE1 HE2 EE1 EE2
```

```
MA PH
1
.5 1
0 0 1
0 0 1 1
0 0 0 0 1
0 0 0 0 .25 1
0 0 0 0 0 0 1
0 0 0 0 0 0 0 1
0 0 0 0 0 0 0 0 1
0 0 0 0 0 0 0 0 .5 1
0 0 0 0 0 0 0 0 0 0 1
0 0 0 0 0 0 0 0 0 0 0 1
0 0 0 0 0 0 0 0 0 0 0 0 1
0 0 0 0 0 0 0 0 0 0 0 0 0 .5 1
0 0 0 0 0 0 0 0 0 0 0 0 0 0 1
0 0 0 0 0 0 0 0 0 0 0 0 0 0 0 1
0 0 0 0 0 0 0 0 0 0 0 0 0 0 0 0 1
0 0 0 0 0 0 0 0 0 0 0 0 0 0 0 0 0 .5 1
0 0 0 0 0 0 0 0 0 0 0 0 0 0 0 0 0 0 0 1
0 0 0 0 0 0 0 0 0 0 0 0 0 0 0 0 0 0 0 0 1
0 0 0 0 0 0 0 0 0 0 0 0 0 0 0 0 0 0 0 0 0 1
0 0 0 0 0 0 0 0 0 0 0 0 0 0 0 0 0 0 0 0 0 0 .5 1
0 0 0 0 0 0 0 0 0 0 0 0 0 0 0 0 0 0 0 0 0 0 0 1
0 0 0 0 0 0 0 0 0 0 0 0 0 0 0 0 0 0 0 0 0 0 0 0 1 /
OU
```

Appendix F

LISREL Script for Sibling Interaction Model

F.1 Sibling Interaction Model

The following LISREL 7 script represents a univariate genetic model incorporating sibling interaction fitted to covariance matrices for two twin groups: 1) MZ pairs reared together, and 2) DZ pairs reared together.

```
;Analysis of maternal ratings of children's externalizing behavior
;problems. Data are based on 24 core items from the Achenbach Child
;Behavior Checklist collected by mail as part of a survey of school
;age twins in Virginia.
;
;These data are for white schoolchildren aged 8-16 years. They are
;age and sex corrected, up to quadratic regression on age, and log
;transformed to approximate normality.
;
;In addition to the traditional decomposition by sex and zygosity
;these families have been sub-divided according to family size:
;sibcat=0 where there are no sibs in the family apart from the twins
;themselves, and sibcat=1 where there is at least one other sibling
;apart from the twins themselves. This is a crude division and takes
;no account of the age structure, for example. Nevertheless, as a
;starting point it is instructive to consider this source of
;environmental heterogeneity for which most models of social
;interaction within families will predict differences.
;
;In  this first program we consider the data
```

413

```
;for boy-boy pairs in larger families (sibcat=1) only.
;
MALE MZ TWINS IN LARGER FAMILIES
DA NG=2 NI=2 NO=171 MA=CM
LA
EXTER1 EXTER2
CM SY
0.923
0.798 0.907
MO NY=2 NE=2 NK=6 LY=ID GA=FU,FR BE=FU,FI PH=FI PS=ZE TE=ZE
LK
At1 Ct1 Et1 At2 Ct2 Et2
LE
Pt1 Pt2
PA GA
1 0 1 0 0 0
0 0 0 1 0 1
EQ GA(1,1) GA(2,4)
EQ GA(1,2) GA(2,5)
EQ GA(1,3) GA(2,6)
VA 1. PH(1,1) PH(2,2) PH(3,3) PH(4,4) PH(5,5) PH(6,6)
VA 1. PH(4,1) PH(5,2)
ST 0.3 GA(1,1)-GA(2,6)
;ADDING SIBLING INTERACTION COMPONENT
;PA BE
;0 1
;1 0
;EQ BE(1,2) BE(2,1)
;ST 0.05 BE(1,2)
OU NS ND=2 AD=OFF
Male DZ twins in larger families
DA NI=2 NO=194 MA=CM
LA
EXTER1 EXTER2
CM SY
0.671
0.448 0.700
MO NY=2 NE=2 NK=6 LY=IN GA=IN BE=IN PH=FI PS=IN TE=IN
VA 1.0 PH(1,1) PH(2,2) PH(3,3) PH(4,4) PH(5,5) PH(6,6)
VA 1.0 PH(5,2)
VA 0.5 PH(4,1)
OU NS ND=2 AD=OFF
```

Appendix G

LISREL Scripts for Sex and G×E Interaction

G.1 General Model for Scalar Sex-Limitation

In this example, we estimate sex-dependent additive genetic effects and fix the sex-dependent dominance effects to zero. Four same-sex groups are used: MZ female, DZ female, MZ male, and DZ male.

```
GENERAL SEX LIMITATION MODEL - U.S. MZ FEMALES BMI (With Dom.)
DA NG=5 NI=2 NO=1802 MA=CM
LA
BMI1 BMI2
CM
.276533 0.203348 0.269922
MO NY=2 NE=12 NK=10 GA=FU,FR LY=FU,FI PH=SY,FI BE=FU,FR PS=ZE TE=ZE
LE
A1_f D1_f E1_f X1_1 X2_1 A2_f D2_f E2_f X1_2 X2_2 P1_f P2_f
LK
A1_f D1_f E1_f X1_1 X2_1 A2_f D2_f E2_f X1_2 X2_2
VA 1.0 PH(1,1) PH(2,2) PH(3,3) PH(4,4) PH(5,5) PH(6,6)
VA 1.0 PH(7,7) PH(8,8) PH(9,9) PH(10,10)
VA 1.0 PH(1,6) PH(2,7)
PA GA
1 0 0 0 0 0 0 0 0 0
0 1 0 0 0 0 0 0 0 0
0 0 1 0 0 0 0 0 0 0
0 0 0 0 0 0 0 0 0 0
0 0 0 0 0 0 0 0 0 0
```

```
0 0 0 0 0 1 0 0 0 0
0 0 0 0 0 0 1 0 0 0
0 0 0 0 0 0 0 1 0 0
0 0 0 0 0 0 0 0 0 0
0 0 0 0 0 0 0 0 0 0
0 0 0 0 0 0 0 0 0 0
0 0 0 0 0 0 0 0 0 0
EQ GA(1,1) GA(6,6)
EQ GA(2,2) GA(7,7)
EQ GA(3,3) GA(8,8)
PA BE
0 0 0 0 0 0 0 0 0 0 0 0
0 0 0 0 0 0 0 0 0 0 0 0
0 0 0 0 0 0 0 0 0 0 0 0
0 0 0 0 0 0 0 0 0 0 0 0
0 0 0 0 0 0 0 0 0 0 0 0
0 0 0 0 0 0 0 0 0 0 0 0
0 0 0 0 0 0 0 0 0 0 0 0
0 0 0 0 0 0 0 0 0 0 0 0
0 0 0 0 0 0 0 0 0 0 0 0
0 0 0 0 0 0 0 0 0 0 0 0
1 1 1 0 0 0 0 0 0 0 0 0
0 0 0 0 0 1 1 1 0 0 0 0
EQ GA(1,1) BE(11,1) BE(12,6)
EQ GA(2,2) BE(11,2) BE(12,7)
EQ GA(3,3) BE(11,3) BE(12,8)
VA 1.0 LY(1,11)
VA 1.0 LY(2,12)
ST 0.5 ALL
OU NS AD=OFF
FEMALE DZ PAIRS
DA NI=2 NO=1142 MA=CM
LA
BMI1 BMI2
CM
.284734 0.098942 0.278211
MO NY=2 NE=12 NK=10 GA=FU,FR LY=FU,FI PH=SY,FI BE=FU,FR PS=ZE TE=ZE
LE
A1_f D1_f E1_f X1_1 X2_1 A2_f D2_f E2_f X1_2 X2_2 P1_f P2_f
LK
A1_f D1_f E1_f X1_1 X2_1 A2_f D2_f E2_f X1_2 X2_2
VA 1.0 PH(1,1) PH(2,2) PH(3,3) PH(4,4) PH(5,5) PH(6,6)
VA 1.0 PH(7,7) PH(8,8) PH(9,9) PH(10,10)
```

```
VA 0.5 PH(1,6)
VA 0.25 PH(2,7)
PA GA
1 0 0 0 0 0 0 0 0 0
0 1 0 0 0 0 0 0 0 0
0 0 1 0 0 0 0 0 0 0
0 0 0 0 0 0 0 0 0 0
0 0 0 0 0 0 0 0 0 0
0 0 0 0 0 1 0 0 0 0
0 0 0 0 0 0 1 0 0 0
0 0 0 0 0 0 0 1 0 0
0 0 0 0 0 0 0 0 0 0
0 0 0 0 0 0 0 0 0 0
0 0 0 0 0 0 0 0 0 0
0 0 0 0 0 0 0 0 0 0
EQ GA(1,1,1) GA(1,1) GA(6,6)
EQ GA(1,2,2) GA(2,2) GA(7,7)
EQ GA(1,3,3) GA(3,3) GA(8,8)
PA BE
0 0 0 0 0 0 0 0 0 0 0 0
0 0 0 0 0 0 0 0 0 0 0 0
0 0 0 0 0 0 0 0 0 0 0 0
0 0 0 0 0 0 0 0 0 0 0 0
0 0 0 0 0 0 0 0 0 0 0 0
0 0 0 0 0 0 0 0 0 0 0 0
0 0 0 0 0 0 0 0 0 0 0 0
0 0 0 0 0 0 0 0 0 0 0 0
0 0 0 0 0 0 0 0 0 0 0 0
0 0 0 0 0 0 0 0 0 0 0 0
1 1 1 0 0 0 0 0 0 0 0 0
0 0 0 0 0 1 1 1 0 0 0 0
EQ GA(1,1,1) BE(11,1) BE(12,6)
EQ GA(1,2,2) BE(11,2) BE(12,7)
EQ GA(1,3,3) BE(11,3) BE(12,8)
VA 1.0 LY(1,11)
VA 1.0 LY(2,12)
OU NS AD=OFF
MALE MZ PAIRS (estimating hp_m)
DA NI=2 NO=750 MA=CM
LA
BMI1 BMI2
CM
0.154669 0.104787 0.144701
```

```
MO NY=2 NE=12 NK=10 GA=FU,FR LY=FU,FI PH=SY,FI BE=FU,FR PS=ZE TE=ZE
LE
A1_m D1_m E1_m AP_1 DP_1 A2_m D2_m E2_m AP_2 DP_2 P1_m P2_m
LK
A1_m D1_m E1_m AP1_1 DP_1 A2_m D2_m E2_m AP_2 DP_2
VA 1.0 PH(1,1) PH(2,2) PH(3,3) PH(4,4) PH(5,5) PH(6,6)
VA 1.0 PH(7,7) PH(8,8) PH(9,9) PH(10,10)
VA 1.0 PH(1,6) PH(2,7)
VA 1.0 PH(4,9) PH(5,10)
PA GA
1 0 0 0 0 0 0 0 0 0
0 1 0 0 0 0 0 0 0 0
0 0 1 0 0 0 0 0 0 0
0 0 0 1 0 0 0 0 0 0
0 0 0 0 0 0 0 0 0 0
0 0 0 0 0 1 0 0 0 0
0 0 0 0 0 0 1 0 0 0
0 0 0 0 0 0 0 1 0 0
0 0 0 0 0 0 0 0 1 0
0 0 0 0 0 0 0 0 0 0
0 0 0 0 0 0 0 0 0 0
0 0 0 0 0 0 0 0 0 0
EQ GA(1,1) GA(6,6)
EQ GA(2,2) GA(7,7)
EQ GA(3,3) GA(8,8)
EQ GA(4,4) GA(9,9)
EQ GA(5,5) GA(10,10)
PA BE
0 0 0 0 0 0 0 0 0 0 0 0
0 0 0 0 0 0 0 0 0 0 0 0
0 0 0 0 0 0 0 0 0 0 0 0
0 0 0 0 0 0 0 0 0 0 0 0
0 0 0 0 0 0 0 0 0 0 0 0
0 0 0 0 0 0 0 0 0 0 0 0
0 0 0 0 0 0 0 0 0 0 0 0
0 0 0 0 0 0 0 0 0 0 0 0
0 0 0 0 0 0 0 0 0 0 0 0
0 0 0 0 0 0 0 0 0 0 0 0
1 1 1 1 0 0 0 0 0 0 0 0
0 0 0 0 0 1 1 1 1 0 0 0
EQ GA(1,1) BE(11,1) BE(12,6)
EQ GA(2,2) BE(11,2) BE(12,7)
EQ GA(3,3) BE(11,3) BE(12,8)
```

```
EQ GA(4,4) BE(11,4) BE(12,9)
EQ GA(5,5) BE(11,5) BE(12,10)
VA 1.0 LY(1,11)
VA 1.0 LY(2,12)
ST 0.5 ALL
OU NS AD=OFF
MALE DZ PAIRS (estimating hp_m)
DA NI=2 NO=553 MA=CM
LA
BMI1 BMI2
CM
0.160091 0.050899 0.168401
MO NY=2 NE=12 NK=10 GA=FU,FR LY=FU,FI PH=SY,FI BE=FU,FR PS=ZE TE=ZE
LE
A1_m D1_m E1_m AP_1 DP1_1 A2_m D2_m E2_m AP_2 DP_2 P1_m P2_m
LK
A1_m D1_m E1_m AP_1 DP_1 A2_m D2_m E2_m AP_2 DP_2
VA 1.0 PH(1,1) PH(2,2) PH(3,3) PH(4,4) PH(5,5) PH(6,6)
VA 1.0 PH(7,7) PH(8,8) PH(9,9) PH(10,10)
VA 0.5 PH(1,6)
VA 0.25 PH(2,7)
VA 0.5 PH(4,9)
VA 0.25 PH(5,10)
PA GA
1 0 0 0 0 0 0 0 0 0
0 1 0 0 0 0 0 0 0 0
0 0 1 0 0 0 0 0 0 0
0 0 0 1 0 0 0 0 0 0
0 0 0 0 0 0 0 0 0 0
0 0 0 0 0 1 0 0 0 0
0 0 0 0 0 0 1 0 0 0
0 0 0 0 0 0 0 1 0 0
0 0 0 0 0 0 0 0 1 0
0 0 0 0 0 0 0 0 0 0
0 0 0 0 0 0 0 0 0 0
0 0 0 0 0 0 0 0 0 0
EQ GA(3,1,1) GA(1,1) GA(6,6)
EQ GA(3,2,2) GA(2,2) GA(7,7)
EQ GA(3,3,3) GA(3,3) GA(8,8)
EQ GA(3,4,4) GA(4,4) GA(9,9)
EQ GA(3,5,5) GA(5,5) GA(10,10)
PA BE
0 0 0 0 0 0 0 0 0 0 0 0
```

```
0 0 0 0 0 0 0 0 0 0 0 0
0 0 0 0 0 0 0 0 0 0 0 0
0 0 0 0 0 0 0 0 0 0 0 0
0 0 0 0 0 0 0 0 0 0 0 0
0 0 0 0 0 0 0 0 0 0 0 0
0 0 0 0 0 0 0 0 0 0 0 0
0 0 0 0 0 0 0 0 0 0 0 0
0 0 0 0 0 0 0 0 0 0 0 0
0 0 0 0 0 0 0 0 0 0 0 0
1 1 1 1 0 0 0 0 0 0 0 0
0 0 0 0 0 1 1 1 1 0 0 0
EQ GA(3,1,1) BE(11,1) BE(12,6)
EQ GA(3,2,2) BE(11,2) BE(12,7)
EQ GA(3,3,3) BE(11,3) BE(12,8)
EQ GA(3,4,4) BE(11,4) BE(12,9)
EQ GA(3,5,5) BE(11,5) BE(12,10)
VA 1.0 LY(1,11)
VA 1.0 LY(2,12)
OU NS AD=OFF
DZO PAIRS - females first, males second - estimating hp_m
DA NI=2 NO=1341 MA=CM
LA
BMI1 BMI2
CM
0.273517 0.054524 0.172811
MO NY=2 NE=12 NK=10 GA=FU,FR LY=FU,FI PH=SY,FI BE=FU,FR PS=ZE TE=ZE
LE
A1_f D1_f E1_f X1_1 X2_1 A2_m D2_m E2_m AP2_m DP2_m P1_f P2_m
LK
A1_f D1_f E1_f X1_1 X2_1 A2_m D2_m E2_m AP2_m DP2_m
VA 1.0 PH(1,1) PH(2,2) PH(3,3) PH(4,4) PH(5,5) PH(6,6)
VA 1.0 PH(7,7) PH(8,8) PH(9,9) PH(10,10)
VA 0.5 PH(1,6)
VA 0.25 PH(2,7)
PA GA
1 0 0 0 0 0 0 0 0 0
0 1 0 0 0 0 0 0 0 0
0 0 1 0 0 0 0 0 0 0
0 0 0 0 0 0 0 0 0 0
0 0 0 0 0 0 0 0 0 0
0 0 0 0 0 1 0 0 0 0
0 0 0 0 0 0 1 0 0 0
0 0 0 0 0 0 0 1 0 0
```

```
0 0 0 0 0 0 0 0 1 0
0 0 0 0 0 0 0 0 0 0
0 0 0 0 0 0 0 0 0 0
0 0 0 0 0 0 0 0 0 0
EQ GA(1,1,1) GA(1,1)
EQ GA(3,1,1) GA(6,6)
EQ GA(1,2,2) GA(2,2)
EQ GA(3,2,2) GA(7,7)
EQ GA(1,3,3) GA(3,3)
EQ GA(3,3,3) GA(8,8)
EQ GA(3,9,9) GA(9,9)
EQ GA(3,5,5) GA(10,10)
PA BE
0 0 0 0 0 0 0 0 0 0 0 0
0 0 0 0 0 0 0 0 0 0 0 0
0 0 0 0 0 0 0 0 0 0 0 0
0 0 0 0 0 0 0 0 0 0 0 0
0 0 0 0 0 0 0 0 0 0 0 0
0 0 0 0 0 0 0 0 0 0 0 0
0 0 0 0 0 0 0 0 0 0 0 0
0 0 0 0 0 0 0 0 0 0 0 0
0 0 0 0 0 0 0 0 0 0 0 0
0 0 0 0 0 0 0 0 0 0 0 0
1 1 1 0 0 0 0 0 0 0 0 0
0 0 0 0 0 1 1 1 1 0 0 0
EQ GA(1,1,1) BE(11,1)
EQ GA(3,1,1) BE(12,6)
EQ GA(1,2,2) BE(11,2)
EQ GA(3,2,2) BE(12,7)
EQ GA(1,3,3) BE(11,3)
EQ GA(3,3,3) BE(12,8)
EQ GA(3,4,4) BE(12,9)
EQ GA(3,5,5) BE(12,10)
VA 1.0 LY(1,11)
VA 1.0 LY(2,12)
OU NS AD=OFF ND=5 IT=100
```

G.2   Scalar Sex-Limitation Model

This script fits a model in which genetic and environmental factors are proportional across the sexes, so that $a_M = ka_F$; $d_M = kd_F$; and $e_M = ke_F$.

```
COMMON MULTIPLIER MODEL - U.S. MZ FEMALES BMI (with dom.)
```

```
DA NG=5 NI=2 NO=1802 MA=CM
LA
BMI1 BMI2
CM
.276533 0.203348 0.269922
MO NY=2 NE=4 NK=6 GA=FU,FR LY=FU,FI PH=SY,FI BE=FU,FI PS=ZE TE=ZE
LE
L11_f L12_f L21_f L22_f
LK
A1 D1 E1 A2 D2 E2
VA 1.0 PH(1,1) PH(2,2) PH(3,3) PH(4,4) PH(5,5) PH(6,6)
VA 1.0 PH(1,4) PH(2,5)
PA GA
1 1 1 0 0 0
0 0 0 0 0 0
0 0 0 1 1 1
0 0 0 0 0 0
EQ GA(1,1) GA(3,4)
EQ GA(1,2) GA(3,5)
EQ GA(1,3) GA(3,6)
VA 1.0 BE(2,1)
VA 1.0 BE(4,3)
VA 1.0 LY(1,2)
VA 1.0 LY(2,4)
ST 0.7 ALL
OU NS AD=OFF
FEMALE DZ PAIRS
DA NI=2 NO=1142 MA=CM
LA
BMI1 BMI2
CM
.284734 0.098942 0.278211
MO NY=2 NE=4 NK=6 GA=IN LY=FU,FI PH=SY,FI BE=FU,FI PS=ZE TE=ZE
LE
L11_f L12_f L21_f L22_f
LK
A1 D1 E1 A2 D2 E2
VA 1.0 PH(1,1) PH(2,2) PH(3,3) PH(4,4) PH(5,5) PH(6,6)
VA 0.5 PH(1,4)
VA 0.25 PH(2,5)
VA 1.0 BE(2,1)
VA 1.0 BE(4,3)
VA 1.0 LY(1,2)
```

```
VA 1.0 LY(2,4)
ST 0.7 ALL
OU NS AD=OFF
MALE MZ PAIRS
DA NI=2 NO=750 MA=CM
LA
BMI1 BMI2
CM
0.154669 0.104787 0.144701
MO NY=2 NE=4 NK=6 GA=IN LY=FU,FI PH=SY,FI BE=FU,FI PS=ZE TE=ZE
LE
L11_m L12_m L21_m L22_m
LK
A1 D1 E1 A2 D2 E2
VA 1.0 PH(1,1) PH(2,2) PH(3,3) PH(4,4) PH(5,5) PH(6,6)
VA 1.0 PH(1,4) PH(2,5)
FR BE(2,1) BE(4,3) LY(1,2) LY(2,4)
EQ BE(2,1) BE(4,3) LY(1,2) LY(2,4)
ST 0.7 ALL
OU NS AD=OFF
MALE DZ PAIRS
DA NI=2 NO=553 MA=CM
LA
BMI1 BMI2
CM
0.160091 0.050899 0.168401
MO NY=2 NE=4 NK=6 GA=IN LY=FU,FI PH=SY,FI BE=FU,FI PS=ZE TE=ZE
LE
L11_m L12_m L21_m L22_m
LK
A1 D1 E1 A2 D2 E2
VA 1.0 PH(1,1) PH(2,2) PH(3,3) PH(4,4) PH(5,5) PH(6,6)
VA 0.5 PH(1,4)
VA 0.25 PH(2,5)
FR BE(2,1) BE(4,3) LY(1,2) LY(2,4)
EQ BE (3,2,1) BE(2,1) BE(4,3) LY(1,2) LY(2,4)
OU NS AD=OFF
DZO PAIRS
DA NI=2 NO=1341 MA=CM
LA
BMI_m BMI_f
CM
0.273517 0.054524 0.172811
```

```
MO NY=2 NE=4 NK=6 GA=IN LY=FU,FI PH=SY,FI BE=FU,FI PS=ZE TE=ZE
LE
L11_f L12_f L21_m L22_m
LK
A1 D1 E1 A2 D2 E2
VA 1.0 PH(1,1) PH(2,2) PH(3,3) PH(4,4) PH(5,5) PH(6,6)
VA 0.5 PH(1,4)
VA 0.25 PH(2,5)
VA 1.0 BE(2,1) LY(1,2)
FR BE(4,3) LY(2,4)
EQ BE (3,2,1) BE(4,3) LY(2,4)
OU NS AD=OFF IT=200
```

G.3   General Model for G × E Interaction

This script fits a G × E interaction model in which the environmental agent is dichotomous. Thus we discriminate between concordant exposed, discordant, and concordant non-exposed pairs of (i) MZ and (ii) DZ twins, giving six groups in total.

```
GxE INTERACTION FULL MODEL.  Depressed Conc Single MZ Australians
DA NG=6 NI=2 NO=254 MA=CM
LA
DEP1 DEP2
CM
0.0968 0.0381 0.0896
MO NY=2 NE=12 NK=10 GA=FU,FI LY=FU,FI PH=SY,FI BE=FU,FI PS=ZE TE=ZE
LE
A1_s D1_s E1_s X1_1 X2_1 A2_s D2_s E2_s X1_2 X2_2 P1_s P2_s
LK
A1_s D1_s E1_s X1_1 X2_1 A2_s D2_s E2_s X1_2 X2_2
VA 1.0 PH(1,1) PH(2,2) PH(3,3) PH(4,4) PH(5,5) PH(6,6)
VA 1.0 PH(7,7) PH(8,8) PH(9,9) PH(10,10)
VA 1.0 PH(1,6) PH(2,7)
PA GA
1 0 0 0 0 0 0 0 0 0
0 1 0 0 0 0 0 0 0 0
0 0 1 0 0 0 0 0 0 0
0 0 0 0 0 0 0 0 0 0
0 0 0 0 0 0 0 0 0 0
0 0 0 0 0 1 0 0 0 0
0 0 0 0 0 0 1 0 0 0
0 0 0 0 0 0 0 1 0 0
```

```
0 0 0 0 0 0 0 0 0 0
0 0 0 0 0 0 0 0 0 0
0 0 0 0 0 0 0 0 0 0
0 0 0 0 0 0 0 0 0 0
EQ GA(1,1) GA(6,6)
EQ GA(2,2) GA(7,7)
EQ GA(3,3) GA(8,8)
PA BE
0 0 0 0 0 0 0 0 0 0 0 0
0 0 0 0 0 0 0 0 0 0 0 0
0 0 0 0 0 0 0 0 0 0 0 0
0 0 0 0 0 0 0 0 0 0 0 0
0 0 0 0 0 0 0 0 0 0 0 0
0 0 0 0 0 0 0 0 0 0 0 0
0 0 0 0 0 0 0 0 0 0 0 0
0 0 0 0 0 0 0 0 0 0 0 0
0 0 0 0 0 0 0 0 0 0 0 0
0 0 0 0 0 0 0 0 0 0 0 0
1 1 1 0 0 0 0 0 0 0 0 0
0 0 0 0 0 1 1 1 0 0 0 0
EQ GA(1,1) BE(11,1) BE(12,6)
EQ GA(2,2) BE(11,2) BE(12,7)
EQ GA(3,3) BE(11,3) BE(12,8)
VA 1.0 LY(1,11)
VA 1.0 LY(2,12)
ST 0.3 ALL
OU NS AD=OFF ND=5 TM=1200 IT=500
CONC SINGLE DZ PAIRS
DA NI=2 NO=155 MA=CM
LA
DEP1 DEP2
CM
0.1087 0.0250 0.1182
MO NY=2 NE=12 NK=10 GA=FU,FI LY=FU,FI PH=SY,FI BE=FU,FI PS=ZE TE=ZE
LE
A1_s D1_s E1_s X1_1 X2_1 A2_s D2_s E2_s X1_2 X2_2 P1_s P2_s
LK
A1_s D1_s E1_s X1_1 X2_1 A2_s D2_s E2_s X1_2 X2_2
VA 1.0 PH(1,1) PH(2,2) PH(3,3) PH(4,4) PH(5,5) PH(6,6)
VA 1.0 PH(7,7) PH(8,8) PH(9,9) PH(10,10)
VA 0.5 PH(1,6)
VA 0.25 PH(2,7)
PA GA
```

```
1 0 0 0 0 0 0 0 0 0
0 1 0 0 0 0 0 0 0 0
0 0 1 0 0 0 0 0 0 0
0 0 0 0 0 0 0 0 0 0
0 0 0 0 0 0 0 0 0 0
0 0 0 0 0 1 0 0 0 0
0 0 0 0 0 0 1 0 0 0
0 0 0 0 0 0 0 1 0 0
0 0 0 0 0 0 0 0 0 0
0 0 0 0 0 0 0 0 0 0
0 0 0 0 0 0 0 0 0 0
0 0 0 0 0 0 0 0 0 0
EQ GA(1,1,1) GA(1,1) GA(6,6)
EQ GA(1,2,2) GA(2,2) GA(7,7)
EQ GA(1,3,3) GA(3,3) GA(8,8)
PA BE
0 0 0 0 0 0 0 0 0 0 0 0
0 0 0 0 0 0 0 0 0 0 0 0
0 0 0 0 0 0 0 0 0 0 0 0
0 0 0 0 0 0 0 0 0 0 0 0
0 0 0 0 0 0 0 0 0 0 0 0
0 0 0 0 0 0 0 0 0 0 0 0
0 0 0 0 0 0 0 0 0 0 0 0
0 0 0 0 0 0 0 0 0 0 0 0
0 0 0 0 0 0 0 0 0 0 0 0
0 0 0 0 0 0 0 0 0 0 0 0
1 1 1 0 0 0 0 0 0 0 0 0
0 0 0 0 0 1 1 1 0 0 0 0
EQ GA(1,1,1) BE(11,1) BE(12,6)
EQ GA(1,2,2) BE(11,2) BE(12,7)
EQ GA(1,3,3) BE(11,3) BE(12,8)
VA 1.0 LY(1,11)
VA 1.0 LY(2,12)
OU NS AD=OFF ND=5
CONC MARRIED MZ PAIRS
DA NI=2 NO=177 MA=CM
LA
DEP1 DEP2
CM
0.1002 0.0336 0.0769
MO NY=2 NE=12 NK=10 GA=FU,FI LY=FU,FI PH=SY,FI BE=FU,FI PS=ZE TE=ZE
LE
A1_m D1_m E1_m AP1_m DP1_m A2_m D2_m E2_m AP2_m DP2_m P1_m P2_m
```

```
LK
A1_m D1_m E1_m AP1_m DP1_m A2_m D2_m E2_m AP2_m DP2_m
VA 1.0 PH(1,1) PH(2,2) PH(3,3) PH(4,4) PH(5,5) PH(6,6)
VA 1.0 PH(7,7) PH(8,8) PH(9,9) PH(10,10)
VA 1.0 PH(1,6) PH(2,7)
VA 1.0 PH(4,9) PH(5,10)
PA GA
1 0 0 0 0 0 0 0 0 0
0 1 0 0 0 0 0 0 0 0
0 0 1 0 0 0 0 0 0 0
0 0 0 1 0 0 0 0 0 0
0 0 0 0 0 0 0 0 0 0
0 0 0 0 0 1 0 0 0 0
0 0 0 0 0 0 1 0 0 0
0 0 0 0 0 0 0 1 0 0
0 0 0 0 0 0 0 0 1 0
0 0 0 0 0 0 0 0 0 0
0 0 0 0 0 0 0 0 0 0
0 0 0 0 0 0 0 0 0 0
EQ GA(1,1) GA(6,6)
EQ GA(2,2) GA(7,7)
EQ GA(3,3) GA(8,8)
EQ GA(4,4) GA(9,9)
EQ GA(5,5) GA(10,10)
PA BE
0 0 0 0 0 0 0 0 0 0 0 0
0 0 0 0 0 0 0 0 0 0 0 0
0 0 0 0 0 0 0 0 0 0 0 0
0 0 0 0 0 0 0 0 0 0 0 0
0 0 0 0 0 0 0 0 0 0 0 0
0 0 0 0 0 0 0 0 0 0 0 0
0 0 0 0 0 0 0 0 0 0 0 0
0 0 0 0 0 0 0 0 0 0 0 0
0 0 0 0 0 0 0 0 0 0 0 0
0 0 0 0 0 0 0 0 0 0 0 0
1 1 1 1 0 0 0 0 0 0 0 0
0 0 0 0 0 1 1 1 1 0 0 0
EQ GA(1,1) BE(11,1) BE(12,6)
EQ GA(2,2) BE(11,2) BE(12,7)
EQ GA(3,3) BE(11,3) BE(12,8)
EQ GA(4,4) BE(11,4) BE(12,9)
EQ GA(5,5) BE(11,5) BE(12,10)
VA 1.0 LY(1,11)
```

```
VA 1.0 LY(2,12)
ST 0.3 ALL
OU NS AD=OFF ND=5
CONC MARRIED  DZ PAIRS
DA NI=2 NO=107 MA=CM
LA
DEP1 DEP2
CM
0.0692 0.0076 0.0882
MO NY=2 NE=12 NK=10 GA=FU,FI LY=FU,FI PH=SY,FI BE=FU,FI PS=ZE TE=ZE
LE
A1_m D1_m E1_m AP1_m DP1_m A2_m D2_m E2_m AP2_m DP2_m P1_m P2_m
LK
A1_m D1_m E1_m AP1_m DP1_m A2_m D2_m E2_m AP2_m DP2_m
VA 1.0 PH(1,1) PH(2,2) PH(3,3) PH(4,4) PH(5,5) PH(6,6)
VA 1.0 PH(7,7) PH(8,8) PH(9,9) PH(10,10)
VA 0.5 PH(1,6)
VA 0.25 PH(2,7)
VA 0.5 PH(4,9)
VA 0.25 PH(5,10)
PA GA
1 0 0 0 0 0 0 0 0 0
0 1 0 0 0 0 0 0 0 0
0 0 1 0 0 0 0 0 0 0
0 0 0 1 0 0 0 0 0 0
0 0 0 0 0 0 0 0 0 0
0 0 0 0 0 1 0 0 0 0
0 0 0 0 0 0 1 0 0 0
0 0 0 0 0 0 0 1 0 0
0 0 0 0 0 0 0 0 1 0
0 0 0 0 0 0 0 0 0 0
0 0 0 0 0 0 0 0 0 0
0 0 0 0 0 0 0 0 0 0
EQ GA(3,1,1) GA(1,1) GA(6,6)
EQ GA(3,2,2) GA(2,2) GA(7,7)
EQ GA(3,3,3) GA(3,3) GA(8,8)
EQ GA(3,4,4) GA(4,4) GA(9,9)
EQ GA(3,5,5) GA(5,5) GA(10,10)
PA BE
0 0 0 0 0 0 0 0 0 0 0 0
0 0 0 0 0 0 0 0 0 0 0 0
0 0 0 0 0 0 0 0 0 0 0 0
0 0 0 0 0 0 0 0 0 0 0 0
```

```
0 0 0 0 0 0 0 0 0 0 0 0
0 0 0 0 0 0 0 0 0 0 0 0
0 0 0 0 0 0 0 0 0 0 0 0
0 0 0 0 0 0 0 0 0 0 0 0
0 0 0 0 0 0 0 0 0 0 0 0
0 0 0 0 0 0 0 0 0 0 0 0
1 1 1 1 0 0 0 0 0 0 0 0
0 0 0 0 0 1 1 1 1 0 0 0
EQ GA(3,1,1) BE(11,1) BE(12,6)
EQ GA(3,2,2) BE(11,2) BE(12,7)
EQ GA(3,3,3) BE(11,3) BE(12,8)
EQ GA(3,4,4) BE(11,4) BE(12,9)
EQ GA(3,5,5) BE(11,5) BE(12,10)
VA 1.0 LY(1,11)
VA 1.0 LY(2,12)
OU NS AD=OFF
DISCORDANT MZ PAIRS
DA NI=2 NO=139 MA=CM
LA
DEP1 DEP2
CM
0.1198 0.0359 0.1009
MO NY=2 NE=12 NK=10 GA=FU,FI LY=FU,FI PH=SY,FI BE=FU,FI PS=ZE TE=ZE
LE
A1_s D1_s E1_s X1_1 X2_1 A2_m D2_m E2_m AP2_m DP2_m P1_s P2_m
LK
A1_s D1_s E1_s X1_1 X2_1 A2_m D2_m E2_m AP2_m DP2_m
VA 1.0 PH(1,1) PH(2,2) PH(3,3) PH(4,4) PH(5,5) PH(6,6)
VA 1.0 PH(7,7) PH(8,8) PH(9,9) PH(10,10)
VA 1.0 PH(1,6)
VA 1.00 PH(2,7)
PA GA
1 0 0 0 0 0 0 0 0 0
0 1 0 0 0 0 0 0 0 0
0 0 1 0 0 0 0 0 0 0
0 0 0 0 0 0 0 0 0 0
0 0 0 0 0 0 0 0 0 0
0 0 0 0 0 1 0 0 0 0
0 0 0 0 0 0 1 0 0 0
0 0 0 0 0 0 0 1 0 0
0 0 0 0 0 0 0 0 1 0
0 0 0 0 0 0 0 0 0 0
0 0 0 0 0 0 0 0 0 0
```

```
0 0 0 0 0 0 0 0 0 0
EQ GA(1,1,1) GA(1,1)
EQ GA(3,1,1) GA(6,6)
EQ GA(1,2,2) GA(2,2)
EQ GA(3,2,2) GA(7,7)
EQ GA(1,3,3) GA(3,3)
EQ GA(3,3,3) GA(8,8)
EQ GA(3,9,9) GA(9,9)
EQ GA(3,5,5) GA(10,10)
PA BE
0 0 0 0 0 0 0 0 0 0 0 0
0 0 0 0 0 0 0 0 0 0 0 0
0 0 0 0 0 0 0 0 0 0 0 0
0 0 0 0 0 0 0 0 0 0 0 0
0 0 0 0 0 0 0 0 0 0 0 0
0 0 0 0 0 0 0 0 0 0 0 0
0 0 0 0 0 0 0 0 0 0 0 0
0 0 0 0 0 0 0 0 0 0 0 0
0 0 0 0 0 0 0 0 0 0 0 0
0 0 0 0 0 0 0 0 0 0 0 0
1 1 1 0 0 0 0 0 0 0 0 0
0 0 0 0 0 1 1 1 1 0 0 0
EQ GA(1,1,1) BE(11,1)
EQ GA(3,1,1) BE(12,6)
EQ GA(1,2,2) BE(11,2)
EQ GA(3,2,2) BE(12,7)
EQ GA(1,3,3) BE(11,3)
EQ GA(3,3,3) BE(12,8)
EQ GA(3,4,4) BE(12,9)
EQ GA(3,5,5) BE(12,10)
VA 1.0 LY(1,11)
VA 1.0 LY(2,12)
OU NS AD=OFF IT=100
DZO PAIRS
DA NI=2 NO=87 MA=CM
LA
DEP1 DEP2
CM
0.1013 0.0050 0.0694
MO NY=2 NE=12 NK=10 GA=FU,FI LY=FU,FI PH=SY,FI BE=FU,FI PS=ZE TE=ZE
LE
A1_s D1_s E1_s X1_1 X2_1 A2_m D2_m E2_m AP2_m DP2_m P1_s P2_m
LK
```

```
A1_s D1_s E1_s X1_1 X2_1 A2_m D2_m E2_m AP2_m DP2_m
VA 1.0 PH(1,1) PH(2,2) PH(3,3) PH(4,4) PH(5,5) PH(6,6)
VA 1.0 PH(7,7) PH(8,8) PH(9,9) PH(10,10)
VA 0.5 PH(1,6)
VA 0.25 PH(2,7)
PA GA
1 0 0 0 0 0 0 0 0 0
0 1 0 0 0 0 0 0 0 0
0 0 1 0 0 0 0 0 0 0
0 0 0 0 0 0 0 0 0 0
0 0 0 0 0 0 0 0 0 0
0 0 0 0 0 1 0 0 0 0
0 0 0 0 0 0 1 0 0 0
0 0 0 0 0 0 0 1 0 0
0 0 0 0 0 0 0 0 1 0
0 0 0 0 0 0 0 0 0 0
0 0 0 0 0 0 0 0 0 0
0 0 0 0 0 0 0 0 0 0
EQ GA(1,1,1) GA(1,1)
EQ GA(3,1,1) GA(6,6)
EQ GA(1,2,2) GA(2,2)
EQ GA(3,2,2) GA(7,7)
EQ GA(1,3,3) GA(3,3)
EQ GA(3,3,3) GA(8,8)
EQ GA(3,9,9) GA(9,9)
EQ GA(3,5,5) GA(10,10)
PA BE
0 0 0 0 0 0 0 0 0 0 0 0
0 0 0 0 0 0 0 0 0 0 0 0
0 0 0 0 0 0 0 0 0 0 0 0
0 0 0 0 0 0 0 0 0 0 0 0
0 0 0 0 0 0 0 0 0 0 0 0
0 0 0 0 0 0 0 0 0 0 0 0
0 0 0 0 0 0 0 0 0 0 0 0
0 0 0 0 0 0 0 0 0 0 0 0
0 0 0 0 0 0 0 0 0 0 0 0
0 0 0 0 0 0 0 0 0 0 0 0
1 1 1 0 0 0 0 0 0 0 0 0
0 0 0 0 0 1 1 1 1 0 0 0
EQ GA(1,1,1) BE(11,1)
EQ GA(3,1,1) BE(12,6)
EQ GA(1,2,2) BE(11,2)
EQ GA(3,2,2) BE(12,7)
```

```
EQ GA(1,3,3) BE(11,3)
EQ GA(3,3,3) BE(12,8)
EQ GA(3,4,4) BE(12,9)
EQ GA(3,5,5) BE(12,10)
VA 1.0 LY(1,11)
VA 1.0 LY(2,12)
OU NS AD=OFF IT=500 ND=5 RS TM=1200
```

G.4   Scalar G × E interaction model

The following script fits a model in which there is a proportionate change of the multifactorial genetic and environmental effect between exposed and non-exposed individuals.

```
GXE INTERACTION "K MODEL" Conc. Single MZF Australian depression
DA NG=6 NI=2 NO=254 MA=CM
LA
DEP1 DEP2
CM
0.0968 0.0381 0.0896
MO NY=2 NE=4 NK=6 GA=FU,FR LY=FU,FI PH=SY,FI BE=FU,FI PS=ZE TE=ZE
LE
L11_s L12_s L21_s L22_s
LK
A1 D1 E1 A2 D2 E2
VA 1.0 PH(1,1) PH(2,2) PH(3,3) PH(4,4) PH(5,5) PH(6,6)
VA 1.0 PH(1,4) PH(2,5)
PA GA
1 0 1 0 0 0
0 0 0 0 0 0
0 0 0 1 0 1
0 0 0 0 0 0
EQ GA(1,1) GA(3,4)
EQ GA(1,2) GA(3,5)
EQ GA(1,3) GA(3,6)
VA 1.0 BE(2,1)
VA 1.0 BE(4,3)
VA 1.0 LY(1,2)
VA 1.0 LY(2,4)
ST 0.4 ALL
OU NS AD=OFF
CONCORDANT SINGLE DZ FEMALES
DA NI=2 NO=155 MA=CM
```

```
LA
DEP1 DEP2
CM
0.1087 0.0250 0.1182
MO NY=2 NE=4 NK=6 GA=IN LY=FU,FI PH=SY,FI BE=FU,FI PS=ZE TE=ZE
LE
L11_s L12_s L21_s L22_s
LK
A1 D1 E1 A2 D2 E2
VA 1.0 PH(1,1) PH(2,2) PH(3,3) PH(4,4) PH(5,5) PH(6,6)
VA 0.5 PH(1,4)
VA 0.25 PH(2,5)
VA 1.0 BE(2,1)
VA 1.0 BE(4,3)
VA 1.0 LY(1,2)
VA 1.0 LY(2,4)
ST 0.4 ALL
OU NS AD=OFF
CONCORDANT MARRIED MZ PAIRS
DA NI=2 NO=177 MA=CM
LA
DEP1 DEP2
CM
0.1002 0.0336 0.0769
MO NY=2 NE=4 NK=6 GA=IN LY=FU,FI PH=SY,FI BE=FU,FI PS=ZE TE=ZE
LE
L11_m L12_m L21_m L22_m
LK
A1 D1 E1 A2 D2 E2
VA 1.0 PH(1,1) PH(2,2) PH(3,3) PH(4,4) PH(5,5) PH(6,6)
VA 1.0 PH(1,4) PH(2,5)
FR BE(2,1) BE(4,3) LY(1,2) LY(2,4)
EQ BE(2,1) BE(4,3) LY(1,2) LY(2,4)
ST 1.0 BE(2,1)
OU NS AD=OFF
CONCORDANT MARRIED DZ PAIRS
DA NI=2 NO=107 MA=CM
LA
DEP1 DEP2
CM
0.0692 0.0076 0.0882
MO NY=2 NE=4 NK=6 GA=IN LY=FU,FI PH=SY,FI BE=FU,FI PS=ZE TE=ZE
LE
```

```
L11_m L12_m L21_m L22_m
LK
A1 D1 E1 A2 D2 E2
VA 1.0 PH(1,1) PH(2,2) PH(3,3) PH(4,4) PH(5,5) PH(6,6)
VA 0.5 PH(1,4)
VA 0.25 PH(2,5)
FR BE(2,1) BE(4,3) LY(1,2) LY(2,4)
EQ BE (3,2,1) BE(2,1) BE(4,3) LY(1,2) LY(2,4)
OU NS AD=OFF
DISCORDANT MZ PAIRS
DA NI=2 NO=139 MA=CM
LA
DEP_m DEP_s
CM
0.1198 0.0359 0.1009
MO NY=2 NE=4 NK=6 GA=IN LY=FU,FI PH=SY,FI BE=FU,FI PS=ZE TE=ZE
LE
L11_s L12_s L21_m L22_m
LK
A1 D1 E1 A2 D2 E2
VA 1.0 PH(1,1) PH(2,2) PH(3,3) PH(4,4) PH(5,5) PH(6,6)
VA 0.5 PH(1,4)
VA 1.00 PH(2,5)
VA 1.0 BE(2,1) LY(1,2)
FR BE(4,3) LY(2,4)
EQ BE (3,2,1) BE(4,3) LY(2,4)
OU NS AD=OFF IT=100
DISCORDANT DZ PAIRS
DA NI=2 NO=87 MA=CM
LA
DEP_m DEP_s
CM
0.1013 0.0050 0.0694
MO NY=2 NE=4 NK=6 GA=IN LY=FU,FI PH=SY,FI BE=FU,FI PS=ZE TE=ZE
LE
L11_s L12_s L21_m L22_m
LK
A1 D1 E1 A2 D2 E2
VA 1.0 PH(1,1) PH(2,2) PH(3,3) PH(4,4) PH(5,5) PH(6,6)
VA 0.5 PH(1,4)
VA 0.25 PH(2,5)
VA 1.0 BE(2,1) LY(1,2)
FR BE(4,3) LY(2,4)
```

```
EQ BE (3,2,1) BE(4,3) LY(2,4)
OU NS AD=OFF IT=500
```

Appendix H

LISREL Script for Rater Bias Model

H.1 Rater Bias Model

The LISREL 7 script below fits a rater bias model to parental ratings of young childrens Child Behavior Checklist internalizing behavior problems. The script represents a five group problem, for MZ-male, MZ-female, DZ-male, DZ-female, and DZ-opposite sex twins.

```
Parents ratings of younger twins
;  Complete families - CBC internalizing MZ boys
DA NO=96 NI=4 NG=5 MA=CM
LA
'MRT1' 'MRT2' 'FRT1' 'FRT2'
CM FU
0.693855 0.568978 0.312244 0.308165
0.568978 0.665695 0.238173 0.293263
0.312244 0.238173  0.63751 0.461195
0.308165 0.293263 0.461195 0.647022
SE
1,2,3,4/
MO NY=4 NX=0 NE=4 NK=8 GA=FR PH=FI LY=FR PS=ZE
EQ TE(1,1) TE(2,2)
EQ TE(3,3) TE(4,4)
PA GA
0 0 0 0 0 0 0 0
0 0 0 0 0 0 0 0
0 0 1 1 1 0 0 0
```

```
0 0 0 0 0 1 1 1
VA 1.0 GA(1,1) GA(2,2)
EQ GA(3,3) GA(4,6)
EQ GA(3,4) GA(4,7)
EQ GA(3,5) GA(4,8)
PA LY
1 0 0 0
1 0 0 0
0 1 1 0
0 1 0 1
EQ LY(1,1) LY(2,1)
EQ LY(3,2) LY(4,2)
VA 1.0  LY(1,3) LY(2,4)
EQ LY(3,3) LY(4,4)
MA PH
1
0 1
0 0 1
0 0 0 1
0 0 0 0 1
0 0 1 0 0 1
0 0 0 1 0 0 1
0 0 0 0 0 0 0 1
ST 0.2 ALL
ST 0.5 GA(3,3) GA(3,4)
OU SE RS SS NS  AD=OFF IT=500 TM=120
Parents ratings of younger twins.
; CBC internalizing data. MZ girls
DA NO=102 NI=4  MA=CM
LA
'MT1' 'MT2' 'FT1' 'FT2'
CM FU
0.674638 0.512857 0.265012 0.291518
0.512857 0.713646 0.236512 0.353789
0.265012 0.236512 0.652153 0.513158
0.291518 0.353789 0.513158 0.675623
SE
1,2,3,4/
MO NY=4 NX=0 NE=4 NK=8 GA=FR PH=FI LY=FR PS=ZE TE=DI
EQ TE(1,1) TE(2,2)
EQ TE(3,3) TE(4,4)
PA GA
0 0 0 0 0 0 0 0
```

```
0 0 0 0 0 0 0 0
0 0 1 1 1 0 0 0
0 0 0 0 0 1 1 1
VA 1.0 GA(1,1) GA(2,2)
EQ GA(3,3) GA(4,6)
EQ GA(3,4) GA(4,7)
EQ GA(3,5) GA(4,8)
PA LY
1 0 0 0
1 0 0 0
0 1 1 0
0 1 0 1
EQ LY(1,1) LY(2,1)
EQ LY(3,2) LY(4,2)
VA 1.0 LY(1,3) LY(2,4)
EQ LY(3,3) LY(4,4)
MA PH
1
0 1
0 0 1
0 0 0 1
0 0 0 0 1
0 0 1 0 0 1
0 0 0 1 0 0 1
0 0 0 0 0 0 0 1
ST 0.2 ALL
OU
Parents ratings of yonger twins.
; CBC internalizing data. DZ boys
DA NO=102 NI=4 MA=CM
LA
'MT1' 'MT2' 'FT1' 'FT2'
CM FU
0.565119 0.291145 0.241471 0.171134
0.291145 0.488443 0.137396 0.285151
0.241471 0.137396  0.60361 0.346618
0.171134 0.285151 0.346618 0.604151
SE
1,2,3,4/
MO NY=4 NX=0 NE=4 NK=8 GA=FR PH=FI LY=FR PS=ZE TE=DI
EQ TE(1,1,1) TE(1,1) TE(2,2)
EQ TE(1,3,3) TE(3,3) TE(4,4)
PA GA
```

```
0 0 0 0 0 0 0 0
0 0 0 0 0 0 0 0
0 0 1 1 1 0 0 0
0 0 0 0 0 1 1 1
VA 1.0 GA(1,1) GA(2,2)
EQ GA(1,3,3) GA(3,3) GA(4,6)
EQ GA(1,3,4) GA(3,4) GA(4,7)
EQ GA(1,3,5) GA(3,5) GA(4,8)
PA LY
1 0 0 0
1 0 0 0
0 1 1 0
0 1 0 1
EQ LY(1,1,1) LY(1,1) LY(2,1)
EQ LY(1,3,2) LY(3,2) LY(4,2)
VA 1.0 LY(1,3) LY(2,4)
EQ LY(1,3,3) LY(3,3) LY(4,4)
MA PH
1
0 1
0 0 1
0 0 0 1
0 0 0 0 1
0 0 .5 0 0 1
0 0 0 1 0 0 1
0 0 0 0 0 0 0 1
ST 0.2 ALL
OU
Parents ratings of younger twins.
; CBC internalizing data. DZ girls
DA NO=97 NI=4   MA=CM
LA
'MT1' 'MT2' 'FT1' 'FT2'
CM FU
0.621255 0.434264 0.315264 0.232753
0.434264 0.623154 0.236398 0.250744
0.315264 0.236398 0.719002  0.53069
0.232753 0.250744  0.53069 0.743137
SE
1,2,3,4/
MO NY=4 NX=0 NE=4 NK=8 GA=FR PH=FI LY=FR PS=ZE TE=DI
EQ TE(2,1,1) TE(1,1) TE(2,2)
EQ TE(2,3,3) TE(3,3) TE(4,4)
```

```
PA GA
0 0 0 0 0 0 0 0
0 0 0 0 0 0 0 0
0 0 1 1 1 0 0 0
0 0 0 0 0 1 1 1
VA 1.0 GA(1,1) GA(2,2)
EQ GA(2,3,3) GA(3,3) GA(4,6)
EQ GA(2,3,4) GA(3,4) GA(4,7)
EQ GA(2,3,5) GA(3,5) GA(4,8)
PA LY
1 0 0 0
1 0 0 0
0 1 1 0
0 1 0 1
EQ LY(2,1,1) LY(1,1) LY(2,1)
EQ LY(2,3,2) LY(3,2) LY(4,2)
VA 1.0 LY(1,3) LY(2,4)
EQ LY(2,3,3) LY(3,3) LY(4,4)
MA PH
1
0 1
0 0 1
0 0 0 1
0 0 0 0 1
0 0 .5 0 0 1
0 0 0 1 0 0 1
0 0 0 0 0 0 0 1
ST 0.2 ALL
OU
Parents ratings of younger twins.
; CBC internalizing data DZ-OS.
DA NO=103 NI=4 MA=CM
LA
'MT1' 'MT2' 'FT1' 'FT2'
CM FU
0.538015 0.243458 0.161654    0.1025
0.243458 0.465392 0.101643 0.191458
0.161654 0.101643 0.729673 0.372469
0.1025 0.191458 0.372469 0.574346
SE
2,1,4,3/
MO NY=4 NX=0 NE=4 NK=8 GA=FR PH=FI LY=FR PS=ZE TE=DI
EQ TE(1,1,1) TE(1,1)
```

```
EQ TE(2,2,2) TE(2,2)
EQ TE(1,3,3) TE(3,3)
EQ TE(2,4,4) TE(4,4)
PA GA
0 0 0 0 0 0 0 0
0 0 0 0 0 0 0 0
0 0 1 1 1 0 0 0
0 0 0 0 0 1 1 1
VA 1.0 GA(1,1) GA(2,2)
EQ GA(1,3,3) GA(3,3)
EQ GA(2,4,6) GA(4,6)
EQ GA(1,3,4) GA(3,4)
EQ GA(2,4,7) GA(4,7)
EQ GA(1,3,5) GA(3,5)
EQ GA(2,4,8) GA(4,8)
PA LY
1 0 0 0
1 0 0 0
0 1 1 0
0 1 0 1
EQ LY(1,1,1) LY(1,1)
EQ LY(2,2,1) LY(2,1)
EQ LY(1,3,2) LY(3,2)
EQ LY(2,4,2) LY(4,2)
VA 1.0 LY(1,3) LY(2,4)
EQ LY(1,3,3) LY(3,3)
EQ LY(2,4,4) LY(4,4)
MA PH
1
0 1
0 0 1
0 0 0 1
0 0 0 0 1
0 0 .5 0 0 1
0 0 0 1 0 0 1
0 0 0 0 0 0 0 1
ST 0.2 ALL
OU
```

H.2   CBC Items for Internalizing Scale Score

Below are the core items of the Child Behavior Checklist (CBC: Achenbach, 1988)
assessing children's internalizing behaviors.

1. Can't get his/her mind off certain thoughts, obsessions (describe):

2. Fears going to school

3. Fears he/she might do something bad

4. Feels he/she has to be perfect

5. Hears sounds or voices that aren't there (describe):

6. Too fearful or anxious

7. Feels dizzy

8. Feels too guilty

9. Overtired

10. Aches or pains

11. Headaches

12. Nausea, feels sick

13. Stomach-aches or cramps

14. Vomiting, throwing up

15. Refuses to talk

16. Secretive, keeps things to self

17. Self-conscious or easily embarassed

18. Stares blankly

19. Strange behavior (describe):

20. Strange ideas (describe):

21. Sulks a lot

22. Unhappy, sad or depressed

23. Worrying

Appendix I

LISREL Scripts for Direction of Causation

I.1 Reciprocal Causation Model

The LISREL 7 script below fits a reciprocal causation model to alcohol consumption and sensitivity assessments from female twin pairs. ξ variables represent additive (A) and dominance (D) genetic factors, and common (C) and unique (E) environment factors for the two traits A and B.

```
Alcohol consumption & sensitivity, MZF RECIPROCAL CAUSATION
DA NG=2 NI=4 NO=43 MA=CM
LA
T1-CONS T1-SENS T2-CONS T2-SENS
CM SY
0.9927
0.5329 0.9829
0.5332 0.4859 0.9134
0.2731 0.5214 0.4285 1.2121
MO NY=4 NE=4 NK=16 GA=FU,Fi LY=id,fi PH=SY,FI TE=di,fi C
PS=ZE BE=fu,fi
LK
ECONS-T1 CCONS-T1 ACONS-T1 DCONS-T1
ESENS-T1 CSENS-T1 ASENS-T1 DSENS-T1
ECONS-T2 CCONS-T2 ACONS-T2 DCONS-T2
ASENS-T2 CSENS-T2 ASENS-T2 DSENS-T2
LE
CONS-T1 SENS-T1 CONS-T2 SENS-T2
MA PH
```

```
1.0
0.0 1.0
0.0 0.0 1.0
0.0 0.0 0.0 1.0
0.0 0.0 0.0 0.0 1.0
0.0 0.0 0.0 0.0 0.0 1.0
0.0 0.0 0.0 0.0 0.0 0.0 1.0
0.0 0.0 0.0 0.0 0.0 0.0 0.0 1.0
0.0 0.0 0.0 0.0 0.0 0.0 0.0 0.0 1.0
0.0 1.0 0.0 0.0 0.0 0.0 0.0 0.0 0.0 1.0
0.0 0.0 1.0 0.0 0.0 0.0 0.0 0.0 0.0 0.0 1.0
0.0 0.0 0.0 1.0 0.0 0.0 0.0 0.0 0.0 0.0 0.0 1.0
0.0 0.0 0.0 0.0 0.0 0.0 0.0 0.0 0.0 0.0 0.0 0.0 1.0
0.0 0.0 0.0 0.0 0.0 1.0 0.0 0.0 0.0 0.0 0.0 0.0 0.0 1.0
0.0 0.0 0.0 0.0 0.0 0.0 1.0 0.0 0.0 0.0 0.0 0.0 0.0 0.0 1.0
0.0 0.0 0.0 0.0 0.0 0.0 0.0 1.0 0.0 0.0 0.0 0.0 0.0 0.0 0.0 1.0
eq be(2,1) be(4,3)
eq be(1,2) be(3,4)
fr be(2,1)
fr be(1,2)
st 0.1 be(2,1)
st 0.1 be(1,2)
PA GA
1 1 1 0 0 0 0 0 0 0 0 0 0 0 0 0
0 0 0 0 1 0 1 1 0 0 0 0 0 0 0 0
0 0 0 0 0 0 0 0 1 1 1 0 0 0 0 0
0 0 0 0 0 0 0 0 0 0 0 0 1 0 1 1
EQ GA(1,1) GA(3,9)
EQ GA(1,2) GA(3,10)
EQ GA(1,3) GA(3,11)
EQ GA(1,4) GA(3,12)
EQ GA(2,1) GA(4,9)
EQ GA(2,2) GA(4,10)
EQ GA(2,3) GA(4,11)
EQ GA(2,4) GA(4,12)
EQ GA(2,5) GA(4,13)
EQ GA(2,6) GA(4,14)
EQ GA(2,7) GA(4,15)
EQ GA(2,8) GA(4,16)
st 0.6 ga(1,1) ga(1,2) ga(1,3)
st 0.6 ga(2,5) ga(2,7) ga(2,8)
eq te(1,1) te(2,2) te(3,3) te(4,4)
fr te(1,1)
```

```
st 0.1 te(1,1)
OU TM=1200 NS
FEMALE DZ PAIRS - baseline consumption & post-alcohol intoxication
DA NO=42 NI=4 MA=CM
LA
T1-A T1-B T2-A T2-B
CM SY
0.839
0.2731 0.7283
0.3578 -0.0584 1.2359
0.0698 -0.0208 0.2157 1.1453
MO NY=4 NE=4 NK=16 LY=IN GA=IN PH=SY,FI TE=IN BE=IN PS=IN
LK
ECONS-T1 CCONS-T1 ACONS-T1 DCONS-T1
ESENS-T1 CSENS-T1 ASENS-T1 DSENS-T1
ECONS-T2 CCONS-T2 ACONS-T2 DCONS-T2
ESENS-T2 CSENS-T2 ASENS-T2 DSENS-T1
LE
CONS-T1 SENS-T1 CONS-T2 SENS-T2
MA PH
1.0
0.0 1.0
0.0 0.0 1.0
0.0 0.0 0.0 1.0
0.0 0.0 0.0 0.0 1.0
0.0 0.0 0.0 0.0 0.0 1.0
0.0 0.0 0.0 0.0 0.0 0.0 1.0
0.0 0.0 0.0 0.0 0.0 0.0 0.0 1.0
0.0 0.0 0.0 0.0 0.0 0.0 0.0 0.0 1.0
0.0 1.0 0.0 0.0 0.0 0.0 0.0 0.0 0.0 1.0
0.0 0.0 0.5 0.0 0.0 0.0 0.0 0.0 0.0 0.0 1.0
0.0 0.0 0.0 0.25 0.0 0.0 0.0 0.0 0.0 0.0 0.0 1.0
0.0 0.0 0.0 0.0 0.0 0.0 0.0 0.0 0.0 0.0 0.0 0.0 1.0
0.0 0.0 0.0 0.0 0.0 0.0 1.0 0.0 0.0 0.0 0.0 0.0 0.0 1.0
0.0 0.0 0.0 0.0 0.0 0.0 0.0 0.5 0.0 0.0 0.0 0.0 0.0 0.0 1.0
0.0 0.0 0.0 0.0 0.0 0.0 0.0 0.25 0.0 0.0 0.0 0.0 0.0 0.0 0.0 1.0
OU ND=5 NS RS it=150 ad=off pc sc ef
```

I.2 Bivariate Genetic Model

This example program for LISREL 8 fits the bivariate genetic model of Figure 13.4a. Features to be noted are: (i) the use of constrained parameters (CO lines); (ii) the use of bounds constraints ('interval restrictions'; IR lines); (iii) declaration of the

PHi matrix as invariant in the second group, then use of VAlue statements and constraints to override some of the elements of the matrix; (iv) identification of free parameters by a numeric value (2, 3, 4 etc.), which allows easier specificiation of equalities between first and second twins than the conventional 0/1 notation to designate fixed and free parameters. All of these new features are implemented in LISREL 8. At the time of writing, the IR command is not working correctly in the β version; we hope these problems will be corrected by the time this book hits the shelves!

```
Habitual consumption (cons) and alcohol sensitivity (sens)
; Australian male pairs (LISREL 8)
DA NG=2 NI=4 NO=42 MA=CM
LA
T1-Cons T1-Sens T2-Cons T2-Sens
CM SY
1.0727
0.6686 0.9773
0.6970 0.5751 0.9093
0.6167 0.5238 0.6794 1.2041
MO NY=4 NE=4 NK=16 GA=FU,FI LY=ID PH=SY,FI TE=ZE PS=ZE BE=ZE
LK
EA-T1 CA-T1 AA-T1 DA-T1 EB-T1 CB-T1 AB-T1 DB-T1 EA-T2 CA-T2
AA-T2 DA-T2 EB-T2 CB-T2 AB-T2 DB-T1
LE
Cons-T1 Sens-T1 Cons-T2 Sens-T2
MA PH
1.0
0.0 1.0
0.0 0.0 1.0
0.0 0.0 0.0 1.0
0.7 0.0 0.0 0.0 1.0
0.0 0.0 0.0 0.0 0.0 1.0
0.0 0.0 0.9 0.0 0.0 0.0 1.0
0.0 0.0 0.0 0.8 0.0 0.0 0.0 1.0
0.0 0.0 0.0 0.0 0.0 0.0 0.0 0.0 1.0
0.0 1.0 0.0 0.0 0.0 0.0 0.0 0.0 0.0 1.0
0.0 0.0 1.0 0.0 0.0 0.0 0.0 0.9 0.0 0.0 0.0 1.0
0.0 0.0 0.0 1.0 0.0 0.0 0.0 0.0 0.8 0.0 0.0 0.0 1.0
0.0 0.0 0.0 0.0 0.0 0.0 0.0 0.0 0.0 0.7 0.0 0.0 0.0 1.0
0.0 0.0 0.0 0.0 1.0 0.0 0.0 0.0 0.0 0.0 0.0 0.0 0.0 0.0 1.0
0.0 0.0 0.9 0.0 0.0 0.0 1.0 0.0 0.0 0.0 0.9 0.0 0.0 0.0 1.0
0.0 0.0 0.0 0.8 0.0 0.0 0.0 1.0 0.0 0.0 0.0 0.8 0.0 0.0 0.0 1.0
FR PH(1,5) PH(3,7) PH(4,8)
EQ PH(1,5) PH(9,13)
```

```
EQ PH(3,7) PH(11,15) PH(3,15) PH(7,11)
EQ PH(2,6) PH(10,14) PH(2,14) PH(6,10)
EQ PH(4,8) PH(12,16) PH(4,16) PH(8,12)
IR PH(4,8) < 1.0
PA GA
·2 0 3 4 0 0 0 0 0 0 0 0 0 0 0 0
 0 0 0 0 5 0 6 7 0 0 0 0 0 0 0 0
 0 0 0 0 0 0 0 0 2 0 3 4 0 0 0 0
 0 0 0 0·0 0 0 0 0 0 0 0 5 0 6 7
ST 0.6 GA(1,1)
ST 0.6 GA(1,3)
ST 0.6 GA(1,4)
ST 0.6 GA(2,5)
ST 0.6 GA(2,7)
ST 0.6 GA(2,8)
OU TM=1200 NS
MALE DZ PAIRS: baseline consumption & post-alcohol intoxication
DA NO=37 NI=4 MA=CM
LA
T1-Cons T1-Sens T2-Cons T2-Sens
CM SY
1.0766
0.571 1.0918
0.2606 0.2732 1.0561
0.0509 0.141  0.3836 0.857
MO NY=4 NE=4 NK=16 LY=IN GA=IN PH=IN TE=IN BE=IN PS=IN
LK
EA-T1 CA-T1 AA-T1 DA-T1 EB-T1 CB-T1 AB-T1 DB-T1 EA-T2 CA-T2
AA-T2 DA-T2 EB-T2 CB-T2 AB-T2 DB-T1
LE
Cons-T1 Sens-T1 Cons-T2 Sens-T2
VA 0.5 PH(3,11) PH(7,15)
VA 0.25 PH(4,12) PH(8,16)
EQ PH(1,1,5) PH(1,5) PH(9,13)
EQ PH(1,2,6) PH(2,6) PH(10,14) PH(2,14) PH(6,10)
EQ PH(1,3,7) PH(3,7) PH(11,15)
CO PH(3,15)=0.5*PH(1,3,7)
CO PH(7,11)=0.5*PH(1,3,7)
EQ PH(1,4,8) PH(4,8) PH(12,16)
CO PH(4,16)=0.25*PH(1,4,8)
CO PH(8,12)=0.25*PH(1,4,8)
OU ND=5 NS RS IT=150 AD=OFF PC SC EF
```

I.3 Bivariate Genetic Cholesky Model

This LISREL 7 script illustrates the application of a genetic cholesky model (Figure 13.4b) to the bivariate case.

```
Alcohol consumption and sensitivity - bivariate Cholesky - MZFs
DA NG=2 NI=4 NO=43 MA=CM
LA
T1-SENS T1-CONS T2-SENS T2-CONS
CM SY
0.9829
0.5329 0.9927
0.5214 0.2731 1.2121
0.4859 0.5332 0.4285 0.9134
MO NY=4 NE=4 NK=16 GA=FU,Fi LY=id PH=SY,FI TE=ze PS=ZE BE=ze
LK
ECOMM-T1 CCOMM-T1 ACOMM-T1 DCOMM-T1
ESPEC-T1 CSPEC-T1 ASPEC-T1 DSPEC-T1
ECOMM-T2 CCOMM-T2 ACOMM-T2 DCOMM-T2
ESPEC-T2 CSPEC-T2 ASPEC-T2 DSPEC-T2
LE
SENS-T1 CONS-T1 SENS-T2 CONS-T2
MA PH
1.0
0.0 1.0
0.0 0.0 1.0
0.0 0.0 0.0 1.0
0.0 0.0 0.0 0.0 1.0
0.0 0.0 0.0 0.0 0.0 1.0
0.0 0.0 0.0 0.0 0.0 0.0 1.0
0.0 0.0 0.0 0.0 0.0 0.0 0.0 1.0
0.0 0.0 0.0 0.0 0.0 0.0 0.0 0.0 1.0
0.0 1.0 0.0 0.0 0.0 0.0 0.0 0.0 0.0 1.0
0.0 0.0 1.0 0.0 0.0 0.0 0.0 0.0 0.0 0.0 1.0
0.0 0.0 0.0 1.0 0.0 0.0 0.0 0.0 0.0 0.0 0.0 1.0
0.0 0.0 0.0 0.0 0.0 0.0 0.0 0.0 0.0 0.0 0.0 0.0 1.0
0.0 0.0 0.0 0.0 0.0 1.0 0.0 0.0 0.0 0.0 0.0 0.0 0.0 1.0
0.0 0.0 0.0 0.0 0.0 0.0 1.0 0.0 0.0 0.0 0.0 0.0 0.0 0.0 1.0
0.0 0.0 0.0 0.0 0.0 0.0 0.0 1.0 0.0 0.0 0.0 0.0 0.0 0.0 0.0 1.0
PA GA
1 0 1 1 0 0 0 0 0 0 0 0 0 0 0 0
1 0 1 1 1 1 1 0 0 0 0 0 0 0 0 0
0 0 0 0 0 0 0 0 1 0 1 1 0 0 0 0
0 0 0 0 0 0 0 0 1 0 1 1 1 1 1 0
```

```
EQ GA(1,1) GA(3,9)
EQ GA(1,2) GA(3,10)
EQ GA(1,3) GA(3,11)
EQ GA(1,4) GA(3,12)
EQ GA(2,1) GA(4,9)
EQ GA(2,2) GA(4,10)
EQ GA(2,3) GA(4,11)
EQ GA(2,4) GA(4,12)
EQ GA(2,5) GA(4,13)
EQ GA(2,6) GA(4,14)
EQ GA(2,7) GA(4,15)
EQ GA(2,8) GA(4,16)
st 0.6 ga(1,1) ga(1,4) ga(1,3)
st 0.45 ga(2,1) ga(2,4) ga(2,3) ga(2,5) ga(2,7) ga(2,6)
OU TM=1200 NS ND=4
FEMALE DZ - average weekly consumption & post-alcohol intoxication
DA NO=42 NI=4 MA=CM
LA
T1-SENS T1-CONS T2-SENS T2-CONS
CM SY
0.7283
0.2731 0.839
-0.0208 0.0698 1.1453
-0.0584 0.3578 0.2157 1.2359
MO NY=4 NE=4 NK=16 LY=IN GA=IN PH=SY,FI TE=IN BE=IN PS=IN
LK
EC-T1 CC-T1 AC-T1 DC-T1 ES-T1 CS-T1 AS-T1 DS-T1
EC-T2 CC-T2 AC-T2 DC-T2 ES-T2 CS-T2 AS-T2 DS-T2
LE
CONS-T1 SENS-T1 CONS-T2 SENS-T2
MA PH
1.0
0.0 1.0
0.0 0.0 1.0
0.0 0.0 0.0 1.0
0.0 0.0 0.0 0.0 1.0
0.0 0.0 0.0 0.0 0.0 1.0
0.0 0.0 0.0 0.0 0.0 0.0 1.0
0.0 0.0 0.0 0.0 0.0 0.0 0.0 1.0
0.0 0.0 0.0 0.0 0.0 0.0 0.0 0.0 1.0
0.0 1.0 0.0 0.0 0.0 0.0 0.0 0.0 0.0 1.0
0.0 0.0 0.5 0.0 0.0 0.0 0.0 0.0 0.0 0.0 1.0
0.0 0.0 0.0 0.25 0.0 0.0 0.0 0.0 0.0 0.0 0.0 1.0
```

```
0.0 0.0 0.0 0.0 0.0 0.0 0.0 0.0 0.0 0.0 0.0 0.0 1.0
0.0 0.0 0.0 0.0 0.0 1.0 0.0 0.0 0.0 0.0 0.0 0.0 0.0 1.0
0.0 0.0 0.0 0.0 0.0 0.0 0.5 0.0 0.0 0.0 0.0 0.0 0.0 0.0 1.0
0.0 0.0 0.0 0.0 0.0 0.0 0.0 0.25 0.0 0.0 0.0 0.0 0.0 0.0 0.0 1.0
OU ND=4 NS RS it=150 ad=off pc sc ef se tv
```

Appendix J

LISREL Script and Data for Simplex Model

J.1 Data Matrix for Phenotypic Simplex Model

The matrix below shows within-person covariances among weight measurements at successive six-month intervals from 66 females obtained from Fischbein's (1977) sample of opposite-sex DZ twin pairs. This matrix is for use in the LISREL script shown in Chapter 14, Section 14.2.1.

```
Weight 1    51.470
Weight 2    53.867   58.150
Weight 3    55.399   59.709   63.658
Weight 4    58.573   63.124   67.071   72.820
Weight 5    56.597   60.644   65.104   70.421   71.634
Weight 6    52.222   55.930   60.485   66.239   67.360   66.855
```

J.2 Genetic Simplex Model

The following LISREL 7 script fits a simplex model to additive genetic (G) and non-shared environmental (E) effects over 5 successive six-month intervals.

```
GROUP1 DZ weight 6 time points
DA NG=2 NI=12 NO=51 MA=CM
<INPUT MATRIX>
MO NY=12 NE=24 PS=ST,FI LY=FU,FI TE=ZE BE=FU,FI
LE
A1T1 A2T1 A3T1 A4T1 A5T1 A6T1 A1T2 A2T2 A3T2 A4T2 A5T2 A6T2
E1T1 E2T1 E3T1 E4T1 E5T1 E6T1 E1T2 E2T2 E3T2 E4T2 E5T2 E6T2
```

```
ST 1 PS 1,1 PS 2,2 PS 3,3 PS 4,4 PS 5,5 PS 6,6 PS 7,7 PS 8,8 PS 9,9
ST 1 PS 10,10 PS 11,11 PS 12,12 PS 13,13 PS 14,14 PS 15,15 PS 16,16
ST 1 PS 17,17 PS 18,18 PS 19,19 PS 20,20 PS 21,21 PS 22,22 PS 23,23
ST 1 PS 24,24
ST 0.5 PS 7,1 PS 8,2 PS 9,3 PS 10,4 PS 11,5 PS 12,6
FR LY 1,1 LY 2,2 LY 3,3 LY 4,4 LY 5,5 LY 6,6 LY 7,7 LY 8,8
FR LY 9,9 LY 10,10 LY 11,11 LY 12,12
EQ LY 1,1 LY 7,7
EQ LY 2,2 LY 8,8
EQ LY 3,3 LY 9,9
EQ LY 4,4 LY 10,10
EQ LY 5,5 LY 11,11
EQ LY 6,6 LY 12,12
FR LY 1,13 LY 2,14 LY 3,15 LY 4,16 LY 5,17 LY 6,18 LY 7,19
FR LY 8,20 LY 9,21 LY 10,22 LY 11,23 LY 12,24
EQ LY 1,13 LY 7,19
EQ LY 2,14 LY 8,20
EQ LY 3,15 LY 9,21
EQ LY 4,16 LY 10,22
EQ LY 5,17 LY 11,23
EQ LY 6,18 LY 12,24
FR BE 2,1 BE 3,2 BE 4,3 BE 5,4 BE 6,5
FR BE 8,7 BE 9,8 BE 10,9 BE 11,10 BE 12,11
FR BE 14,13 BE 15,14 BE 16,15 BE 17,16 BE 18,17
FR BE 20,19 BE 21,20 BE 22,21 BE 23,22 BE 24,23
EQ BE 2,1 BE 8,7
EQ BE 3,2 BE 9,8
EQ BE 4,3 BE 10,9
EQ BE 5,4 BE 11,10
EQ BE 6,5 BE 12,11
EQ BE 14,13 BE 20,19
EQ BE 15,14 BE 21,20
EQ BE 16,15 BE 22,21
EQ BE 17,16 BE 23,22
EQ BE 18,17 BE 24,23
ST 4 ALL
ST 0.4 BE 2,1 BE 3,2 BE 4,3 BE 5,4 BE 6,5
ST 0.4 BE 14,13 BE 15,14 BE 16,15 BE 17,16 BE 18,17
OU NS SS SE AD=OFF IT=200
GROUP2 MZ DATA
DA NI=12 NO=32 MA=CM
<INPUT MATRIX>
MO PS=ST,FI LY=IN TE=ZE BE=IN
```

```
LE
A1T1 A2T1 A3T1 A4T1 A5T1 A6T1 A1T2 A2T2 A3T2 A4T2 A5T2 A6T2
E1T1 E2T1 E3T1 E4T1 E5T1 E6T1 E1T2 E2T2 E3T2 E4T2 E5T2 E6T2
ST 1 PS 1,1 PS 2,2 PS 3,3 PS 4,4 PS 5,5 PS 6,6 PS 7,7 PS 8,8 PS 9,9
ST 1 PS 10,10 PS 11,11 PS 12,12 PS 13,13 PS 14,14 PS 15,15 PS 16,16
ST 1 PS 17,17 PS 18,18 PS 19,19 PS 20,20 PS 21,21 PS 22,22 PS 23,23
ST 1 PS 24,24
ST 1 PS 7,1 PS 8,2 PS 9,3 PS 10,4 PS 11,5 PS 12,6
OU NS AD=OFF
```

J.3   Data Matrices for Genetic Simplex Model

DZ COVARIANCE MATRIX

	Twin1 T1	Twin1 T2	Twin1 T3	Twin1 T4	Twin1 T5	Twin1 T6
Twin1 T1	28.873					
Twin1 T2	29.423	31.546				
Twin1 T3	31.087	33.341	38.996			
Twin1 T4	30.395	32.557	37.267	38.366		
Twin1 T5	30.987	32.649	37.896	38.620	41.418	
Twin1 T6	29.880	31.727	36.752	37.826	40.317	42.379

	Twin1 T1	Twin1 T2	Twin1 T3	Twin1 T4	Twin1 T5	Twin1 T6
Twin2 T1	16.157	15.524	16.402	16.393	16.040	16.231
Twin2 T2	16.319	15.992	16.393	16.431	15.513	15.809
Twin2 T3	15.946	15.356	16.315	15.873	15.253	15.175
Twin2 T4	16.367	15.565	16.465	17.038	15.913	14.977
Twin2 T5	15.763	14.633	16.289	15.970	16.144	14.905
Twin2 T6	13.692	12.443	13.782	13.592	13.583	12.886

	Twin2 T1	Twin2 T2	Twin2 T3	Twin2 T4	Twin2 T5	Twin2 T6
Twin2 T1	20.032					
Twin2 T2	20.140	21.577				
Twin2 T3	21.600	22.822	26.738			
Twin2 T4	21.730	23.331	26.453	28.948		
Twin2 T5	21.520	22.878	26.361	27.891	30.103	
Twin2 T6	20.940	22.117	25.784	27.361	29.373	31.204

MZ COVARIANCE MATRIX

	Twin1 T1	Twin1 T2	Twin1 T3	Twin1 T4	Twin1 T5	Twin1 T6

```
Twin1 T1    30.347
Twin1 T2    33.096   37.443
Twin1 T3    33.993   38.210   42.319
Twin1 T4    34.778   39.356   44.020   47.606
Twin1 T5    34.703   39.403   44.038   48.239   50.931
Twin1 T6    33.202   37.419   41.574   45.373   47.971   48.154
```

	Twin1 T1	Twin1 T2	Twin1 T3	Twin1 T4	Twin1 T5	Twin1 T6
Twin2 T1	33.469	36.124	36.005	36.979	38.484	37.885
Twin2 T2	35.551	39.813	39.439	41.009	42.988	41.554
Twin2 T3	37.010	40.972	42.773	44.962	46.657	45.031
Twin2 T4	38.504	42.658	45.377	48.841	50.994	49.015
Twin2 T5	38.829	42.866	46.065	49.803	53.449	51.444
Twin2 T6	38.266	42.058	44.320	47.550	50.958	51.082

	Twin2 T1	Twin2 T2	Twin2 T3	Twin2 T4	Twin2 T5	Twin2 T6
Twin2 T1	44.188					
Twin2 T2	45.593	49.280				
Twin2 T3	46.284	49.359	52.083			
Twin2 T4	47.113	50.631	54.266	58.924		
Twin2 T5	48.183	51.669	55.154	59.748	63.154	
Twin2 T6	48.319	51.284	53.965	57.913	61.290	62.310

J.4   Output from Genetic Simplex Model

The tables below show parameter estimates and standard errors obtained from fitting the simplex model shown in Appendix J.2 to the longitudinal MZ and DZ weight covariances in Appendix J.3.

```
LAMBDA Y
        A1T1        A2T1        A3T1        A4T1        A5T1        A6T1
     --------    --------    --------    --------    --------    --------
        4.794       1.121       1.498       1.235       1.389       1.387
         .349        .098        .146        .147        .134        .148

LAMBDA Y
        E1T1        E2T1        E3T1        E4T1        E5T1        E6T1
     --------    --------    --------    --------    --------    --------
        1.815        .563        .980        .955        .814        .999
         .220        .069        .115        .110        .099        .118
```

BETA

	A1T1	A2T1	A3T1	A4T1	A5T1	A6T1
	---------	---------	---------	---------	---------	---------
	.000	4.503	.781	1.235	.910	.973
	.000	.524	.105	.197	.144	.142

BETA

	E1T1	E2T1	E3T1	E4T1	E5T1	E6T1
	---------	---------	---------	---------	---------	---------
	.000	2.962	.605	.872	.987	.824
	.000	.540	.117	.163	.183	.158

CHI-SQUARE WITH 134 DEGREES OF FREEDOM = 161.00 (P = .056)

J.5 Output from Genetic Factor Model

The tables below show parameter estimates and standard errors from a genetic common factor model fit to Fishbein's (1977) longitudinal weight measurements for MZ and DZ twins (see Chapter 12 for a description of this model in LISREL).

LAMBDA X:	Estimates		Standard Errors	
	AT1	ET1	AT1	ET1
	---------	-----	--------	-----
Weight 1	3.841	3.735	.410	.261
Weight 2	4.200	3.909	.431	.269
Weight 3	5.114	3.390	.444	.275
Weight 4	5.674	2.908	.446	.270
Weight 5	6.190	2.402	.447	.260
Weight 6	6.084	2.264	.449	.278

THETA DELTA	Weight 1	Weight 2	Weight 3	Weight 4	Weight 5	Weight 6
	--------	--------	--------	--------	--------	--------
Estimates	1.086	.587	1.466	1.449	.933	2.786
SE	.198	.170	.189	.197	.191	.374

CHI-SQUARE WITH 138 DEGREES OF FREEDOM = 359.11 (P = .000)

Appendix K

LISREL Scripts for Assortment Models

K.1 Social Homogamy Model

This LISREL 7 script specifies a social homogamy model of assortative mating for twins and their parents (Eaves et al., 1989).

```
SOCIAL HOMOGAMY MODEL; DZ TWINS AND PARENTS
DA NG=2 NI=4 NO=144
LA
DZ1 DZ2 Mother Father
CM
1.21
0.29 1.03
0.23 0.16 0.91
0.13 0.09 0.21 1.08
MO NY=2 NX=2 NE=3 NK=4 GA=FU,FI PS=SY,FI PH=SY,FI LY=FI
PA LX
1 1 0 0
0 0 1 1
LK
AM CM AF CF
MA PH
1.
0. 1.
0. 0. 1.
0. 0. 0. 1.
FR PH(4,2)
```

```
MA GA
0.5  0.   0.5  0.
0.   0.   0.   0.
0.5  0.   0.5  0.
FR GA(2,2) GA(2,4)
MA PS
0.5
0.   0.1
0.   0.   0.5
FR PS(2,2)
EQ LX(1,1) LX(2,3) LY(1,1) LY(2,3)
EQ LX(1,2) LX(2,4) LY(1,2) LY(2,2)
EQ TE(1,1) TE(2,2) TD(1,1) TD(2,2)
LE
AT1 CT AT2
ST .3 ALL
OU AD=OFF NS SE PC
SOCIAL HOMOGAMY MODEL; MZ TWINS AND PARENTS
DA NO=106
LA
MZ1 MZ2 Mother Father
CM
0.95
0.54 0.89
0.08 0.21 1.11
0.28 0.18 0.11 0.90
MO LX=IN TD=IN PH=IN GA=IN PS=IN TE=IN LY=FI
EQ LY(1,1,1) LY(1,1) LY(2,1)
EQ LY(1,1,2) LY(1,2) LY(2,2)
OU
```

K.2   Phenotypic Assortment Model

The following LISREL 8 script fits a reverse path model of phenotypic assortment with "P to C" cultural transmission to twin/parent data on fear of social criticism.

```
ASSORTMENT AND CULTURAL TRANSMISSION REVERSE PATH MODEL;
MZ TWINS AND PARENTS
DA NG=2 NI=4 NO=144
LA
MZ1 MZ2 Mother Father
CM FI=MZ.DAT
```

```
MO NY=2 NX=2 NE=5 NK=2 LX=ID TD=ZE BE=FU GA=FI PS=DI
LK
PM PF
LE
AM AF AT1 CT AT2
FR LY(1,4) GA(1,1) GA(4,1) PH(2,1) TE(1,1)
EQ LY(1,4) LY(2,4)
CO
LY(1,3)=GA(1,1)-LY(1,4)*GA(4,1)*GA(1,1)- C
LY(1,4)*GA(4,1)*GA(1,1)*PH(2,1)
CO
LY(2,3)=GA(1,1)-LY(1,4)*GA(4,1)*GA(1,1)- C
LY(1,4)*GA(4,1)*GA(1,1)*PH(2,1)
VA .5 BE(3,1) BE(3,2) BE(5,1) BE(5,2)
EQ GA(1,1) GA(2,2)
EQ GA(4,1) GA(4,2)
CO
PH(1,1)=LY(1,4)**2+TE(1)+GA(1,1)**2- C
GA(1,1)**2*LY(1,4)**2*GA(4,1)**2- C
     2*GA(1,1)**2*LY(1,4)**2*GA(4,1)**2*PH(2,1)- C
     GA(1,1)**2*LY(1,4)**2*GA(4,1)**2*PH(2,1)**2
CO PH(2,2)=LY(1,4)**2+TE(1)+GA(1,1)**2- C
GA(1,1)**2*LY(1,4)**2*GA(4,1)**2- C
     2*GA(1,1)**2*LY(1,4)**2*GA(4,1)**2*PH(2,1)- C
     GA(1,1)**2*LY(1,4)**2*GA(4,1)**2*PH(2,1)**2
CO PS(1,1)=1-GA(1,1)**2
CO PS(2,2)=1-GA(1,1)**2
CO PS(3,3)=.5-.5*PH(2,1)*GA(1,1)**2
CO PS(5,5)=.5-.5*PH(2,1)*GA(1,1)**2
CO PS(4,4)=1-2*GA(4,1)**2-2*PH(2,1)*GA(4,1)**2
EQ TE(1,1) TE(2,2)
ST .5 ALL
OU AD=OFF SE TV RS
ASSORTMENT AND CULTURAL TRANSMISSION REVERSE PATH MODEL;
DZ TWINS AND PARENTS
DA NO=106
LA
DZ1 DZ2 Mother Father
CM  FI=DZ.DAT
MO BE=IN GA=IN PS=DI TE=IN
LE
AM AF AT1 CT AT2
LK
```

```
PM PF
EQ LY(1,1,4) LY(1,4) LY(2,4)
EQ PH(1,2,1) PH(2,1)
CO LY(1,3)=GA(1,1,1)-LY(1,1,4)*GA(1,4,1)*GA(1,1,1)- C
      LY(1,1,4)*GA(1,4,1)*GA(1,1,1)*PH(1,2,1)
CO LY(2,5)=GA(1,1,1)-LY(1,1,4)*GA(1,4,1)*GA(1,1,1)- C
      LY(1,1,4)*GA(1,4,1)*GA(1,1,1)*PH(1,2,1)
CO PH(1,1)=LY(1,1,4)**2+TE(1)+GA(1,1,1)**2- C
      GA(1,1,1)**2*LY(1,1,4)**2*GA(1,4,1)**2- C
      2*GA(1,1,1)**2*LY(1,1,4)**2*GA(1,4,1)**2*PH(1,2,1)- C
      GA(1,1,1)**2*LY(1,1,4)**2*GA(1,4,1)**2*PH(1,2,1)**2
CO PH(2,2)=LY(1,1,4)**2+TE(1)+GA(1,1,1)**2- C
      GA(1,1,1)**2*LY(1,1,4)**2*GA(1,4,1)**2- C
      2*GA(1,1,1)**2*LY(1,1,4)**2*GA(1,4,1)**2*PH(1,2,1)-C
      GA(1,1,1)**2*LY(1,1,4)**2*GA(1,4,1)**2*PH(1,2,1)**2
CO PS(1,1)=1-GA(1,1,1)**2
CO PS(2,2)=1-GA(1,1,1)**2
CO PS(3,3)=.5-.5*PH(1,2,1)*GA(1,1,1)**2
CO PS(5,5)=.5-.5*PH(1,2,1)*GA(1,1,1)**2
CO PS(4,4)=1-2*GA(1,4,1)**2-2*PH(1,2,1)*GA(1,4,1)**2
OU
```

Bibliography

Achenbach, T. M. & Edelbrock, C. S. (1981). *Behavior problems and competencies reported by parents of normal and disturbed children age four through sixteen. Monographs of the Society for Research in Child Development.* Number 188 in 46.

Achenbach, T. M. & Edelbrock, C. S. (1983). *Manual for the Child Gehavior Checklist and Revised Child Behavior Profile.* Burlington, VT: University of Vermont Dept. of Psychiatry.

Achenbach, T. M., McConaughy, S. H., & Howell, C. T. (1987). Child/adolescent behavioral and emotional problems: Implications of cross-informant correlations for situational specificity. *Psychological Bulletin, 101,* 213–232.

Aitken, A. C. (1934). Note on selection from a multivariate normal population. *Proceedings of the Edinburgh Mathematical Society B, 4,* 106–110.

Akaike, H. (1987). Factor analysis and aic. *Psychometrika, 52,* 317–332.

Anderson, T. W. & Amemiya, Y. (1985). The asymptotic normal distribution of estimators in factor analysis under general conditions. *The Annals of Statistics, 16,* 759–771.

Annett, M. (1978). Handedness in human families. *Annals Human Genetics, 37,* 93–105.

Arnold, S. J. (1990). Inheritance and the evolution of behavioral ontogenies. In M. Hahn, J. Hewitt, N. Henderson, & R. Benno (Eds.), *Developmental Behavior Genetics. Neural, Biometrical, and Evolutionary Approaches,* (pp. 167–189). Oxford University Press: Oxford.

Australian Bureau of Statistics (1977). *Alcohol and tobacco consumption patterns: February 1977* (catalogue no. 4312.0. ed.). Australian Bureau of Statistics.

Bedford, A., Foulds, G. A., & Sheffield, B. F. (1976). A new personal disturbance scale (DSSI/SAD). *British Journal of Social Clinical Psychology, 15,* 387–394.

463

Bem, S. L. (1974). The measurement of psychological androgyny. *Journal of Consulting and Clinical Psychology*, *42*, 155–162.

Bentler, P. M. (1989). *EQS: Structural equations program manual.* Los Angeles: BMDP Statistical Software.

Biddle, B. J., Slavings, R. L., & Anderson, D. S. (1985). Methodological observations on applied behavioral science. *Journal of Applied Behavioral Science*, *21*, 79–93.

Bock, R. D. & Vandenberg, S. G. (1968). Components of heritable variation in mental test scores. In S. G. Vandenberg (Ed.), *Progress in human behavior genetics*, (pp. 233–260). The Johns Hopkins Press: Baltimore.

Bodmer, W. F. (1987). HLA, immune response, and disease. In F. Vogel & K. Sperling (Eds.), *Human Genetics: Proceedings of the 7th international congress*, (pp. 107–113). Springer-Verlag: New York.

Bollen, K. A. (1989). *Structural Equations with Latent Variables*. New York: John Wiley.

Boomsma, A. (1983). *On the robustness of LISREL (maximum likelihood estimation) against small sample size and non-normality.* Unpublished doctoral dissertation, University of Groningen, Groningen, The Netherlands.

Boomsma, D. I., Martin, N. G., & Molenaar, P. C. M. (1989a). Factor and simplex models for repeated measures: Application to two psychomotor measures of alcohol sensitivity in twins. *Behavior Genetics*, *19*, 79–96.

Boomsma, D. I. & Molenaar, P. C. M. (1986). Using lisrel to analyze genetic and environmental covariance structure. *Behavior Genetics*, *16*, 237–250.

Boomsma, D. I. & Molenaar, P. C. M. (1987). The genetic analysis of repeated measures. *Behavior Genetics*, *17*, 111–123.

Boomsma, D. I., Van Den Bree, M. B., Orlebeke, J. F., & Molenaar, P. C. M. (1989b). Resemblances of parents and twins in sports participation and heart rate. *Behavior Genetics*, *19*, 123–141.

Boyer, C. B. (1985). *A history of mathematics.* Princeton, New Jersey: Princeton University Press.

Bray, J. A. (1976). *The Obese Patient.* Philadelphia: W. B. Saunders.

Brown, G. W. & Harris, T. O. (1978). *Social Origins of Depression: A Study of Psychiatric Disorder in Women.* London: Tavistock.

Browne, M. W. (1974). Generalized least squares estimators in the analysis of covariance structures. *South African Statistical Journal*, *8*, 1–24.

Browne, M. W. (1982). Covariance structures. In D. M. Hawkins (Ed.), *Topics in applied multivariate analysis*, (pp. 72–141). Cambridge University Press: Cambridge.

Browne, M. W. (1984). Asymptotically distribution-free methods for the analysis of covariance structures. *British Journal of Mathematical and Statistical Psychology*, *37*, 62–83.

Browne, M. W. (1987). Robustness of statistical inference in factor analysis and related models. *Biometrika*, *74*, 375–384.

Browne, M. W. (1990). *RAMONA User's Guide*. Ohio: Ohio State University.

Browne, M. W. & Cudeck, R. (1990). Single sample cross-validation indices for covariance structures. *Multivariate Behavioral Research*, *24*, 445–455.

Bulmer, M. G. (1980). *The Mathematical Theory of Quantitative Genetics*. Oxford: Clarendon Press.

Cadoret, R. J., Cain, C. A., & Grove, W. M. (1980). Development of alcoholism in adoptees raised apart from alcoholic biologic relatives. *Archives General Psychiatry*, *37*, 561–563.

Campbell, D. T. (1963). From description to experimentation: Interpreting trends from quasi-experiments. In C. Harris (Ed.), *Problems in Measuring Change*, (pp. 212–242). University of Wisconsin Press: Madison, WI.

Cantor, R. M. (1983). A multivariate genetic analysis of ridge count data from the offspring of monozygotic twins. *Acta Geneticae Medicae et Gemellologiae*, *32*, 161–208.

Cardon, L. R. (1992). *Multivariate Path Analysis of Specific Cognitive Abilities in the Colorado Adoption Project*. Unpublished doctoral dissertation, University of Colorado, Boulder, Colorado.

Cardon, L. R. & Fulker, D. W. (1991). Sources of continuity in infant predictors of adult IQ. *Intelligence*, *15*, 279–293.

Cardon, L. R. & Fulker, D. W. (1992). Genetic influences on body fat from birth to age 9. *Genetic Epidemiology*. (in press).

Cardon, L. R., Fulker, D. W., DeFries, J. C., & Plomin, R. (1992). Continuity and change in general cognitive ability from 1 to 7 years. *Developmental Psychology*. (in press).

Cardon, L. R., Fulker, D. W., & Jöreskog, K. G. (1991). A LISREL model with constrained parameters for twin and adoptive families. *Behavior Genetics*, *21*, 327–350.

Carey, G. (1986a). A general multivariate approach to linear modeling in human genetics. *American Journal of Human Genetics, 39*, 775–786.

Carey, G. (1986b). Sibling imitation and contrast effects. *Behavior Genetics*, (pp. 319–341).

Carey, G. (1988). Inference about genetic correlations. *Behavior Genetics, 18*, 329–338.

Casti, L. (1989). *Alternate Realities: Mathematical Models of Nature and Man.* New York: John Wiley & Sons.

Castle, W. E. (1903). The law of heredity of Galton and Mendel and some laws governing race improvement by selection. *Proceedings of the American Academy of Sciences, 39*, 233–242.

Cattell, R. B. (1963). Theory of fluid and crystallized intelligence: A critical experiment. *Journal of Educational Psychology, 54*, 1–22.

Cavalli-Sforza, L. L. & Feldman, M. (1981). *Cultural Transmission and Evolution: A Quantitative Approach.* Princeton: Princeton University.

Cederloff, R., Friberg, L., & Lundman, T. (1977). The interactions of smoking, environment and heredity and their implications for disease etiology: A report of epidemiological studies on the Swedish twin registries. *Acta Med Scand Supplement, 612*, 1–128.

Clifford, C. A., Fulker, D. W., Gurling, H. M. D., & Murray, R. M. (1981). Preliminary findings from a twin study of alcohol use. In L. Gedda, P. Parisi, & W. E. Nance (Eds.), *Twin Research 3: Epidemiological and Clinical Studies (Progress in Clinical and Biological Research)*, volume 69C, (pp. 47–52). Alan R. Liss: New York.

Cloninger, C. R. (1980). Interpretation of intrinsic and extrinsic structural relations by path analysis: Theory and application to assortative mating. *Genetic Research, 36*, 133–145.

Cloninger, C. R. (1987). Neurogenetic adaptive mechanisms in alcoholism. *Science, 236*, 410–416.

Cloninger, C. R., Bohman, M., & Sigvardsson, S. (1981). Inheritance of alcohol abuse: Cross-fostering analysis of adopted men. *Archives General Psychiatry, 38*, 861–868.

Cloninger, C. R., Rice, J., & Reich, T. (1979a). Multifactorial inheritance with cultural transmission and assortative mating. II. A general model of combined polygenic and cultural inheritance. *American Journal of Human Genetics, 31*, 176–198.

Cloninger, C. R., Rice, J., & Reich, T. (1979b). Multifactorial inheritance with cultural transmission and assortative mating. III. Family structure and the analysis of separation experiments. *American Journal of Human Genetics, 31,* 366–388.

Corey, L. A., Eaves, L. J., Mellen, B. G., & Nance, W. E. (1986). Testing for developmental changes in gene expression on resemblance for quantitative traits in kinships of monozygotic twins. *Genetic Epidemiology, 3,* 73–83.

Cox, A. & Rutter, M. (1985). Diagnostic appraisal and interviewing. In M. Rutter & L. Hersor (Eds.), *Child and adolescent psychiatry.* Blackwell: Oxford, (2nd ed.).

Crow, J. F. & Kimura, M. (1970). *Introduction to Population Genetics Theory.* New York: Harper and Row.

Cudeck, R. (1989). Analysis of correlation matrices using covariance structure models. *Psychological Bulletin, 105,* 317–327.

Darlington, C. D. (1971). Axiom and process in genetics. *Nature, 234,* 131–133.

Dawkins, R. (1982). *The Extended Phenotype: The Gene as the Unit of Selection.* Oxford: Oxford University Press.

Dennis, J. E. & Schnabel, R. B. (1983). *Numerical Methods for Unconstrained Optimization and Nonlinear Equations.* Englewood Cliffs, N.J.: Prentice Hall.

Dolan, C. V. & Molenaar, P. C. M. (1991). A comparison of four methods of calculating standard errors of maximum likelihood estimates in the analysis of covariance structure. *British Journal of Mathematical and Statistical Psychology, 44,* 359–368.

Dolan, C. V., Molenaar, P. C. M., & Boomsma, D. I. (1991). Longitudinal genetic analysis of longitudinal means and covariance structure in the simplex model using LISREL. *Behavior Genetics, 21,* 49–61.

Duffy, D. L. & Martin, N. G. (1992). Inferring the direction of causation in cross-sectional twin data: theoretical and empirical considerations. *Genetic Epidemiology, In press.*

Duffy, D. L., Martin, N. G., Battistutta, D., Hopper, J. L., & Mathews, J. D. (1990). Genetics of asthma and hayfever in australian twins. *American Review of Respiratory Disease, 142,* 1351–1358.

Duncan, O. D. (1969). Some linear models for two-wave, two-variable panel analysis. *Psychological Bulletin, 72,* 177–182.

Eaves, L. J. (1969). The genetic analysis of continuous variation: A comparison of experimental designs applicable to human data. *British Journal of Mathematical and Statistical Psychology, 22*, 131–147.

Eaves, L. J. (1970). *Aspects of Human Psychogenetics.* Unpublished doctoral dissertation, University of Birmingham, Birmingham, England.

Eaves, L. J. (1976a). The effect of cultural transmission on continuous variation. *Heredity, 37*, 41–57.

Eaves, L. J. (1976b). A model for sibling effects in man. *Heredity, 36*, 205–214.

Eaves, L. J. (1982). The utility of twins. In V. Anderson, et al (Ed.), *Genetic Bases of the Epilepsies.* New York: Raven Press.

Eaves, L. J. & Eysenck, H. J. (1975). The nature of extraversion: A genetical analysis. *Journal of Personality and Social Psychology, 32*, 102–112.

Eaves, L. J., Eysenck, H. J., & Martin, N. G. (1989a). *Genes, Culture and Personality: An Empirical Approach.* London: Oxford University Press.

Eaves, L. J., Fulker, D. W., & Heath, A. C. (1989b). The effects of social homogamy and cultural inheritance on the covariances of twins and their parents. *Behavior Genetics, 19*, 113–122.

Eaves, L. J., Heath, A. C., Neale, M. C., Hewitt, J. K., & Martin, N. G. (1992). Sex differences and non-additivity in the effects of genes on personality. *Psychological Science.* (in press).

Eaves, L. J., Hewitt, J. K., Meyer, J. M., & Neale, M. C. (1990a). Approaches to quantitative genetic modeling of development and age-related changes. In M. E. Hahn, J. K. Hewitt, N. D. Henderson, & R. Benno (Eds.), *Developmental Behavior Genetics. Neural, Biometrical and Evolutionary Approaches*, (pp. 266–277). Oxford University Press: Oxford.

Eaves, L. J., Last, K. A., Martin, N. G., & Jinks, J. L. (1977). A progressive approach to non-additivity and genotype-environmental covariance in the analysis of human differences. *British Journal of Mathematical and Statistical Psychology, 30*, 1–42.

Eaves, L. J., Last, K. A., Young, P. A., & Martin, N. G. (1978). Model-fitting approaches to the analysis of human behavior. *Heredity, 41*, 249–320.

Eaves, L. J., Long, J., & Heath, A. C. (1986). A theory of developmental change in quantitative phenotypes applied to cognitive development. *Behavior Genetics, 16*, 143–162.

Eaves, L. J., Martin, N. G., & Heath, A. C. (1990b). Religious affiliation in twins and their parents: testing a model of cultural inheritance. *Behavior Genetics*, *20*, 1–22.

Eaves, L. J., Neale, M. C., & Meyer, J. M. (1991). A model for comparative ratings in studies of within-family differences. *Behavior Genetics*, *21*, 531–536.

Falconer, D. S. (1960). *Quantitative Genetics*. Edinburgh: Oliver and Boyd.

Falconer, D. S. (1990). *Introduction to Quantitative Genetics* (3rd ed.). New York: Longman Group Ltd.

Fischbein, S. (1977). Intra-pair similarity in physical growth of monozygotic and of dizygotic twins during puberty. *Annals of Human Biology*, *4*, 417–430.

Fischbein, S., Molenaar, P. C. M., & Boomsma, D. I. (1990). Simultaneous genetic analysis of longitudinal means and covariance strucutre using the simplex model: Application to repeatedly measured weight in a sample of 164 female twins. *Acta Geneticae Medicae et Gemellologiae*, *39*, 165–172.

Fisher, R. A. (1918). The correlation between relatives on the supposition of Mendelian inheritance. *Translations of the Royal Society, Edinburgh*, *52*, 399–433.

Fisher, R. A. (1920). A mathematical examination of the methods of determining the accuracy of an observation by the mean error, and by the mean square error. *Monthly Notices of the Royal Astronomical Society*, *80*, 758–770.

Fraser, C. (1988). *COSAN User's Guide. Unpublished documentation*. Centre for Behavioural Studies in Education, University of England, Armidale NSW, Australia 2351: Unpublished documentation.

Friedrich, J., Kierniesky, N., & Cardon, L. R. (1989). Drawing moral inferences from descriptive science: The impact of attitudes on naturalistic fallacy errors. *Personality and Social Psychology Bulletin*, *15*, 414–425.

Fulker, D. W. (1982). Extensions of the classical twin method. In *Human genetics, part A: The unfolding genome* (pp. 395–406). New York: Alan R. Liss.

Fulker, D. W. (1988). Genetic and cultural transmission in human behavior. In B. S. Weir, E. J. Eisen, M. M. Goodman, & G. Namkoong (Eds.), *Proceedings of the second international conference on quantitative genetics* (pp. 318–340). Sunderland, MA: Sinauer.

Fulker, D. W., Baker, L. A., & Bock, R. D. (1983). Estimating components of covariance using LISREL. *Data Analyst*, *1*, 5–8.

Fuller, J. L. & Thompson, W. R. (1978). *Foundations of Behavior Genetics*. St. Louis: C. V. Mosby.

Geer, J. H. (1965). The development of a scale to measure fear. *Behavioral Research Therapy, 3*, 45–53.

Gill, P. E., Murray, W., , & Wright, M. H. (1981). *Practical Optimization*. New York: Academic Press.

Goodman, L. A. & Kruskal, W. H. (1979). *Measures of association for cross-classification*. New York: Springer-Verlag.

Goodwin, D. W., Schulsinger, F., Moller, N., Hermansen, L., Winokur, G., & Guze, S. B. (1974). Drinking problems in adopted and nonadopted sons of alcoholics. *Archives General Psychiatry, 31*, 164–169.

Gorsuch, R. L. (1983). *Factor Analysis* (2nd ed.). Hillsdale, NJ: Lawrence Erlbaum.

Graybill, F. A. (1969). *Introduction to Matrices with Applications in Statistics*. Belmont, CA: Wadsworth Publishing Company.

Grayson, D. A. (1989). Twins reared together: Minimizing shared environmental effects. *Behavior Genetics, 19*, 593–603.

Grilo, C. M. & Pogue-Guile, M. F. (1991). The nature of environmental influences on weight and obesity: A behavior genetic analysis. *Psychological Bulletin, 110*, 520–537.

Guttman, L. (1954). A new approach to factor analysis: The radex. In P. F. Lazarsfeld (Ed.), *Mathematical thinking in the social sciences*, (pp. 258–349). Free Press: Glencoe, Ill.

Haley, C. S., Jinks, J. L., & Last, K. (1981). The monozygotic twin half-sib method for analyzing maternal effects and sex-linkage in humans. *Heredity, 46*, 227–238.

Hao, B. (1984). *Chaos*. Singapore: World Scientific.

Harlow, L. L. (1985). *Behavior of some elliptical theory estimators with nonnormal data in a covariance structures framework: A Monte Carlo study*. Unpublished doctoral dissertation, University of California, Los Angeles, Los Angeles.

Harman, H. H. (1976). *Modern Factor Analysis*. Chicago: University of Chicago Press.

Hayduk, L. A. (1987). *Structural equation modelling with LISREL*. Baltimore: John Hopkins Press.

Heath, A. C. (1983). *Human Quantitative Genetics: Some Issues and Applications.* Unpublished doctoral dissertation, University of Oxford, Oxford, England.

Heath, A. C. (1987). The analysis of marital interaction in cross-sectional twin data. *Acta Geneticae Medicae et Gemellologiae, 36,* 41–49.

Heath, A. C. & Eaves, L. J. (1985). Resolving the effects of phenotype and social background on mate selection. *Behavior Genetics, 15,* 15–30.

Heath, A. C., Eaves, L. J., & Martin, N. G. (1989a). The genetic structure of personality. iii. multivariate genetic item analysis of the epq scales. *Personality and Individual Differences, 10,* 877–888.

Heath, A. C., Jardine, R., & Martin, N. G. (1989b). Interactive effects of genotype and social environment on alcohol consumption in female twins. *Journal of Studies on Alcohol, 50,* 38–48.

Heath, A. C., Kendler, K. S., Eaves, L. J., & Markell, D. (1985). The resolution of cultural and biological inheritance: Informativeness of different relationships. *Behavior Genetics, 15,* 439–465.

Heath, A. C., Kessler, R. C., Neale, M. C., Hewitt, J. K., Eaves, L. J., & Kendler, K. S. (1992). Testing hypotheses about direction-of-causation using cross-sectional family data. (manuscript in review).

Heath, A. C. & Martin, N. G. (1986). Detecting the effects of genotype × environment interaction on personality and symptoms of anxiety and depression. *Behavior Genetics, 16,* 622.

Heath, A. C. & Martin, N. G. (1991a). The inheritance of alcohol sensitivity and of patterns of alcohol use. *Alcohol and Alcoholism, Supplement 1,* 141–145.

Heath, A. C. & Martin, N. G. (1991b). Intoxication after an acute dose of alcohol. An assessment of its association with alcohol consumption patterns by using twin data. *Alcoholism: Clinical and Experimental Research, 15,* 122–128.

Heath, A. C., Meyer, J., Eaves, L. J., & Martin, N. G. (1991a). The inheritance of alcohol consumption patterns in a general population twin sample I. Multidimensional scaling of quantity/frequency data. *Journal of Studies on Alcohol, 52,* 345–352.

Heath, A. C., Meyer, J., Jardine, R., & Martin, N. G. (1991b). The inheritance of alcohol consumption patterns in a general population twin sample II. Determinants of consumption frequency and quantity consumed. *Journal of Studies on Alcohol, 52,* 425–433.

Heath, A. C., Meyer, J. M., & Martin, N. G. (1990). Inheritance of alcohol consumption patterns in the Australian twin survey, 1981. In C. R. Cloninger & H. Begleiter (Eds.), *Genetics and Biology of Alcoholism.* Cold Spring Harbor Laboratory Press: New York.

Heath, A. C., Neale, M. C., Hewitt, J. K., Eaves, L. J., & Fulker, D. W. (1989c). Testing structural equation models for twin data using LISREL. *Behavior Genetics, 19,* 9–36.

Heise, D. R. (1975). *Causal Analysis.* New York: Wiley-Interscience.

Helzer, J. E., Robins, L. N., Taibleson, M., Woodruff, R. A., Reich, T., & Wish, E. D. (1977). Reliability of psychiatric diagnosis. *Archives of General Psychiatry, 34,* 129–133.

Hewitt, J. K. (1989). Of biases and more in the study of twins reared together: A reply to Grayson. *Behavior Genetics, 19,* 605–610.

Hewitt, J. K., Eaves, L. J., Neale, M. C., & Meyer, J. M. (1988). Resolving causes of developmental continuity or "tracking." I. Longitudinal twin studies during growth. *Behavior Genetics, 18,* 133–151.

Hewitt, J. K., Silberg, J. L., & Erickson, M. (1990). Genetic and environmental influences on internalizing and externalizing behavior problems in childhood and adolescence. *Behavior Genetics, 20,* 725. (abstract).

Hewitt, J. K., Silberg, J. L., Neale, M. C., Eaves, L. J., & Erickson, M. (1992). The analysis of parental ratings of children's behavior using LISREL. *Behavior Genetics.* (in press).

Hopper, J. L. (1988). *Review of FISHER, volume* 5.

Hopper, J. L. & Mathews, J. D. (1983). *Extensions to multivariate normal models for pedigree analysis. II. Modeling the effect of shared environments in the analysis of variation in blood lead levels, volume* 117.

Hrubec, Z. & Omenn, G. S. (1981). Evidence of genetic predisposition to alcoholic cirrhosis and psychosis: Twin concordances for alcoholism and its biological end points by zygosity among male veterans. *Alcohol Clinical Experimental Research, 11,* 349–356.

IMSL (1987). *IMSL User's Manual. Version 1.0.* Houston, Texas: IMSL, Inc.

Jardine, R. (1985). *A twin study of personality, social attitudes, and drinking behavior.* Unpublished doctoral dissertation, Australian National University, Australia.

Jeffrey, D. B. & Knauss, M. R. (1981). The etiologies, treatments, and assessments of obesity. In S. N. Haynes & L. Gannon (Eds.), *Psychosomatic disorders: A psychophysiological apprach to etiology and treatment.* New York: Praeger.

Jencks, C. (1972). *Inequality: A Reassessment of the Effect of Family and Schooling in America.* New York: Basic Books.

Jinks, J. L. & Fulker, D. W. (1970). Comparison of the biometrical genetical, MAVA, and classical approaches to the analysis of human behavior. *Psychological Bulletin, 73,* 311–349.

Johnston, J. J. (1972). *Econometric Methods* (2nd ed.). New York: McGraw-Hill.

Jöreskog, K. G. (1967). Some contributions to maximum likelihood factor analysis. *Psychometrika, 32,* 443–482.

Jöreskog, K. G. (1970). Estimation and testing of simplex models. *British Journal of Mathematical and Statistical Psychology, 23,* 121–145.

Jöreskog, K. G. (1973). A general method for estimating a linear structural equation system. In A. Goldberger & O. Duncan (Eds.), *Structural equation models in the social sciences,* (pp. 85–112). Seminar Press: New York.

Jöreskog, K. G. (1977). Structural equation models in the social sciences: Specification, estimation and testing. In P. Krishnaiah (Ed.), *Applications of statistics,* (pp. 265–287). North-Holland Publishing Co.: Amsterdam.

Jöreskog, K. G. (1978). Structural analysis of covariance and correlation matrices. *Psychometrika, 43,* 443–477.

Jöreskog, K. G. (1981). Analysis of covariance structures. *Scandinavian Journal of Statistics, 8,* 65–92.

Jöreskog, K. G. (1988). Analysis of covariance structures. In J. R. Nesselroade & R. B. Cattell (Eds.), *Handbook of Multivariate Experimental Psychology.* Plenum Press: New York, (2nd ed.).

Jöreskog, K. G. & Goldberger, A. S. (1972). Factor analysis by generalized least squares. *Psychometrika, 37,* 243–250.

Jöreskog, K. G. & Sörbom, D. (1986a). *LISREL: Analysis of Linear Structural Relationships by the Method of Maximum Likelihood.* Chicago: National Educational Resources.

Jöreskog, K. G. & Sörbom, D. (1986b). *PRELIS: A Preprocessor for LISREL.* Mooresville, Ind: Scientific Software.

Jöreskog, K. G. & Sörbom, D. (1988). *PRELIS - A Program for Multivariate Data Screening and Data Summarization. A Preprocessor for LISREL* (second ed.). Mooresville, Indiana: Scientific Software, Inc.

Jöreskog, K. G. & Sörbom, D. (1989). *LISREL 7: A Guide to the Program and Applications* (2nd ed.). Chicago: SPSS, Inc.

Jöreskog, K. G. & Sörbom, D. (1992). New features in LISREL 8. Manuscript in preparation.

Kaij, L. (1960). *Alcoholism in Twins: Studies on the Etiology and Sequelae of Abuse of Alcohol.* Stockholm: Almquist and Wiksell International.

Kaplan, D. (1990). Evaluating and modifying covarainace structure models: A review and recommendation. *Multivariate Behavioral Research, 25,* 137–155.

Kaprio, J., Koskenvuo, M., & Sarna, S. (1981). Cigarette smoking, use of alcohol, and leisure-time physical activity among same-sexed adult twins. In L. Gedda, P. Parisi, & W. Nance (Eds.), *Twin Research 3: Epidemiological and Clinical Studies (Progress in Clinical and Biological Research), volume 69C,* (pp. 47–52). Alan R. Liss: New York.

Kaprio, J., Koskenvuo, M. D., Langinvainio, H., Romanov, K., Sarna, S., & Rose, R. J. (1987). Genetic influences on use and abuse of alcohol: A study of 5638 adult Finnish brothers. *Alcohol Clinical Experimental Research, 11,* 349–356.

Kempthorne, O. (1960). *Biometrical Genetics.* New York: Pergammon Press.

Kendler, K. S., Heath, A. C., Martin, N. G., & Eaves, L. J. (1986). Symptoms of anxiety and depression in a volunteer twin population: The etiologic role of genetic and environmental factors. *Archives General Psychiatry, 43,* 213–221.

Kendler, K. S., Heath, A. C., Martin, N. G., & Eaves, L. J. (1987). Symptoms of anxiety and symptoms of depression: Same genes, different environments? *Archives General Psychiatry, 44,* 451–457.

Kendler, K. S., Kessler, R. C., Heath, A. C., Neale, M. C., & Eaves, L. J. (1991a). Coping: A genetic epidemiologic investigation. *Psychological Medicine, 21,* 337–346.

Kendler, K. S. & Kidd, K. K. (1986). Recurrence risks in an oligogenic threshold model: The effect of alterations in allele frequency. *Annals Human Genetics, 50,* 83–91.

Kendler, K. S., Neale, M. C., Heath, A. C., Kessler, R. C., & Eaves, L. J. (1991b). Life events and depressive symptoms: A twin study perspective. In P. McGuffin & R. Murray (Eds.), *The New Genetics of Mental Illness* (pp. 144–162). London: Butterworth-Heinemann.

Kendler, K. S., Neale, M. C., Kessler, R. C., Heath, A. C., & Eaves, L. J. (1992a). Childhood parental loss and adult psychopathology in women: A twin study perspective. *Archives General Psychiatry, 49*, 109–116.

Kendler, K. S., Neale, M. C., Kessler, R. C., Heath, A. C., & Eaves, L. J. (1992b). Generalized anxiety disorder in women: A population based twin study. *Archives General Psychiatry.* (in press).

Kendler, K. S., Neale, M. C., Kessler, R. C., Heath, A. C., & Eaves, L. J. (1992c). Major depression and generalized anxiety disorder: Same genes, (partly) different environments? *Archives General Psychiatry.* (in press).

Kendler, K. S., Neale, M. C., Kessler, R. C., Heath, A. C., & Eaves, L. J. (1992d). A twin study of recent life events and difficulties: The genetics of the environment. (manuscript in review).

Kenny, D. A. (1975). Cross-lagged panel correlation: A test for spuriousness. *Psychological Bulletin, 82*, 887–903.

Kenny, D. A. (1979). *Correlation and Causality.* New York: Wiley-Interscience.

Kenny, D. A. & Judd, C. M. (1984). Estimating the nonlinear and interactive effects of latent variables. *Psychological Bulletin, 96*, 201–210.

Kessler, R. C. (1983). Methodological issues in the study of psychosocial stress. In H. Kaplan (Ed.), *Psychosocial Stress: Trends in Theory and Research.* Academic Press: New York.

Kessler, R. C. & Greenberg, D. F. (1981). *Linear Panel Analysis: Quantitative Models of Change.* New York: Academic Press.

Kessler, R. C., Kendler, K. S., Heath, A. C., Neale, M. C., & Eaves, L. J. (1992). Social support, depressed mood, and adjustment to stress: A genetic epidemiologic investigation. *Journal of Personality and Social Psychology.* (in press).

Lange, K., Weeks, D., & Boehnke, M. (1988). Programs for pedigree analysis: Mendel, fisher and dgene. *Genetic Epidemiology, 5*, 471–472.

Lange, K., Westlake, J., & Spence, M. A. (1976). Extensions to pedigree analysis: III. Variance components by the scoring method. *Annals of human genetics, 39*, 485–491.

Lawley, D. N. & Maxwell, A. E. (1971). *Factor Analysis as a Statistical Method.* London: Butterworths.

Li, C. C. (1975). *Path Analysis: A Primer.* Pacific Grove, CA: Boxwood Press.

Little, R. J. A. & Rubin, D. B. (1987). *Statistical analysis with missing data.* New York: Wiley and Son.

Loeber, R., Green, S. M., Lahey, B., & Stouthamer-Loeber, M. (1989). Optimal informants on childhood disruptive behaviors. *Developmental Psychopathology*, *1*, 317–337.

Loehlin, J. C. (1987). *Latent Variable Models*. Baltimore: Lawrence Erlbaum.

Loehlin, J. C. & Nichols, R. C. (1976). *Heredity, Environment, and Personality*. Austin: University of Texas Press.

Loehlin, J. C. & Vandenberg, S. G. (1968). Genetic and environmental components in the covariation of cognitive abilities: An additive model. In S. G. Vandenberg (Ed.), *Progress in human behavior genetics*, (pp. 261–285). Johns Hopkins University Press: Baltimore.

Long, J. S. (1983). *Confirmatory Factor Analysis: A Preface to LISREL*. Beverly Hills: Sage Publications.

Longini, I. M., Higgins, M. W., Hinton, P. C., Moll, P. P., & Keller, J. B. (1991). Genetic and environmental sources of familial aggregation of body mass in tucumseh, michigan. *Human Biology*, *56*, 733–757.

Lykken, D. T., McGue, M., & Tellegen, A. (1987). Recruitment bias in twin research: the rule of two-thirds reconsidered. *Behavior Genetics*, *17*, 343–362.

Lytton, H. (1977). Do parents create, or respond to differences in twins? *Developmental Psychology*, *13*, 456–459.

MacDonald, A. & Stunkard, A. J. (1990). Body-mass indexes of British separated twins. *New England Journal of Medicine*, *322*, 1530.

Mardia, K. V., Kent, J. T., & Bibby, J. M. (1979). *Multivariate Analysis*. New York: Academic Press.

Marsh, H. W., Balla, J. R., & McDonald, R. P. (1988). Goodness-of-fit indexes in confirmatory factor analysis: The effect of sample size. *Psychological Bulletin*, *103*, 391–410.

Martin, N. G. & Boomsma, D. I. (1989). Willingness to drive when drunk and personality: A twin study. *Behavior Genetics*, *9*, 97–112.

Martin, N. G. & Eaves, L. J. (1977). The genetical analysis of covariance structure. *Heredity*, *38*, 79–95.

Martin, N. G., Eaves, L. J., Heath, A. C., Jardine, R., Feindgold, L. M., & Eysenck, H. J. (1986). Transmission of social attitudes. *Proceedings of the National Academy of Science*, *83*, 4364–4368.

Martin, N. G., Eaves, L. J., Kearsey, M. J., & Davies, P. (1978). The power of the classical twin study. *Heredity*, *40*, 97–116.

Martin, N. G., Eaves, L. J., & Loesch, D. Z. (1982). A genetical analysis of covariation between finger ridge counts. *Annals Human Biology, 9,* 539–552.

Martin, N. G. & Jardine, R. (1986). Eysenck's contribution to behavior genetics. In S. Modgil & C. Modgil (Eds.), *Hans Eysenck: Consensus and Controversy.* Falmer Press: Lewes, Sussex.

Martin, N. G., Oakeshott, J. G., Gibson, J. B., Starmer, G. A., Perl, J., & Wilks, A. V. (1985). A twin study of psychomotor and physiological responses to an acute dose of alcohol. *Behavior Genetics, 15,* 305–347.

Martin, N. G. & Wilson, S. R. (1982). Bias in the estimation of heritability from truncated samples of twins. *Behavior Genetics, 12,* 467–472.

Mather, K. & Jinks, J. L. (1971). *Biometrical Genetics.* London: Chapman and Hall.

Mather, K. & Jinks, J. L. (1977). *Introduction to Biometrical Genetics.* Ithaca, New York: Cornell University Press.

Mather, K. & Jinks, J. L. (1982). *Biometrical genetics: The Study of Continuous Variation* (3rd ed.). London: Chapman and Hall.

Maxwell, A. E. (1977). *Multivariate Analysis in Behavioral Research.* New York: John Wiley.

McArdle, J. J. (1986). Latent variable growth within behavior genetic models. *Behavior Genetics, 16,* 163–200.

McArdle, J. J. & Boker, S. M. (1990). *RAMpath path diagram software.* Denver, CO: Data Transforms Inc.

McArdle, J. J., Connell, J. P., & Goldsmith, H. H. (1980). Structural modeling of stability and genetic influences: Some results from a longitudinal study of behavioral style. *Behavior Genetics, 10,* 487.

McArdle, J. J. & Goldsmith, H. H. (1990). Alternative common-factor models for multivariate biometric analyses. *Behavior Genetics, 20,* 569–608.

McArdle, J. J. & McDonald, R. P. (1984). Some algebraic properties of the reticular action model. *British Journal of Mathematical and Statistical Psychology, 37,* 234–251.

McDonald, R. P. (1980a). A simple comprehensive model for the analysis of covariance structures. *British Journal of Mathematical and Statistical Psychology, 31,* 59–72.

McDonald, R. P. (1980b). A simple comprehensive model for the analysis of co-variance structures: Some remarks on applications. *British Journal of Mathematical and Statistical Psychology*, *33*, 161–183.

McManus, I. C. (1980). Handedness in twins: A critical review. *Neuropsychologia*, *18*, 347–355.

Meyer, J. M. & Eaves, L. J. (1988). Estimating genetic parameters of survival distributions: A multifactorial model. *Genetic Epidemiology*, *5*, 265–276.

Meyer, J. M., Eaves, L. J., Heath, A. C., & Martin, N. G. (1991). Estimating genetic influences on the age-at-menarche: A survival analysis approach. *American Journal of Medical Genetics*, *39*, 148–154.

Molenaar, P. C. M. & Boomsma, D. I. (1987). Application of nonlinear factor analysis to genotype-environment interaction. *Behavior Genetics*, *17*, 71–80.

Molenaar, P. C. M., Boomsma, D. I., Neeleman, D., & Dolan, C. V. (1990). Using factor scores to detect g×e interactive origin of "pure" genetic or environmental factors obtained in genetic covariance structure analysis. *Genetic Epidemiology*, *7*, 83–100.

Mood, A. M. & Graybill, F. A. (1963). *Introduction to the Theory of Statistics* (2nd ed.). New York: McGraw-Hill.

Morton, N. E. (1982). *Outline of Genetic Epidemiology*. New York: Karger.

Moss, H. B., Yao, J. K., & Maddock, J. M. (1989). Responses by sons of alcoholic fathers to alcoholic and placebo drinks: Perceived mood, intoxication, and plasma prolactin. *Alcohol Clinical Experimental Research*, *13*, 252–257.

Mulaik, S. A., James, L. R., VanAlstine, J., Bennett, N. Lind, S., & Stilwell, C. D. (1989). Evaluation of goodness-of-fit indices for structural equations models. *Psychological Bulletin*, *105*, 430–445.

Murray, J. D. (1989). *Mathematical Biology*. Berlin: Springer-Verlag.

Muthen, B. O. (1987). *LISCOMP: Analysis of Linear Structural Equations with a Comprehensive Measurement Model*. Mooresville, IN: Scientific Software, Inc.

NAG (1990). *The NAG Fortran Library Manual, Mark 14*. Oxford: Numerical Algorithms Group.

Nance, W. E. & Corey, L. A. (1976). Genetic models for the analysis of data from the families of identical twins. *Genetics*, (pp. 811–825).

Neale, M. C. (1988). Handedness in a sample of volunteer twins. *Behavior Genetics*, *18*, 69–79.

Neale, M. C. (1991). *Mx: Statistical Modeling.* Box 3 MCV, Richmond, VA 23298: Department of Human Genetics.

Neale, M. C. & Eaves, L. J. (1992). Estimating and controlling for the effects of volunteer bias with pairs of relatives. *Behavior Genetics, in press.*

Neale, M. C., Eaves, L. J., Kendler, K. S., & Hewitt, J. K. (1989a). Bias in correlations from selected samples of relatives: the effects of soft selection. *Behavior Genetics, 19*, 163–169.

Neale, M. C. & Fulker, D. W. (1984). A bivariate path analysis of fear data on twins and their parents. *Acta Geneticae Medicae et Gemellologiae, 33*, 273–286.

Neale, M. C., Heath, A. C., Hewitt, J. K., Eaves, L. J., & Fulker, D. W. (1989b). Fitting genetic models with LISREL: Hypothesis testing. *Behavior Genetics, 19*, 37–69.

Neale, M. C., Hewitt, J. K., Heath, A. C., & Eaves, L. J. (1989c). The power of multivariate and categorical twin studies. Presented at the 6th International Congress of Twin Studies, Rome.

Neale, M. C. & Martin, N. G. (1989). The effects of age, sex and genotype on self-report drunkenness following a challenge dose of alcohol. *Behavior Genetics, 19*, 63–78.

Neale, M. C., Rushton, J. P., & Fulker, D. W. (1986). The heritability of items from the eysenck personality questionnaire. *Personality and Individual Differences, 7*, 771–779.

Neale, M. C. & Stevenson, J. (1989). Rater bias in the EASI temperament scales: A twin study. *Journal of Personality and Social Psychology*, (pp. 446–455).

Neale, M. C., Walters, E. W., Heath, A. C., Kessler, R. C., Pérusse, D., Eaves, L. J., & Kendler, K. S. (1992). Depression and parental bonding: cause, consequence, or genetic covariance? *Genetic Epidemiology, In press.*

O'Malley, S. S. & Maisto, S. A. (1989). The effects of family drinking history on responses to alcohol: Expectancies and reactions to intoxication. *Journal Studies Alcohol, 46*, 289–297.

Ott, J. (1985). *Analysis of Human Genetic Linkage.* Baltimore, MD: Johns Hopkins University Press.

Parker, G. (1983). *Parental Overprotection: A Risk Factor in Psychosocial Development.* New York: Grune and Stratton.

Parker, G. (1990). The Parental Bonding Instrument: Psychometric properties reviewed. *Psychiatric Developments, 4*, 317–335.

Pearson, E. S. & Hartley, H. O. (1972). *Biometrika Tables for Statisticians, volume* 2. Cambridge: Cambridge University Press.

Pearson, K. (1904). On a generalized theory of alternative inheritance, with special references to Mendel's laws. *Phil. Trans. Royal Society A, 203,* 53–86.

Phillips, K. & Fulker, D. W. (1989). Quantitative genetic analysis of longitudinal trends in adoption designs with application to IQ in the Colorado Adoption Project. *Behavior Genetics, 19,* 621–658.

Pickens, R. W., Svikis, D. S., McGue, M., Lykken, D. T., Heston, L. L., & Clayton, P. J. (1991). Heterogeneity in the inheritance of alcoholism: A study of male and female twins. *Archives General Psychiatry, 48,* 19–28.

Plomin, R. & Bergeman, C. S. (1991). The nature of nurture: Genetic influence on environmental measures. *Behavior and Brain Sciences, 14,* 373–397.

Plomin, R., DeFries, J. C., & Loehlin, J. L. (1977). Genotype-environment interaction and correlation in the analysis of human variation. *Psychological Bulletin, 84,* 309–322.

Pollock, V. E., Teasdale, T. W., Gabrielli, W. F., & Knop, J. (1986). Subjective and objective measures of response to alcohol among young men at risk for alcoholism. *Journal Studies Alcohol, 47,* 297–304.

Popper, K. R. (1961). *The logic of scientific discovery.* Science Editions. (Translation; Original work published 1934).

Price, A. J. & Gottesman, I. I. (1991). Body fat in identical twins reared apart: Roles for genes and environment. *Behavior Genetics, 21,* 1–7.

Rao, D. C., Laskarzewski, P. M., Morrison, J. A., Khoury, P., Kelly, K., Wette, R., Russell, J. M., & Glueck, C. J. (1982). Cincinnati lipid research clinic family study: Cultural and biological determinants of lipids and lipoprotein concentrations. *American Journal of Human Genetics, 34,* 888–903.

Rao, D. C., Morton, N. E., & Yee, S. (1974). Analysis of family resemblance II. A linear model for familial correlation. *American Journal of Human Genetics, 26,* 331–359.

Rice, J., Cloninger, C. R., & Reich, T. (1978). Multifactorial inheritance with cultural transmission and assortative mating. I. Description and basic properties of the unitary models. *American Journal of Human Genetics, 30,* 618–643.

Rigdon, E. E. & Ferguson, C. E. (1991). The performance of the polychoric correlation coefficient and selected fitting functions in confirmatory factor analysis with ordinal data. *Journal of Marketing Research, 28,* 491–497.

Rindskopf, D. A. (1984). The use of phantom and imaginary latent variables to parameterize constraints in linear structural models. *Psychometrika, 49*, 37–47.

Riskind, J. H., Beck, A. T., Berchick, R. J., Brown, G., & Steer, R. A. (1987). Reliability of DSM-III diagnoses for major depression and generalized anxiety disorder using the Structured Clinical Interview for DSM-III. *Archives General Psychiatry, 44*, 817–820.

Rogosa, D. A. (1980). A critique of cross-lagged correlation. *Psychological Bulletin, 88*, 245–258.

Rose, R., Kaprio, J., Williams, C., Viken, R., & Obremski, K. (1990). Social contact and sibling similarity: facts, issues. and red herrings. *Behavior Genetics, 20*, 763–778.

Rose, R. J. & Ditto, W. B. (1983). A developmental-geneic analysis of common fears from early adolescence to early childhood. *Child Development, 54*, 361–368.

SAS (1985). *SAS/IML User's Guide, Version 5 edition.* Cary, NC: SAS Institute.

SAS (1988). *SAS/STAT User's guide: Release 6.03.* Cary, NC: SAS Institute, Inc.

SAS (1990). *User's Guide, Version 6, Volume 1* (4th ed.). Cary, NC: SAS Institute.

Scarr, S. & McCartney, K. (1983). How people make their own environments: A theory of genotype–environment effects. *Child Development, 54*, 424–435.

Schieken, R. M., Eaves, L. J., Hewitt, J. K., Mosteller, M., Bodurtha, J. M., Moskowitz, W. B., & Nance, W. E. (1989). Univariate genetic analysis of blood pressure in children: the mcv twin study. *American Journal of Cardiology, 64*, 1333–1337.

Schuckit, M. A. (1984a). Differences in plasma cortisol after ingestion of ethanol in relatives of alcoholics and controls: Preliminary results. *Journal Clinical Psychiatry, 45*, 374–376.

Schuckit, M. A. (1984b). Subjective responses to alcohol in sons of alcoholics and control subjects. *Archives General Psychiatry, 41*, 879–884.

Schuckit, M. A. & Gold, E. O. (1988). A simultaneous evaluation of multiple markers of ethanol/placebo challenges in sons of alcoholics and controls. *Archives General Psychiatry, 45*, 211–216.

Schuckit, M. A., Goodwin, D. W., & Winokur, G. (1972). A study of alcoholism in half siblings. *American Journal Psychiatry, 128*, 1132–1136.

Searle, S. R. (1982). *Matrix Algebra Useful for Statistics*. New York: John Wiley.

Silberg, J. L., Erickson, M. T., Eaves, L. J., & Hewitt, J. K. (1992). The contribution of environmental factors to maternal ratings of behavioral and emotional problems in children and adolescents. (manuscript in preparation).

Spence, J. E., Corey, L. A., Nance, W. E., Marazita, M. L., Kendler, K. S., & Schieken, R. M. (1988). Molecular analysis of twin zygosity using VNTR DNA probes. *American Journal of Human Genetics, 43(3)*, A159 (Abstract).

Spitzer, R. L., Williams, J. B., & Gibbon, M. (1987). *Structured Clinical Interview for DSM-III-R*. New York: Biometrics Research Dept. and New York State Psychiatric Institute.

SPSS (1988). *SPSS-X User's Guide* (3rd ed.). Chicago: SPSS Inc.

Steiger, J. H. (1989). *EzPATH: A supplementary module for SYSTAT and SY-GRAPH*. Evanston, IL: SYSTAT Inc.

Steiger, J. H. & Lind, J. (1980). Statistically based tests for the number of common factors. *Paper presented at the annual meeting of the Psychometric Society, Iowa City*.

Stunkard, A. J., Foch, T. T., & Hrubec, Z. (1986). The body-mass index of twins who have been reared apart. *New England Journal of Medicine, 314*, 193–198.

Stunkard, A. J., Harris, J. R., Pedersen, N. L., & McClearn, G. E. (1990). The body-mass index of twins who have been reared apart. *New England Journal of Medicine, 322*, 1483–1487.

Tartar, R. E., Alterman, A. I., & Edwards, K. I. (1985). Vulnerability to alcoholism in men: A behavior genetic perspective. *Journal Studies Alcohol, 46*, 259–261.

Truett, K. R., Eaves, L. J., Heath, A. C., Hewitt, J. K., Meyer, J. M., Silberg, J., Neale, M. C., Martin, N. G., Walters, E. E., & Kendler, K. S. (1992). A model system for analysis of family resemblance in extended kinships of twins. *American Journal of Human Genetics, In review*.

van Eerdewegh, P. (1982). *Statistical selection in multivariate systems with applications in quantitative genetics*. Unpublished doctoral dissertation, Washington University, St. Louis.

Vandenberg, S. G. (1965). Multivariate analysis of twin differences. In S. G. Vandenberg (Ed.), *Methods and goals in human behavior genetics*, (pp. 29–43). Academic Press: New York.

Vlietinck, R., Derom, R., Neale, M. C., Maes, H., Van Loon, H., Van Maele, G., Derom, C., & Thiery, M. (1989). Genetic and environmental variation in the birthweight of twins. *Behavior Genetics, 19*, 151–161.

Vogler, G. P. (1985). Multivariate path analysis of familial resemblance. *Genetic Epidemiology, 2*, 35–53.

Waller, N. G. & Reise, S. P. (1992). Genetic and environmental influences on item response pattern scalability. *Behavior Genetics, in press.*

Wohlwill, J. F. (1973). *The Study of Behavioral Development.* New-York: Academic Press.

Wolfram, S. (1986). *Theory and Applications of Cellular Automata.* Singapore: World Scientific.

Wright, S. (1921a). Correlation and causation. *Journal of Agricultural Research, 20*, 557–585.

Wright, S. (1921b). Systems of mating. *Genetics, 6*, 111–173.

Wright, S. (1931). Statistical methods in biology. *Journal of the American Statistical Association, 26*, 155–163.

Wright, S. (1934). The method of path coefficients. *Annals of Mathematical Statistics, 5*, 161–215.

Wright, S. (1960). The treatment of reciprocal interaction, with or without lag, in path analysis. *Biometrics, 16*, 189–202.

Wright, S. (1968). *Evolution and the Genetics of Populations. Volume 1. Genetic and Biometric Foundations.* Chicago: University of Chicago Press.

Yamane, Y. (1968). *Mathematics for Economists.* Englewood Cliffs, N.J: Prentice Hall.

Young, P. A., Eaves, L. J., & Eysenck, H. J. (1980). Intergenerational stability and change in the causes of variation in personality. *Personality and Individual Differences, 1*, 35–55.

Yule, G. U. (1902). Mendel's laws and their probable relation to intra-racial heredity. *New Phytology, 1*, 192–207.

Index